Rethinking physical
and rehabilitation medicine

Springer

Paris
Berlin
Heidelberg
New York
Hong Kong
Londres
Milan
Tokyo

Jean-Pierre Didier
Emmanuel Bigand

Rethinking physical and rehabilitation medicine

New technologies induce new learning strategies

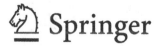 Springer

Jean-Pierre Didier

Professeur émérite de médecine physique et de réadaptation
Université de Bourgogne
Pôle de rééducation-réadaptation
23, rue Gaffarel
BP 77908
21034 Dijon Cedex

Emmanuel Bigand

Institut universitaire de France / Université de Bourgogne
LEAD UMR 5022 CNRS Pôle AAFE
Esplanade Erasme / BP 26513
21065 Dijon Cedex

ISBN 978-2-8178-0033-2 Springer Paris Berlin Heidelberg New York

© Springer-Verlag France, Paris, 2010

Springer is a part of Springer Science + Business Media
springer.com

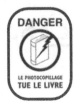

Design of cover : Jean-François Montmarché
Lay-out : Nord-Compo - Villeneuve d'Ascq (59)

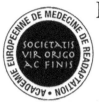

Members of the European Academy of Rehabilitation Medicine

Pr ALARANTTA Hannu
Helsinki (Finlande)

Pr ANDRE Jean-Marie
Nancy (France)

Pr BARAT Michel
Bordeaux (France)

Pr BARDOT André
Marseille (France)

Pr BARNES M. Ph.
Newcastle upon Tyne (Grande-Bretagne)

Pr BERTOLINI Carlo
Rome (Italie)

Pr CHAMBERLAIN M. Anne
Leeds (Grande-Bretagne)

Pr CHANTRAINE Alex
Genève (Suisse)

Pr CONRADI Eberhard
Berlin (Allemagne)

Pr DELARQUE Alain
Marseille (France)

Pr DELBRÜCK Hermann
Wuppertal (Allemagne)

Pr DIDIER Jean-Pierre
Dijon (France)

Pr EKHOLM Jan
Stockholm (Suède)

Dr EL MASRY Wagih
Oswestry Shropshire (Grande-Bretagne)

Pr EYSSETTE Michel
Saint Genis-Laval (France)

Pr FIALKA-MOSER Veronika
Vienne (Autriche)

Pr FRANCHIGNONI Franco
Veruno (Italie)

Pr Garcia-Alsina Joan
Barcelona (Espagne)

Pr GATCHEVA Jordanka
Sofia (Bulgarie)

Pr GOBELET Charles
Sion (Suisse)

Pr HEILPORN André
Bruxelles (Belgique)

Pr LANKHORST Gustaaf J.
Amsterdam (Pays-Bas)

Dr MAIGNE Robert
Paris (France)

Pr MARINCEK Curt
Ljubljana (Slovenia)

Pr McLELLAN Lindsay
Hampshire (Grande-Bretagne)

Dr McNAMARA Angela
Dublin (Irlande)

Pr MEGNA Gianfranco
Bari (Italie)

Pr MICHAIL Xanthi
Athènes (Grèce)

Dr OELZE Fritz
Hamburg (Allemagne)

Pr RODRIGUEZ Luis-Pablo
Madrid (Espagne)

Pr SJÖLUND Bengt H.
Umea (Suède)

Pr STAM Hendrik Jan
Rotterdam (Pays-Bas)

Pr STUCKI Gerold
Munic (Germany)

Pr TONAZZI Amadeo
Saint-Raphaël (France)

Pr VANDERSTRAETEN Guy
Gent (Belgique)

Dr WARD Anthony
Stoke on Trent (Grande-Bretagne)

Dr ZÄCH Guido A.
Nottwil (Suisse)

CONTRIBUTORS

Christophe AVENA
Service d'anesthésie-réanimation
CHU de Dijon
Hôpital Général
3, rue du Faubourg-Raines
BP 1519
21033 Dijon Cedex
France

Michel BARAT
Équipe d'accueil 4136 – Handicap
et système Nerveux
Université Victor Segalen Bordeaux II
Service de médecine physique
et réadaptation
CHU de Bordeaux
Hôpital Pellegrin
Place Amélie-Raba-Léon
33076 Bordeaux Cedex

Emmanuel BIGAND
Institut universitaire de France
Université de Bourgogne
LEAD-CNRS UMR 5022
Pôle AAFE, Esplanade Erasme
Université de Bourgogne
BP 26513
21065 Dijon Cedex
France

Elodie BONNETAIN
LEAD UMR 5022 CNRS
Pôle AAFE, Esplanade Erasme
Université de Bourgogne
BP 26513
21065 Dijon Cedex
France

Jean-Michel BOUCHEIX
LEAD-CNRS UMR 5022
Pôle AAFE, Esplanade Erasme
Université de Bourgogne
BP 26513
21065 Dijon Cedex
France

Patrick DEHAIL
Équipe d'accueil 4136 – Handicap
et système Nerveux
Université Victor Segalen Bordeaux II
Service de médecine physique
et réadaptation
CHU de Bordeaux
Hôpital Pellegrin
Place Amélie Raba-Léon
33076 Bordeaux Cedex
France

Charles DELBÉ
Institut universitaire de France
Université de Bourgogne
LEAD-CNRS UMR 5022
Pôle AAFE, Esplanade Erasme
Université de Bourgogne
BP 26513
21065 Dijon Cedex
France

Jean-Pierre DIDIER
Professeur émérite de médecine
physique et de réadaptation
Université de Bourgogne
Pôle de rééducation-réadaptation
23, rue Gaffarel
BP 77908
21034 Dijon Cedex

Marc FREYSZ
Service d'anesthésie-réanimation
CHU de Dijon
Hôpital Général
3, rue du Faubourg-Raines
BP 1519
21033 Dijon Cedex
France

Rémi GOASDOUÉ
Éducation et apprentissages, EA 4071
Université Paris-Descartes
45, rue des Saints-Pères
75006 Paris
France

Pierre-Alain JOSEPH
Équipe d'accueil 4136 – Handicap
et système Nerveux
Université Victor Segalen Bordeaux II
Service de médecine physique
et réadaptation

CHU de Bordeaux
Hôpital Pellegrin
Place Amélie-Raba-Léon
33076 Bordeaux Cedex
France

Evelyne KLINGER
Arts et Métiers ParisTech Angers
LAMPA
4, rue de l'Ermitage
53000 Laval
France

Jean-Michel MAZAUX
Équipe d'accueil 4136 – Handicap
et système Nerveux
Université Victor Segalen Bordeaux II
Service de médecine physique
et réadaptation
CHU de Bordeaux
Hôpital Pellegrin
Place Amélie-Raba-Léon
33076 Bordeaux Cedex
France

Jean-Marc MOUILLIE PhD
Professeur de philosophie
Département sciences humaines
Faculté de médecine
Université d'Angers
1, rue Haute-de-Reculée
49045 Angers Cedex 01
France

Aline MOUSSARD
LEAD-CNRS UMR 5022
Pôle AAFE, Esplanade Erasme
Université de Bourgogne
BP 26513
21065 Dijon Cedex
France

BRAMS – Suite O-120
Pavillon 1420 boul. Mont Royal
Université de Montréal
C.P. 6128 – Station Centre ville
Montréal (QC) H3C 3J7
Québec, Canada

Sébastien PACTON
Université de Paris-Descartes, LPNC
CNRS UMR 8189
45, rue des Saints-Pères
75006 Paris
France

Pierre PERRUCHET
LEAD-CNRS UMR 5022
Pôle AAFE, Esplanade Erasme
Université de Bourgogne
BP 26513
21065 Dijon Cedex
France

Alexandra RAUCH
Swiss Paraplegic Research (SPF)
Postfach
CH-6207 Nottwil
Switzerland

ICF Research Branch
WHO FIC CC Germany (DIMDI) at SPF
And at Institute for Health
and Rehabilitation Sciences (IHRS)
Ludwig-Maximilian University
Marchioninistr. 17
81377 Munich
Germany

Isabelle RICHARD PhD MD
Service de médecine physique
et de réadaptation
C3RF
Rue des Capucins
BP 2449
49024 Angers Cedex 02
France

Faculté de médecine
Université d'Angers
1, rue Haute-de-Reculée
49045 Angers Cedex 01
France

Johanna V.G. ROBERTSON
Laboratoire de Neurophysique
et Physiologie
Université Paris-Descartes
CNRS UMR 8119
45, rue des Saints-Pères
75006 Paris
France

Agnès ROBY-BRAMI
Labororatoire Neurophysique
et Physiologie
Université Paris-Descartes
CNRS UMR 8119
45, rue des Saints-Pères
75006 Paris
France

Service de médecine physique
et réadaptation
Hôpital Raymond-Poincaré
104, boulevard Raymond-Poincaré
92380 Garches
France

Françoise ROCHETTE
LEAD-CNRS UMR 5022
Pôle AAFE, Esplanade Erasme
Université de Bourgogne
BP 26513
21065 Dijon Cedex
France

Virginie SAOÛT MD
Service de médecine physique
et de réadaptation
C3RF
Rue des Capucins
BP 2449
49024 Angers Cedex 02
France

Faculté de médecine
Université d'Angers
1, rue Haute-de-Reculée
49045 Angers Cedex 01
France

Gerold STUCKI
Department of Health Sciences
and Health Policy
University of Lucerne
Lucerne and SPF
Switzerland

Swiss Paraplegic Research (SPF)
Postfach
CH-6207 Nottwil
Switzerland
ICF Research Branch
WHO FIC CC Germany (DIMDI) at SPF
And at Institute for Health
and Rehabilitation Sciences (IHRS)
Ludwig-Maximilian University
Marchioninistr. 17
81377 Munich
Germany

Patrice L. (Tamar) WEISS
Laboratory for Innovations
in Rehabilitation Technology
University of Haifa
Mount Carmel
Haifa 31905
Israel

Annie WINTER
LEAD-CNRS UMR 5022
Pôle AAFE, Esplanade Erasme
Université de Bourgogne
BP 26513
21065 Dijon Cedex
France

Arnaud WITT
LEAD-CNRS UMR 5022
Pôle AAFE, Esplanade Erasme
Université de Bourgogne
BP 26513
21065 Dijon Cedex
France

CONTENTS

PART III
LEARNING, MEDICAL TRAINING, AND REHABILITATION

EXECUTIVE SUMMARY

Part I – Learning and education into rehabilitation strategy

Chapter I – Learning and teaching: two processes to bear in mind when rethinking physical and rehabilitation medicine

The PRM (physical and rehabilitation medicine) specialist has to develop the functioning of the person in accordance with the life project, as it is defined into the CIF (International Classification of Functioning, Disability and Health). He or she appears as a "medical coach" in terms of health and functioning. The patient commonly has to learn by practice and/or by instruction how to do or how to perform a task, using implicit or explicit learning procedures, and the caregiver is the teacher who has to know and to understand the principles of teaching and learning. Is this indeed the case? We can discuss about when the caregiver's instructions could be summarized as follows:

"Do it like that."

"Do it like I do it."

"Do it in a way that feels right for you."

Thus learning and teaching are most often used in a context of empiricism with its relative ignorance of the paradigms and mechanisms involved. However, it is of great importance to take into account this relative ignorance when the array of resources used in rehabilitation, notably robotics and virtual reality, is providing new opportunities for learning and teaching.

Both learning and teaching are not only essential approaches in the rehabilitation process conducted by the PRM practitioner but also approaches that allow practitioners to reconsider PRM when new technologies present particularly attractive opportunities.

Chapter II – The International Classification of Functioning, Disability and Health (ICF), a unifying model for physical and rehabilitation medicine (PRM)

A unifying scientific model is of utmost importance for any professional, academic and scientific discipline. To be able to rely on a unifying model for functioning is essential for PRM, which can be understood as the "medicine of functioning." The ICF is thus a promising starting point for the development of rehabilitation practice and research.

In this chapter, the development of the ICF in the context of the United Nations system and its specialty agency the World Health Organization is explained. It is then reviewed how the ICF can be used both as reference standard and starting point for the classification and the measurement of functioning. Finally, it is shown how the ICF can serve as a unifying framework for the conceptualization of rehabilitation understood as a public health strategy and the medical specialty PRM and how it may serve as a basis for the organization and development of human functioning and rehabilitation research relevant for PRM.

Chapter III – Rehabilitation and norms

Medical practice aims at creating a norm; as such it is both normalizing and standardizing. It implies evaluations that draw a distinction between what is "normal" and what is pathological: this traditionally defines both its goals and its field of practice. Rehabilitation medicine is both on the margin and at the very heart of this founding distinction, and therefore also of the concepts or representations that underlie the definition of the norm and the actions triggered when a deviation from this norm is observed.

Associating "rehabilitation" and "physical medicine" leads to the use of a "global concept" involving all the various aspects of the patient's situation that are affected by the handicap. In its various fields of practice, from functional rehabilitation to long-term follow-up care within the community, the practice of PRM is at the junction between medicine and society at large. Its field of analysis and intervention is therefore shifted from compensating for an impairment or restoring a function to adapting to a given set of social situations, with the risk that it will rely on, or even contribute to define, a set of "normal" social roles and situations.

Historical shifts in the uses of the word "rehabilitation," occasionally in combination with "camp," are a reminder – assuming one was needed – of the conceptual pitfalls involved, such as the fact that adaptation to the patient's social environment is never in itself a "normal" sign of health, in the sense that it is "desirable."

The process of learning new gestures and new ways of living therefore becomes central to the therapeutic process. Depending on whether goals and references will have been set by the patient within the framework of a process of normativity or defined externally, the patient will be able to call on his or her own motivational resources or depend on the feedback provided by the therapist.

Part II – Implicit learning: a basic learning process

Chapter IV – A historical perspective on learning: the legacy and actuality of I. M. Pavlov and N. A. Bernstein

Learning is defined as a relatively permanent modification of the organism's activity resulting from its interactions with the external environment. There are two theoretical streams: the main stream that we may call very schematically computo-representational neurosciences, which aims to improve understanding of the physiology of the nervous system, and various alternative approaches that share a more systemic or dynamical point of view, with strong references to psychology and a common aim to understand human activity. These streams differ on some important points, particularly on the question of the mechanisms of learning.

This debate would necessitate an extensive and detailed review of the experimental, theoretical and modeling evidences supporting or refuting both approaches, which are well beyond the scope of this chapter. We chose to tackle the question *from a historical point of view*, through the controversy that occurred between Pavlov and Bernstein during the 1930s.

The impressive legacy of Pavlov has fertilized very different fields in psychology, neuroscience, and formal neurons. It is commonly accepted in the community and very largely applied for learning, teaching, and therapy with unquestionable efficiency. It remains nowadays the mainstream paradigm for learning and adaptation and has received much evidence from basic and integrated neuroscience.

Although quite varied, the approaches in Bernstein's tradition share common principles that differ markedly from the tradition of conditioning inherited from Pavlov. The drive for learning is action itself and not stimuli. The focus is put on dynamical processes and not on representation (called traces by Pavlov) and on the sensorimotor history of each individual. All the elements of interaction are considered, including the characteristics of the body structure and the multiple facets of the physical, social, and cultural environment. The theories of reference are more related to physical models of auto-organization and autopoiesis than to neuronal models developed by computational neuroscience.

However, rather than being alternative, these two streams of research should be presented as complementary approaches since they do not really share the same object of research.

Chapter V – Introducing implicit learning: from the laboratory to the real life

What and how do we learn implicitly?

Researches on implicit learning recently lead to revisit basic assumptions about human cognition. Human brains manage to internalize highly sophisticated structures of the environment through mere exposure to these structures in everyday life. One of the main issues of research remains to understand how these structures may be psychologically represented? According to some authors, the knowledge acquired implicitly may be represented in an abstract way. According to some others, the acquired knowledge rests on local organizations, statistically relevant in the environment. A supplementary issue of interest deals with the very implicate nature of this knowledge. For some authors, there is a continuum between implicit and explicit knowledge. Others argue that both types of knowledge do not confound, and some even suggest that knowledge is never entirely implicit. This chapter reviews these two main issues of research by considering the most influential studies in this domain.

Chapter VI – Implicit learning, development, and education

Implicit learning processes have been largely explored in adults, and some studies have been devoted to normally developing children as well as to disabled children. We will review the main developmental studies in this area of research in a first section of the chapter. Most of them have revealed that implicit learning processes operate efficiently from a very early age, and that they are also active in disabled children, while, in the latter, explicit learning processes are known to be impaired.

These results can legitimately elicit new hopes with respect to remediation activities with disabled children. The second section of the chapter addresses the benefits of using implicit learning processes as a way to remediate for behavioral impairments.

Chapter VII – Implicit learning and implicit memory in moderate to severe memory disorders

A lot of studies have shown that implicit learning is a very robust function that can be preserved, despite heavy explicit learning and memory disorders. Such capacities have been highlighted with amnesic patients and in Alzheimer's disease through several lab situations, as artificial grammar learning for an example. In this task, participants see a number of pseudowords (such as MVTMX), composed by a combination of letters following a complex grammar that determines their association rules. After this learning period, participants see new pseudowords; half of them follow the same conception rules, while the others do not. Participants have to determine which of these new words are "correct," according to this artificial grammar. Results show that patients have the same percentage of correct responses than normal control participants. However, when participants have to do an explicit task with this material, for example, to generate new pseudowords that follow the same grammar, patients have impaired performances, which confirm their memory disorders. These results show that new learning is possible despite cognitive disorders, and open new prospects for rehabilitation of heavy memory disorders. We will discuss how further studies could use these preserved capacities for helping amnesic or Alzheimer patients in their everyday life.

Chapter VIII – Learning process and recovery of higher functions after brain damage

Developmental psychology has long since shown the reality of changes in brain activity under the influence of intensive and systematic training and the influence of external stimuli on the structuring and function of the brain.

Learning processes work on the brain in different ways, operating through brain plasticity. In response to a new experience or new stimulation, neuroplasticity induces either changes in an already existing structure or the creation of new connections between neurones. The latter process leads to an increase in the density of synapses, while the former simply reinforces the most efficient or best adapted of the existing pathways. In both cases, it is a matter of «remodeling» the brain in order to acquire these new data and, if required, to preserve them.

Practitioners confronted by patients suffering from cognitive deficiencies are faced with many methodological constraints: evaluation and especially the impact of deficiencies on the functioning of daily life and restriction of participation, and the choice of retraining method. The issue at stake here is nothing less than the credibility of reeducation in neuropsychology. Theoretical models have developed remarkably, thanks to our knowledge of cerebral function and to the concept of post-lesional plasticity. The fundamental problem is to reduce the effect of fragmentation of the functions assessed by analytical or cognitive neuropsychology and to clarify the transfer of abilities derived from reeducation to everyday life, beyond simply measuring learning of the items involved. The issue at stake in such training, whatever the theoretical modality, is to facilitate the functioning of preserved capacities and means of substitution put into action by patients themselves and their entourage.

Part III – Learning, medical training, and rehabilitation practice

Chapter IX – Benefits of learning technologies in medical training, from full-scale simulators to virtual reality and multimedia presentation

Emerging technology for medical training, including interactive animated images in anatomy, 3-D models, full-scale patient simulator, and virtual reality, is claimed to have great potential to enhance learning.

The literature presents many qualitative descriptions of technologies, but there is still little scientific research concerning the real benefits of these tools for professional training. In the first part of this chapter, we will present a review of the main recent studies on the ergonomics of technologies for learning and training.

In the second part of the chapter, we will report on a series of our experimental and empirical studies that concern the benefits of a full-scale patient simulator in emergency medical procedure training.

In previous research, full-scale simulators have been used in order to train operators working with complex systems presenting a great amount of risk such as power plants and aircraft piloting and to prevent serious errors or accidents. Training with a full-scale simulator in medical emergency is new.

The results of our studies revealed that full-scale patient simulators have been found to be very effective in emergency procedure training. Benefits were not limited to improved performance in the resuscitation tasks involved during the learning period. Benefits rather included the acquisition of relevant medical reasoning, deeper comprehension of dynamic events, better control, and awareness of the crucial features of the simulated scenario.

Chapter X – Auditory training in deaf children

The acquisition of the verbal language in childhood is commonly considered as a result of an implicit learning but supposes the efficiency of input system (auditory perception) and a repetitive and abundant exposure to language materials before the end of the sensitive period. In prelingually deaf children, as the rehabilitation of the input system (hearing aid or cochlear implant) depends on several factors, particularly the age of diagnosis, the first auditory stimulations are rare before 18 months (mean: 2 years). To develop verbal communication, the indispensable speech therapy focuses on salient multimodal perceptive oppositions in sounds and uses linguistic stimuli as soon as possible in discrimination and identification tasks.

When considering the underlying perceptive operations in language acquisition, a program including different kinds of nonlinguistic auditory stimuli (but sharing acoustic saliencies with language) in all perceptive tasks should improve language skills.

Chapter XI – Virtual reality for learning and rehabilitation

Given the high incidence of brain injury in the population and the need for additional rehabilitation tools, it is important to explore the possibilities brought by innovative technologies. Virtual reality (VR) has the potential to assist current rehabilitation techniques by offering new opportunities for learning. By providing a safe setting in which users may interact and develop goal-oriented activities within a virtual environment, VR allows the delivery of controlled multisensory stimuli and the creation of innovative learning approaches. VR assets in learning have already been used and proved, leading to their exploitation in rehabilitation. In this chapter, we will present some fundamental VR basic issues; we will give details about some VR-based learning approaches used in cognitive and motor rehabilitation and discuss assets and limits of VR for learning and rehabilitation.

Chapter XII – Augmented feedback, virtual reality, and robotics for designing new rehabilitation methods

Neuro-rehabilitation is currently undergoing a technological revolution! Groups of engineers and rehabilitation specialists are working on designing and testing a great variety of rehabilitation devices and systems. The reason for this is that, although it is generally accepted that rehabilitation improves outcome after stroke, patients are still left with impairments causing various levels of handicap and limiting their integration in community life. Comparison of traditional rehabilitation techniques has failed to show superiority of one over another, and concepts for rehabilitation have been changing over the last 20 years, with the biggest change being evaluation. There is a move to make rehabilitation techniques more evidence based. As such, numerous research teams have set about to create more effective rehabilitation techniques based on the principles of motor control and learning and incorporating new technology to fulfil the principal goals of rehabilitation: increased functional ability and increased participation in the community. The aim of this chapter is to discuss applications for augmented feedback (AF) in the rehabilitation of motor skills of patients with neurological disorders, in particular within VR environments associated or not with mechatronic devices (robotics). First, we will examine some motor learning principles relevant to rehabilitation and how AF fits into these concepts. We will then go on to review applications of AF used for the rehabilitation of specific movement parameters. We will also discuss the use of feedback distortion to manipulate action–perception coupling and systems based on movement observation.

FOREWORD

It is a great pleasure to write the preface to this book "Rethinking Physical and Rehabilitation Medicine." Learning and teaching are introduced in this book as fundamental concepts in Rehabilitation Medicine.

In Rehabilitation Medicine we deal with patients who have permanent disabilities as a result of congenital disorders, injury, or disease. We generally use three types of interventions. The first type concerns medical interventions, for instance treatment of spasticity in order to create a better starting point for functional movements. The second type is teaching the patient new or modified functional movements. The third type is to compensate for lost functions, for instance supplying a wheelchair when walking is impossible.

Teaching functional movements requires teaching skills. However, medical specialists in Rehabilitation Medicine have no specific training in education and teaching. This book gives a very comprehensive overview of the principles of learning and teaching. It helps to understand the underlying neurophysiological mechanisms of learning, which is a special form of plasticity of the nervous system. It probably also helps to design better and more effective rehabilitation programs.

Nowadays, new technologies, for instance robotics and virtual reality, have been introduced in Rehabilitation Medicine. This book discusses principles of motor learning in relation to the opportunities offered by the use of robotics and virtual reality. "Implicit learning" is another important topic that is discussed in depth.

"Rehabilitation and norms" is an interesting chapter of this book. Assessing people with disabilities, as we regularly do as part of our rehabilitation practice, implies having a concept of "normality" and being able to draw a line between normal and abnormal. It is interesting to think about various definitions of normality, their application in

Rehabilitation Medicine, and how the concept of normality can be used for inclusion or exclusion of people with disabilities.

This book is highly recommended to any reader involved in Rehabilitation Medicine or care for people with disabilities.

Gustaaf J Lankhorst
President
Académie Européenne de Médicine de Réadaptation
European Academy of Rehabilitation Medicine

PART I

LEARNING AND EDUCATION INTO REHABILITATION STRATEGY

Learning and teaching: two processes to bear in mind when rethinking physical medicine and rehabilitation

J.-P. Didier

Rehabilitation, a clear objective; PRM, an ambiguous term for the medical specialty

Rehabilitation has been defined by the WHO as a *process aimed at enabling people with disabilities to reach and maintain their optimal physical, sensory, intellectual, psychiatric and/or social functional levels, providing them with the tools to change their lives towards a higher level of independence* (13). *Rehabilitation includes all measures aimed at reducing the impact of disabling and handicapping conditions and enabling the disabled and handicapped to achieve social integration* (14).

This definition is in agreement with the new International Classification of Functioning, Disability and Health (ICF) (40).

This definition makes it possible to distinguish between the medical specialty, which is able to take charge of this objective, and the so-called organ specialties, which concern one organ or a group of organs involved in the same function, such as cardiology, pneumology, or endocrinology.

It is difficult, however, to find a name that clearly identifies this medical specialty. The term physical and rehabilitation medicine (PRM) was chosen at the European level. It is certainly not the best choice insofar as it gives no indication of the principal methods that it uses to optimize a person's ability to function. In particular, it does not emphasize the two essential strategies that are used, learning and teaching, which at the end of the day provide the structure of the specialty.

Thus, for the public at large, the Internet site MedlinePlus had to provide additional information concerning the notion of learning: "After a serious injury, illness, or surgery, you may recover slowly. You may need to regain your strength, relearn skills or find new ways of doing things you did before. This process is rehabilitation," as if rehabilitation had no other ambition than to return to the prior situation. More professionally, the white book on PRM, written by three European bodies that represent this discipline, underlined the fundamental role of learning and teaching in rehabilitation strategies, thus conferring on PRM specialist doctors the new function of teacher (18):

"Learning is a modern part of the rehabilitation process. The PRM specialist is a teacher, especially when new concepts of adaptation (e.g., plasticity) and motor learning have to support rehabilitation programmes." This approach is still not enough to realize that learning and teaching in PRM need to be reconsidered, given the arrival of new technologies, particularly robotics and virtual reality, which have raised new particularly interesting prospects.

PRM appears to be the medical specialty most concerned with teaching, even though the WHO particularly underlined the importance of teaching in the context of chronic diseases, by recommending "therapeutic teaching." In both cases, the lesion and the subsequent deficit are not so much important, but the consequences on the person's everyday life are. Disabled people expect the PRM team, if they choose to consult them, to enable them to function and have a social life in accordance with their physiological, physical, and cognitive capacities, with their environment and with the life they wish to lead.

The difficulties of implementing "therapeutic teaching" have still not been overcome (17), as if the justification for this new mission handed to carers is poorly understood. The same applies to PRM, and we can wonder what has led to this situation.

Learning and teaching: the two pillars of PRM strategy

In French, the term for rehabilitation is "reeducation" and from an etymologic point of view, the verb educate comes from the Latin «educare», which means «train, give instruction», derived from the verb «educere», composed of ducere, which means «conduct, lead», with the prefix ex, which means out.

Learning in French is "apprendre," from the Latin "prehendere," which means "take, seize," preceded by the prefix ad, which means from.

In English neither learn nor teach is derived from Latin; however, the basic meaning is similar. Learn is to get knowledge, by following or finding the track, while teach is "to show, point out also to give instruction."

Thus teaching and rehabilitation play an important role in the work of PRM practitioners; they must help lead patients from their initial situation characterized by the presence of certain disabilities that impair function toward a situation characterized by abilities that allow them to function in accordance with the life they wish to lead. This mission is implicitly included in the professional activity of PRM specialists, the earlier name of the discipline, *Reeducation Fonctionnelle et Readaptation*, in French, notably reflects the teaching role.

There is also a notion of reciprocal teaching. Victims of disability-causing lesions, in the sense of the classical WOOD trilogy (39), seek to compensate for the functional modifications due to the lesion. In order to do this, they must "take on board" new solutions that are likely to enable them to acquire the desired function. Either they can adopt solutions immediately from their environment or everyday practices, or they can benefit from the mediation of a teacher/rehabilitation therapist who, in order to fulfill his or her mission, must in turn "take on board" the information provided by patients, to personalize the mediation.

In such a context, the program proposed cannot be one that is imposed on the other person on the pretext that one knows best what is good for someone else, but it must be the result of reciprocal learning, and each in turn must both learn and teach (12). Far too often, patients are not satisfied with the way doctors listen to them. They describe a doctor who is too confined within medical theory and who imposes his or her theoretical solution on their physical condition instead of first taking into account observations of the patient and the patient's discourse before establishing links with the theories (16). The question about the authority of the experts thus arises.

The practitioner is indeed supposed to be the expert. His or her knowledge stems from the skills acquired, thanks to appropriate training, and from the information obtained from a complete clinical and biological examination, including diagnostic assessment tools, in order to assess all the aspects concerning the abilities of the patient, the characteristics of his family, the social and architectural environment and the main options in the life he or she wishes to lead. The medical assessment is established by the different members of the PRM team, which gives the practitioner additional legitimacy. Given the above, the practitioner may be unconsciously led to propose, if not impose, his or her point of view and prescriptions, or those of the team.

In such conditions, the relationship between the doctor and the patient may become a one-way street – all the more so when "the patient" is in an inferior or defensive situation. This one-way street can be reinforced by the presence of disorders of superior functions. Such an approach may contribute to a violent reaction from the patient (19), and is incompatible with dialogue in which the practitioner and the patient need to learn from each other.

This issue was clearly described in a WHO report (30) on "Therapeutic Patient Teaching," which "is a set of practices that aims to allow patients to acquire skills so that they can actively cope with their disease, the treatments and surveillance, in a partnership with the health care team." To achieve this goal, it should meet the following conditions:

- it must allow patients to acquire and maintain abilities that are essential to the optimal management of their life and illness;
- it must be progressive and incorporated within the treatment plan;
- it is centered on patients and their needs while taking into account their social and family environment;
- it must help patients and their families to understand the disease and the therapeutic strategy while building a harmonious relationship with the health care team in order to maintain and if possible improve the quality of life.

Many of the above aspects can also be applied to disabled people, however, with one essential difference concerning the reference to the word "disease." This is particularly important in French because the word "le malade" (sick person) is frequently used instead of "le patient."

The term "le malade," as the sick person is already contestable when it refers to those with a chronic disease: it is easy to understand that such people wish, with reason, not to be considered sick since the disease has been diagnosed and treatment implemented, and relative stabilization of their condition can reasonably be expected; on the contrary, they wish to be considered normal citizens, whose essential objective is to learn to live a new life.

The term "le malade" as the sick person is totally inappropriate when used to refer to disabled people who suffer from a stable or only slightly progressive lesion. For these people, their essential problem is to learn to live a new life, often with a modified body; it is a question of learning and developing a new corporal potential (16) with which they will have to learn to function, making the most of the various capacities they had before the lesion was acquired. They are not "sick" because of this situation.

The term "le malade" as the sick person is also inappropriate when people are born with such differences. They aspire to, or sometimes resign themselves to, living with them, as they are, often with a body they have become attached to but always, like the above, standing up to for the right to demand an environment that is not hostile because it was created by and for a non-disabled majority, considered and living as "normal" citizens.

In any case, disabled people will learn to live with their condition, to cope with it, but without ever accepting it (32) and without being "abnormal" or "pathological." They are all the more justified to reject the stigmatization of their condition since it is not only unethical but also contrary to biological reality expressed in Canguilhem's tenet: "…in the life of an organism, what is normal is defined by the organism itself, and contained in its own existence" (9). That is clearly expressed in the UN Convention on the Rights of Persons with Disabilities.

Normality will be tackled in another chapter, but we wish to underline here the danger engendered by the overwhelming power of normality and standards in the learning and teaching process.

The overwhelming power of normality and standards

In order to structure the therapeutic strategy, the practitioner will establish an objective based on normality and standards. It is logical for the practitioner to refer to data validated by a evidence-based medicine in order to define the objective that rehabilitation should aim to achieve. These standards also bring comfort, thanks to the certainty of experimental proof, but with the risk of possible fascination due to the scientific connotations.

The notions of what is normal and standard are based on presumably healthy subjects, controls, or normal people in laboratory conditions that are far removed from the conditions of everyday life; such statistical standards can be controversial. The only prospect they validate is the return to intangible normality or the need to tend towards "the situation before the lesion," which may be the only conceivable eventuality.

The risks of such practices are illustrated by a number of caricatural examples of rehabilitation of an impaired locomotor system.

Thanks to modern methods of movement analysis, standards for "normal gait" have been defined. Given the precision of these standards, they cannot be used as references to be applied to subjects who no longer have a "normal" biomechanical system because of the lesions, which in most cases can never disappear. On this point, the example of the subject fitted with prosthesis for an amputated lower limb is particularly relevant (28).

Similarly, anthropomorphic prostheses of the shoulder have shown their limits in advanced degenerative lesions. The efficacy of equipment designed with no intention to reproduce anatomic normality, but with the aim to provide form-function efficiency, has been shown with the shoulder reverse prosthesis. Biomechanical analyses of the degenerative scapulohumeral joint have validated this design of prosthesis, which is fundamentally different from the "normal" biomechanical system. The ball becomes the socket, and the socket becomes the ball, because the implant is designed so that the ball portion is attached to the scapula and the socket is placed at the upper end of the humerus. These clinical results have confirmed the superiority of this anatomically "abnormal" prosthesis compared to its anthropomorphically "normal" equivalent (10). These findings from clinical research encourage the rehabilitation practitioner to take a second look at the concept of normality and to question the authority of what is supposed to be obvious, whether it stems from empiricism and dogma or to habit and received wisdom.

The weight of empiricism and dogma

Empiricism sometimes reinforced by references to physiological and/or to providential anatomical schemas may have led to questionable excesses.

We will not insist on certain methods of "rehabilitation" that stem from this process, most of which derive from empirical practices, validated by pseudoscientific knowledge, which also lends credibility to the practices and provides justification for the development of schools, sometimes "sects" devoted to the training of new followers and the perpetuation of dogmatic approaches incorporated into questionable alternative medicines.

The same cannot be said of certain approaches used in rehabilitation for neurological disorders, which after being derived from empirical discovery of effective strategies also gave rise to methods and schools. The methods of Kabat, Bobath, and Brunstrom are examples. These methods were created by remarkable clinicians, but they have been taken to excess, thanks to the dogmatic approach of some of their followers. By supposing that their methods were based on intangible scientific considerations and by neglecting their relativism because the science was evolving, they tended to impose their prerogatives without justification.

In his day, Cajal was right: "Once development is complete, the sources of growth and regeneration of axons and dendrites are irretrievably lost. In the adult brain, the nerve paths are fixed and immutable: everything can die, nothing can be regenerated" (8). With this in mind, following a cerebral lesion, it is logical to expect no reorganization of neuronal circuits and no post-lesion reorganization of the remaining cerebral structures. For this reason, rehabilitation was based exclusively on the psychomotor development of the infant according to the hierarchical reflex model. It used to be legitimate to discourage walking in hemiplegic patients until the reflex circuits responsible for the spasticity were once again under control, but continuing such practices in the ignorance of the biological function of plasticity has become reprehensible (27).

Paillard distinguished between:
– evolving plasticity, linked to phylogenetic evolution;
– genetic plasticity, linked to ontogenetic evolution;
– adaptative plasticity, linked to experience.

The latter involves processes of memory and learning, which are responsible for mechanisms that establish new programming, thanks to the creation of new neuronal arrangements and new neuronal networks. It also involves the plasticity of structures that transmit commands and sensory information as well as effector structures that control the locomotor system. Together they make up a whole, the plasticity of motor function, which corresponds to a concept that structures the rehabilitation process (11).

Today, we know that the rehabilitation for neurological disorders can benefit from the remarkable possibilities offered by plasticity. The concept of the immutable nature of neuronal networks has been completely demolished by the facts (4). Many methods have thus been developed to restore walking in patients as quickly as possible (20, 21, 38), since walking can be improved through it; that is, "we become a bricklayer by laying bricks" (41), but we will have to shake the beliefs of the many rehabilitation practitioners who systematically use methods that are now recognized as dogmatic.

Moreover, when it is a question of teaching, beware of all dogmas whatever they are, and never accept them at face value without discussion, or worse without taking into account the clinical data that contradict them. Kesselring clearly stated the problem of neurological rehabilitation: "Whereas a main objective of neurology earlier was to describe the deficits and their pathogenesis as precisely as possible according to lesions, interest today has shifted more to pinpointing the functional potential still available and promoting it in a learning process" (24).

The weight of habit and received wisdom

We will use a single particularly illustrative example; it concerns physical exercise. Physical exercise and training have long been studied from a physiological point of view in the context of the practice of sports and/or military activities, but no clinical research has ever been devoted to this issue.

From a clinical point of view, the perception of physical exercise has always appeared complex, since bed rest was considered essential in the treatment of a disease. For a long time, therefore, physical activity was contraindicated in patients with heart disease. Yet, as early as 1802, Heberden reported the observation of a patient who had suffered from angina, but whose condition improved simply by sawing wood for half an hour every day. However, we had to wait almost 150 years to implement rehabilitation based on effort training in patients with heart disease. Proof of the efficacy of this approach first of all concerned the extent of the physiological characteristics of the capacity to adapt to effort. This evidence has been completed only very recently in studies involving significant series of patients, which reported improvements in morbidity and mortality.

Similarly, it was only after clinical research had been conducted that effort training was progressively accepted as quotable as a therapy in arteriopathy and heart failure.

Routine and the feeling of security that it procures have therefore had a powerful influence on the durability of recourse to these methods that have "stood the test of time"; the impact of habit and received wisdom can be measured by referring to the worrying situation recently reported by Thompson (36): "it is surprising to observe that exercise training is rarely prescribed for cardiac patients, as evidenced by the fact that only ≈20% of qualified patients are referred to formal cardiac rehabilitation programs."

Today, physical exercise is recommended both as a method of prevention (5) and as a therapeutic agent in practically every area of disease (33). Using the keywords "physical exercise," the number of papers referenced in the PubMed database is huge and has been soaring over the last 15 years. When "therapeutic effects" is associated with these keywords, it appears that the number of papers selected is drastically reduced, even though the number per year is also increasing (**Fig. 1**).

It is therefore possible to consider that exercise is a dynamic and productive field in biomedical research, but that physicians do not currently consider it a therapeutic agent.

One probable explanation is that we are not able to know the "pharmacology" of this agent. Indeed, if exercise is a therapeutic agent, its prescription should be defined as a pharmacological agent; unfortunately, we have to recognize that it is not yet the case.

We could think that PRM is exemplary because it is the daily use of physical activity as a therapeutic agent, but in current practice it is not yet the case; the prescription of physical activity has not yet been perfectly defined.

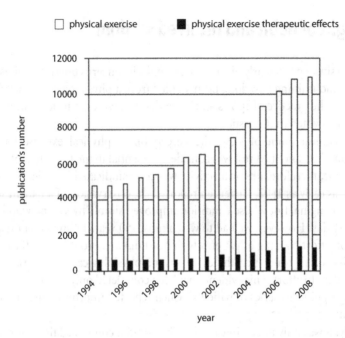

Fig. 1 - Evolution of the number of publications referenced in the Pubmed database from 1994 to 2008 using different keywords.

Of course, the lack of knowledge of the mechanisms involved in the action of physical exercise may explain this paradox; nevertheless, a supplementary difficulty is that it is necessary to teach the patient to do different kinds of exercise. This raises questions concerning learning, which considered a rehabilitation strategy.

Learning and teaching, toward new paradigms

There are many definitions of learning depending on whether we give priority to one of the classical approaches:
- *functionalist* resumed by the expression "learning by doing";
- *behaviorist* expressed by a succession of "trial and error";
- *gestaltist*, which recognizes the central role played by the subject's mental activity "insight" leading to a mental configuration of the environment prior to learning.

Overlap between the different currents has diminished opposition between the different paradigms by recognizing the importance of two major dimensions in learning: the subject's cognitive activity and the impact of social and cultural factors.

Learning and teaching make up two inseparable aspects, most often tackled in the context of learning at school (6), comprising three complementary approaches:
- understand and call upon cognitive mechanisms of learning to learn;

– incorporate the influence of the social context into the learning process;

– know how to motivate and self-motivate to learn.

In any case, it appears that it is about establishing or modifying the ability to carry out a task under the effect of a programmed interaction with the environment. This definition highlights the role played by environmental factors whether they interact directly with the individual immediately or via a third party engaged to teach.

We will not develop here these different aspects, which are covered elsewhere in other chapters of the book. We will, however, point out at this stage the insufficiency of the training for rehabilitation professionals, especially doctors, who are not only unfamiliar with the learning process but also on top of that have not been made aware of the appearance of new paradigms imposed by the introduction of a new technology in rehabilitation.

As they have no specific information on the above points, in most cases, the rehabilitation practitioner is destined to teach using empirical procedures. This can be resumed schematically by formulating a number of the most-often-used instructions, but showing partial understanding of the mechanisms brought into play by each, whether with regard to those involved in explicit or implicit learning:

– do what I say;

– do what I do;

– do it how you like.

We could also add to these frequently used instructions two other instructions that call upon mechanisms that are even less well understood even though they appear able to buttress the interest of certain new technologies such as robotics and virtual reality in the learning process. These instructions may be expressed thus:

– don't do anything and let yourself go;

– don't do anything – just watch the person doing it.

The first of these two instructions corresponds to passive mobilization; yet certain mechanisms of its action are surprising and open the way to new learning practices and the necessary adaptation of teaching methods.

It was long used for "peripheral" purposes, wearing in joints or relaxation of soft tissues, before it was realized that peripheral stimulation performed in this way engendered powerful "central" effects on (re)formatting cerebral structures in a process of reciprocal interaction characteristic of functional plasticity (2). Today, it is regularly used together with imagined movement, which aims to call more strongly upon this biological function.

However, the introduction of robotics opens up new applications by substituting passive manual mobilization with sophisticated instrumental active/passive mobilization, associating the positive constraint of aided mobilization (25) and the negative constraint of resisting mobilization or immobilization; the latter has been recommended notably in rehabilitation of the upper limb in the context of hemiplegia due to stroke (15, 35). Instructions that involve the "person undergoing rehabilitation" as an actor may also become complex by bringing into play new teaching paradigms.

In another area, passive mobilization has been used for "preparation" for movement without imagining that it was able to exert surprising effects on the vasomotor system. Today, it has been shown that stretching vascular walls by the mobilization of body segments can have an effect on endothelial function by releasing mediators of local vasodilatation, notably *no* (26), which supports the use of passive mobilization and validates the instruction *Don't do anything and let yourself go*. However, more details are needed to adapt the instruction in order to exploit the actions of this particular mechanism.

With regard to the instruction that simply requires patients to observe someone else to benefit from the work he or she is doing, without having to do anything themselves, apart from observe, we can easily imagine that it should not be too difficult to motivate someone or to motivate oneself to learn without effort, but we can just as easily imagine that it will be more difficult to learn how to observe in order to see what is supposed to be seen at the right moment. The observation strategy used is apparently not so bereft of interest and may provide information to the rehabilitation practitioner about the cognitive modalities employed by the patient.

In a recent article, it was shown that the muscular strength in any muscle group could be significantly increased in a subject when the subject simply watches another subject actively performing a series of contractions in the same muscle group (29). This surprising effect could bring into play networks of mirror neurons discovered by Rizzolati (31), thus opening the way to new methods of rehabilitation that may, moreover, benefit from the still almost unexplored possibilities offered notably by virtual reality technology.

One chapter of this book is devoted to this particularly stimulating aspect, but already, teaching someone to strengthen a muscle in a muscle group, simply by watching, supposes that the procedure cannot be reduced to simply giving the instruction *Don't do anything – just watch the person doing it*. On the contrary, observing the person who is learning by watching may be an excellent source of information about the cognitive strategies employed by that person, enabling the practitioner to select and, if necessary, reinforce those that prove to be the most effective. The final chapter of this book describes an interesting experiment on this issue.

These comments strongly suggest that clinical practices in PRM involve recourse to an educational approach that will become more and more sophisticated. The approach must evolve in line with better understanding of the mechanisms of action of the procedures and the agents used. It must evolve along with progress in the development of new usable technologies, opening the way for new paradigms in the teaching process.

Learning and teaching without going overboard

The overall aim of rehabilitation is to enable people with disabilities to lead the life that they would wish, given any inevitable restrictions imposed on their activities by impairments resulting from illness or injury. In practice this is often best achieved by a combination of measures to:

– overcome or work around their impairments;

– remove or reduce the barriers to participation in the person's environments;

– support their reintegration in society (18).

According to this definition, the rehabilitation practitioner intervenes in order to enable the person concerned to live and to function with capacities that are different from those he or she would have had without the acquired or congenital lesion, in such a way to allow the person to have a social life that corresponds to the life he or she wishes to lead with the best possible quality of life. The practitioner also intervenes with regard to the person's entourage and, more generally, with regard to society at large in order to promote better understanding and acceptance of the differences, and to implement measures able to make the environment less hostile to disabled people.

Depending on the culture, political choices and the resources made available, it is clear that learning and teaching will prove to be more or less difficult and related to the degree of international harmonization in legislation in favor of disabled people. At the UN, it was thus decided to harmonize the right of disabled people to have access to rehabilitation (37). Individual states are now responsible for the ratification of these provisions. In Europe, a majority of states have still not ratified these provisions, which does not make the task of rehabilitation practitioners any easier. Moreover, the difficulties encountered by disabled people in areas such as respect of the right to work, to be trained, to have access, and to have a minimum revenue are still present in many European states. In these conditions, rehabilitation practitioners may often have the feeling that they are not doing enough.

However, an unexpected difficulty may arise when practitioners, wishing to do their best, may go too far by proposing a program that is overambitious or inappropriate for learning and teaching.

In this context, going overboard may correspond to a lack of objectivity vis-à-vis an unrealistic life project, leading the practitioner to minimize the impact of the subject's functional limits. Ecological analyses of the person's ability to function in everyday life situations – thanks to activity-monitoring devices – considerably reduce this risk (7, 34).

Rehabilitation practitioners may be accused of going too far when they give way to the desires of disabled people or their immediate entourage by testing possible solutions they have proposed even though the practitioner a priori does not agree. This attitude, however, may bear fruit, when it concerns testing an adjustment to therapy or new equipment, or if it involves a consultation with another specialist. These tests may lead to the person adhering to an initially unacceptable rehabilitation program or to revise an initially utopian life project, and in their absence, the necessary motivation to learn may not have been forthcoming.

There are, however, conditions in which "going too far" is inappropriate: learning that results in aggravation of the lesions, the persistence of inappropriate habits and/or the onset of adverse effects.

Aggravation of cerebral lesions linked to the excessively early implementation of overly intensive stimulation or learning in an evolving cerebral lesion has been described in an experimental animal model (22). The sudden massive release of glutamate due to cell death and inflammation engendered by the cerebral lesion has been implicated in the extension of the initial lesions (23). This excitation-related toxicity cannot be ignored even though its effects are local in the immediate post-lesion period.

Learned non-use first described by Meige in 1905 under the name "motor amnesia," then more recently described by Taub in 1993 and termed «learned non-use phenomenon», is an adverse effect of plasticity (3). Inactivity triggers a number of modifications that lead to functional disadaptation, which is self-maintaining and results in a format of inactivity in which nerve structures and effectors adopt an «inactive» mode. Immobilization of a limb segment for therapeutic purposes may perpetuate non-use even though there is no joint stiffness or muscle weakness. In these conditions, inappropriate exploitation functional plasticity may contribute to the learning of misuse by perpetuating genu recurvatum, for example, in hemiplegics.

"Dysplasticity" is another expression to describe inappropriate learning. Repeating an activity in order to learn by mimicking a precise movement identically may lead to segment function dystonia as seen in certain musicians: pianists, violinists, and flutists or other professionals (1). This disorder principally affects the hand when learning is too long and too stereotyped.

Conclusion

Both learning and teaching are not only essential approaches in the rehabilitation process conducted by the PRM practitioner but also approaches that allow practitioners to reconsider PRM when new technologies present particularly attractive opportunities, and when UN has adopted the Convention on the Rights of Persons with Disabilities. The array of resources used in rehabilitation, notably robotics and virtual reality, is providing new opportunities for learning and teaching.

However, learning and teaching are most often used in a context of empiricism with its relative ignorance of the paradigms and mechanisms involved, thus aggravating the risk of seeing habit, and unjustified dogma continue unabated.

The need to resort to validated standards and norms is in line with the modernity of "evidence based medicine," and these norms are the objectives rehabilitation programs aim to achieve. Yet normality, reduced to its statistical dimension, is inappropriate, given the singularity of the disabled person. The needs and the particular conditions of everyday life of such people are not sufficiently taken into account in the learning corpus. Moreover, disabled people cannot be considered sick, whereas the PRM, because it is medical, cannot come to terms with a situation defined according to the distinction between normal and pathological. It thus follows that there is a need to redefine PRM according to the concepts of normality and evidence-based medicine in the light of the particular aspects that differentiate it from other medical specialties.

Finally, those who benefit from rehabilitation and those who implement the process are both actors involved in the same action. They are interdependent on one another and are therefore jointly responsible for the success or failure of the action. The aim of this book is to promote better understanding of the processes involved in learning and teaching so that rehabilitation will be successful more often.

References

1. Altenmuller EO and Jabusch HC (2008) Focal dystonia: diagnostic, therapy, rehabilitation. In: Martin Grunwald (ed) Human haptic perception, Birhäuser, Basel.
2. Andre JM, Didier JP, Paysant J (2004) Plasticité et activité: l'activité musculaire médiatrice réciproque de la plasticité post-lésionnelle du système nerveux et de ses effecteurs. La plasticité de la fonction motrice. Springer, Paris, pp. 341-383
3. André JM, Didier JP, Paysant J (2004) "Functional motor amnesia" in stroke (1904) and "learned non-use phenomenon" (1966). J Rehabil Med 36(3):138-1401. Disability and Rehabilitation Status. Disability and Rehabilitation Team, WHO, Geneva, 2004, p. 11
4. Barbeau H, Norma K, Fung J, Visintin M, Ladouceur M (1998) Does neurohabilitation play a role in the recovery of walking in neurological populations? Ann N Y Acad Sci 860:377-3922. Disability Prevention and Rehabilitation, WHO Technical Report Series 668, Geneva, 1981, p. 9
5. Booth FW, Gordon SE, Carlson CJ, Hamilton MT (2000) Waging war on modern chronic diseases: primary prevention through exercise biology. J Appl Physiol 88;774-7873
6. Bourgeois E, Chapelle G (2006) Apprendre et faire apprendre. Presses Universitaires de France, Paris
7. Bussmann JB, Culhane KM, Horemans HL, *et al.* (2004) Validity of the prosthetic activity monitor to assess the duration and spatio-temporal characteristics of prosthetic walking. IEEE Trans Neural Syst Rehabil Eng 12(4):379-386
8. Cajal R (1928) Degeneration and regeneration of the nervous system. Oxford University Press, London
9. Canguilhem G (1966) Le normal et la pathologique. Ed Presses Universitaires de France, Paris
10. Capon D, Nerot C, Ekelund A, *et al.* (2004) La prothèse d'épaule inversée Delta. A plus de 5 ans de recul. Ann Orthop Ouest 36:41-464. Gutenbrunner C, Ward AB, Chamberlain MA (2007) White book on physical and rehabilitation medicine in Europe. J Rehab Med suppl 45:18
11. Didier JP (2004) La plasticité de la fonction motrice un concept structurant en Médecine Physique et de Réadaptation. In: La plasticité de la fonction motrice. Ed Springer, Paris
12. Didier JP (2007) L'apprentissage, une technique de rééducation, mais apprendre quoi, comment, en évitant quoi? Kinésithérapie Scientifique 39(482):39-45

13. Disability and Rehabilitation Team (2004) Disability and rehabilitation status. WHO, Geneva, p. 11

14. World Health Organization (1981) Disability prevention and rehabilitation. Technical Report Series 668. WHO, Geneva, p. 9

15. Dromerick AW, Edwards DF, Hahn M (2000) Does the application of constraint-induced movement therapy during acute rehabilitation reduce arm impairment after ischemic stroke? Stroke 31:2984-2988

16. Gardien E (2008) L'apprentissage du corps après l'accident. Presses Universitaires de Grenoble

17. Gunn SWA, Mansourian PB, Davies AM, et al. (2005) Understanding the global dimensions of health. Ed Springer, pp. 147-156

18. Gutenbrunner C, Ward AB, Chamberlain MA (2007) White book on physical and rehabilitation medicine in Europe. J Rehab Med suppl 45:18

19. Heilporn A, André JM, Didier JP, Chamberlain MA (2006) Violence to and maltreatment of people with disabilities. A short review. J Rehabil Med 38:1-3

20. Hesse SA, Bertelt C, Jahnke MT, (1995) Treadmill training with partial body weight support compared with physiotherapy in non-ambulatory hemiplegic patients. Stroke 26:976-981

21. Hesse SA, Uhlenbrock D (1999) Gait pattern of severely disabled hemiparetic subjects on a new controlled gait trainer as compared to assisted treadmill walking will partial body weight support. Clin Rehabil 93:401-410

22. Humm JL, Kozlowski DA, James DC, et al. (1998) Use-dependent exacerbation of brain damage occurs during an early post-lesion vulnerable period. Brain Res 783:286-292

23. Humm JL, Kozlowski DA, Bland ST, et al. (1999) Use-dependent exaggeration of brain injury: is glutamate involved? Exp Neurol 157:349-358. 10 – Rapport de l'OMS-Europe1996, Therapeutic Patient Teaching – Continuing Teaching Programmes for Health Care Providers in the field of Chronic Disease

24. Kesselring J (2001) A bridge between basic science and clinical practice. Neurorehabilitation 8(3):221-225

25. Mayr A, Kofler M, Quirbach E (2007) Prospective, blinded, randomized crossover study of gait rehabilitation in stroke patients using the Lokomat gait orthosis. Neurorehabil Neural Repair 21(4):307-314

26. Moyna NM, Thompson PD (2004) The effect of physical activity on endothelial function in man. Acta Physiol Scand 180(2):113-123

27. Paillard J (1976) Réflexions sur l'usage d u concept de plasticité en. Neurobiologie Journal de Psychologie Normale et Pathologique 1:33-47

28. Paysant J, Beyaert C, Datie AM, et al. (2006) Influence of terrain on metabolic and temporal gait characteristics of unilateral transtibial amputees. J Rehabil Res Dev 43(2):153-160

29. Porro CA, Facchin P, Fusi S, et al. (2007) Enhancement of force after action observation. Behavioural and neurophysiological studies. Neuropsychologica 4:3114-3121

30. Rapport de l'OMS-Europe (1996) Therapeutic patient teaching – continuing teaching programmes for health care providers in the field of chronic disease

31. Rizzolati G, Fadiga L, Fogassi L, Gallese V (1996) Premotor cortex and the recognition of motor actions. Cogn Br Res 3:131-141

32. Rondal JA, Comblain A, Bazier G (2001) Manuel de psychologie des handicaps. Sémiologie et principes de remédiation. Ed Mardaga, Hayen-Sprimont.

33. Singh R (2002) The importance of exercise as a therapeutic agent. Malays J Med Sci 9.2:7-16

34. Stam HJ, Bussmann JB (2004) Evaluation et monitoring de la fonction motrice: mesures des activités physiques par accélérométrie embarquée. Ed Springer, Paris, pp. 285-315

35. Taub E, Uswatte G, Pidikiti R (1999) Constraint-induced movement therapy: a new family of techniques with broad application to physical rehabilitation. A clinical review. J Rehabil Res Dev 36(3):237-251

36. Thompson PD (2005) Exercise prescription and proscription for patients with coronary artery disease. Circulation 112:2354-2363

37. United Nations Inter-Agency Support Group for the Convention on the Rights of Persons with Disabilities, December 13, 2006

38. Visintin M, Barbeau H, Korner-Bitensk NK, Mayo NE (1998) A new approach to retrain gait in stroke patient through body weight support and treadmill stimulation. Stroke 29:1122-1128

39. Wood PN (1989) Measuring the consequences of illness. World Health Stat Q 42:115-121

40. World Health Organization (2001) International Classification of Functioning, Disability and Health (ICF). WHO, Geneva

41. Yelnick A (2005) Evolution des concepts en rééducation du patient hémiplégique. Annales de rééducation de médecine Physique 48:270-277

The International Classification of Functioning, Disability and Health (ICF), a unifying model for physical and rehabilitation medicine (PRM)

G. Stucki and A. Rauch

Introduction

A unifying scientific model is of utmost importance for any professional, academic, and scientific discipline. It provides a conceptual link between disparate parts that might appear superficially to lack an intellectual relationship. Thus, it ensures communication and exchange among practitioners and scientists. To be able to rely on a common model seems to be of even more importance for a professional discipline, such as physical medicine and rehabilitation (internationally now called physical and rehabilitation medicine (PRM)), that is not defined by a disease or an organ system. Instead, PRM is concerned with limitations of functioning and disability associated with health conditions and with the complex interaction with personal factors and the environment (45). Indeed, PRM can be understood as the "medicine of functioning."

Until recently, a main barrier to the development of practice and research in relation to PRM was the lack of a globally agreed model and classification of human functioning (20). This unfortunate situation has changed with the International Classification of Functioning, Disability and Health (ICF) (53). With the ICF, the WHO provides for the first time a universal and internationally accepted framework and classification (35). The ICF is a promising starting point for the integrative understanding of functioning, disability, and health and the overcoming of Cartesian dualism of body and mind as well as both sociological and biomedical reductionism (21). The ICF, as a universally applicable and integrative model of human functioning and disability, is thus a promising starting point for the development of rehabilitation practice and research (20, 35).

In this chapter, we first review the development of the ICF in the context of the United Nations (UN) system and its specialty agency the World Health Organization (WHO). We will then review how the ICF can be used both as a reference standard and as a starting point for the classification and measurement of functioning. Next we will outline how the ICF can serve as a unifying framework for the conceptualization of rehabilitation understood as a public health strategy and the medical specialty PRM (39, 45), and how it may serve as the basis for the organization and development of human functioning and rehabilitation research relevant for PRM. Finally, we will summarize how the ICF can be used in rehabilitation management.

The ICF

The ICF in the Perspective of the WHO and the UN System

Recognizing the importance of functioning and disability as a major public health issue both in the developed and in the developing world, the WHO has developed the ICF to provide a unified international and standardized language for describing and classifying health and health-related domains and hence a common framework for health outcome measurement. The ICF thus complements indicators that have traditionally focused on deaths and diseases (52). To complement mortality or diagnostic data on morbidity and diseases is important since they alone do not adequately capture health outcomes of individuals and populations (e.g., diagnosis alone does not explain what patients can do, what their prognosis is, what they need, and what treatment costs are) (4, 50).

The ICF, which is coordinated by the WHO's Classification, Terminology and Standards (CTS) team serves as a reference framework throughout the WHO. Most importantly, the ICF is the reference framework of the WHO's Disability and Rehabilitation (DAR) team under the Department of Violence and Injury Prevention and Disability. The World Health Assembly's (WHA) Resolution 58.23 on "disability, including prevention, management and rehabilitation," approved in May 2005 by the 58th World Health Assembly (51) and coordinated by the DAR team, thus recalls the ICF as its framework (20). As requested by the resolution, the WHO is currently developing a "World Report on Disability and Rehabilitation" whose structure is based on the ICF framework. The International Society of Physical and Rehabilitation Medicine (ISPRM), which is the international PRM organization in official relation with the WHO, is represented on the advisory board of the report and is supporting the DAR team in this development.

While the ICF has been developed by the WHO, the specialty agency responsible for health within the UN system, the ICF has been accepted as one of the UN social classifications (53). It thus now serves as reference framework for the UN and its other specialty agencies, including the UN Statistics Division (UNSTAT), the UN Educational, Scientific and Cultural Organization (UNESCO), and the International Labour Organization (ILO).

Although the ICF is not explicitly mentioned, the understanding of its functioning as a universal experience according to the ICF framework is the basis for the characterization of disability in the UN Convention on the Rights of Persons with Disabilities (49), approved on December 13, 2006, at the UN Headquarters in New York. While the convention does not establish new human rights, it does define the obligations on states to promote, protect, and ensure the rights of persons with disabilities. Most importantly, it sets out the many steps that states must take to create an enabling environment, so that persons with disabilities can enjoy inclusion and equal participation in society.

Development of the ICF

The ICF was developed in a worldwide collaborative process through the network of collaboration centers for the family of international classifications, especially the North American Collaboration Center (NACC) for the Family of International Classifications. After three preliminary drafts and extensive international field testing including linguistic and cultural applicability research, the successor classification, the ICF, which was first tentatively named ICIDH-2, was finalized in 2000 and approved by the 54th World Health Assembly in 2001 (53). The ICF for Children and Youth (ICF-CY) was finalized and officially launched in 2007. Until March 2008, the ICF has been translated in several languages.

Similar to the ICD, which is now undergoing its 11th revision, the ICF will undergo updates and ultimately a revision process. The update is prepared by the WHO's CTS team in collaboration with the relevant committees and the Functioning and Disability Reference Group (FDRG) of the Network of the Collaboration Centers for the Family of International Classifications (WHO FIC CC Network), of whom the NACC is a member.

According to the ICF, functioning is the lived experience of people (2). It is a universal human experience (2, 56) in which body, person, and society are intertwined (13, 53). Over the life span, people may experience a variation in the level of functioning associated with congenital disorders, injuries, acute and chronic health conditions, and ageing. The experience of a limitation of functioning or disability is thus part of the human condition (2).

The ICF not only addresses Western concepts but also has worldwide cultural applicability. The ICF follows the principle of a universal as opposed to a minority model. Accordingly, it covers the entire life span. It is integrative and not merely medical or social. Similarly, it addresses human functioning and not merely disability. It is multidimensional and interactive and rejects the linear linkage between health condition and functioning. It is also etiologically neutral, which means functioning is understood descriptively and not caused by diagnosis. It adopts the parity approach, which does not recognize an inherent distinction or asymmetry between mental and physical functioning.

These principles address many of the criticisms of previous conceptual frameworks and integrate concepts established during the development of the Nagi model (26, 27) and the Institute of Medicine model of 1991 (3, 28). Most importantly, the inclusion of environmental and personal factors, together with the health condition, reflects the integration of the two main conceptual paradigms that had been used previously to understand and explain functioning and disability, i.e., the medical model and the social model. The ICF and its framework achieve a synthesis, thereby providing a coherent view of different perspectives of health (2).

The Structure of the ICF

As shown in **Fig. 1**, the ICF consists of three components making up functioning and the contextual personal and environmental factors. In short, the first component, body functions and structures, refers to physiologic functions and anatomic parts, respectively; loss or deviations from normal body functions and structures are referred to as impairments. The second component, activity, refers to task execution by the individual. "Activity limitations" are thus difficulties the individual may have in executing activities. The third component, participation, refers to involvement in life situations. "Participation restrictions" are thus problems the individual may experience with such involvement. These three components are summarized under the umbrella terms "functioning" and "disability." They are related to and may interact with the health condition (e.g., disorder or disease) and the contextual personal and environmental factors.

The components of body functions and structures, activities and participation, and environmental factors are classified based on the ICF categories. The ICF contains a total of 1424 meaningful and discrete or mutually exclusive categories. Taken together, the mutually exclusive ICF categories are cumulative and exhaustive, and hence cover the whole spectrum of human experience. The categories are organized within a hierarchically nested structure with up to four different levels. The ICF categories are denoted by unique alphanumeric codes with which it is possible to classify functioning and disability, both on the individual and on the population level.

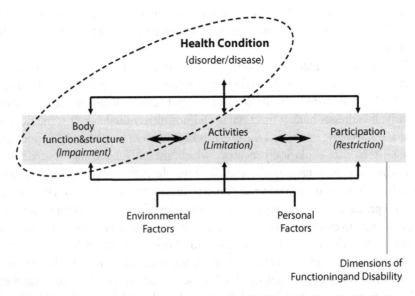

Fig. 1 - The model of functioning and disability on which the ICF is based. The dotted circle illustrates the focused perspective based on the biomedical model versus the comprehensive perspective based on the integrative model of functioning (whole figure).

Validity of the ICF

A wide range of studies across world regions and user perspectives that have been examined have provided empirical and theoretical evidence supporting different aspects of the validity of the ICF framework (12). To the surprise of many clinicians and scientists, the ICF has been shown to be a highly comprehensive classification covering virtually all aspects of the patient experience. More specifically, the ICF has covered the spectrum of problems encountered by people with a wide range of conditions and along the continuum of care within the context of the ICF Core Set development described later in this chapter (12, 44). Further proof as to the comprehensiveness of the ICF is the finding that items of a wide range of measurement instruments can be mapped to the ICF. Most importantly, the ICF broadly represents the contents of health-related quality of life measures (16). The validity of the ICF framework is also strengthened by the fact that the majority of the concepts from three conceptual occupational therapy models could be linked to the ICF (23, 32, 33), and that there is a strong conceptual connection between the ICF and occupational therapy models (32).

ICF-based classification and measurement

ICF categories: building blocks and reference units

Ideally, measures of human functioning or aspects of it are based on a common and universally shared framework and classification. The categories of such a classification can serve as reference standards for the reporting of functioning across a wide range of measures. They can also serve as building blocks for the development of clinical and self-reported measurement instruments tailored to the need of prospective users and suitable for varying purposes. Since its launch in 2001, the ICF has thus attracted wide interest in the health sciences and particularly in the field of measurement and outcomes research (12).

The ICF categories are the discrete, meaningful, universally shared and understood elements that allow users to comprehensively classify and measure functioning of individuals and populations. In this context, it is important to recall the difference between ICF categories and measurement items, e.g., of self-reported health status measures. As meaningful and universally shared elements, ICF categories represent constructs while measurement items are stimuli that allow the quantification of attributes in relation to a construct, e.g., an ICF category.

As discrete elements of functioning, the ICF categories serve as building blocks for the development of ICF-based practical tools such as the ICF Checklist (55) and the ICF Core Sets (6, 17, 42, 48, 50). They also serve as building blocks for the construction of clinical measurement instruments such as the ICF Core Set Indices currently under development for ankylosing spondylitis (9) and osteoarthritis (10) and self-reported measurement instruments such as the WHODAS II (WHO Disability Assessment Schedule II) (14).

ICF-based practical tools: ICF Checklist and ICF Core Sets

To implement the ICF in clinical medicine, service provision, and policy, practical tools need to be developed (41, 50). In this context, it is important to recall that the ICF has been developed as a reference classification and is not intended to be a practical tool. The main challenge to the application of the ICF is the size of the classification system with its 1424 categories. Dr. Üstün, the leader of WHO's CTS team, has pointed out that "a clinician cannot easily take the main volume of the ICF and consistently apply it to his or her patients. In daily practice, clinicians will only need a fraction of the categories found in the ICF" (50).

ICF Checklist

The ICF Checklist is a 12-page "short" version of the ICF, with 125 second-level categories. All information from written records, primary respondent, other informants, and direct observation can be used (55). It takes around one hour to complete but may take much longer in patients with multiple impairments, activity limitations, and participation restrictions. It has been applied in a wide range of surveys and in studies in the process of developing ICF Core Sets (15).

ICF Core Sets

ICF Core Sets are parsimonious and hence practical sets of ICF categories for clinical practice, service provision and payment, research, and health statistics. They link the ICF to health conditions as coded with the ICD (42, 48, 50). The ICF Core Sets serve first as practical tools for the documentation of functioning and second as international reference standards for the reporting of functioning irrespective of measurement instruments used. They are also the starting point for the development of clinical and self-reported measurement instruments (9, 10, 19).

The ICF Core Set Project is a joint project of the ICF Research Branch of the WHO FIC CC Germany (DIMDI) at the Institute of Health and Rehabilitation Sciences at the Ludwig-Maximilian-University in Munich, Germany, and at Swiss Paraplegic Research in Nottwil, Switzerland, together with WHO's CTS team, ISPRM, and a large number of partner organizations and associated institutions as well as committed clinicians and scientists (42, 48, 50).

The conceptual approach for the development of the ICF Core Sets is based on two perspectives: [1] the perspective of people who share the experience of the same condition (e.g., multiple sclerosis) or condition group (e.g., neurological conditions) and [2] the perspective of the health service context along the continuum of care or the life span. Table 1 shows a list of the ICF Core Sets currently available or under development. A full list of references relevant for the ICF Core Set development can be found on the web page of the ICF Research Branch (www.icf-research-branch.org) or in a recent publication summarizing the current state of the ICF-based classification and measurement of functioning (44).

Table 1 - ICF Core Set development.

ICF Core Sets	
Acute context	Neurological conditions Musculoskeletal conditions Cardiopulmonary conditions
Early post-acute Context	Neurological conditions Musculoskeletal conditions Cardiopulmonary conditions Geriatric patients
Long-term context	Chronic widespread pain Low back pain Osteoarthritis Osteoporosis Rheumatoid arthritis Chronic ischemic heart disease Diabetes Obesity Obstructive pulmonary diseases Depression Breast cancer Stroke Psoriasis and psoriatic arthritis Ankylosing spondylitis Spinal cord injury Systemic lupus erythematosus Multiple sclerosis Head and neck cancer Bipolar disorders

Sources: (6, 37, 39, 44, 50)

Mapping the world of measures to the ICF and vice versa

Since the ICF is the universal and standardized language to classify, describe, and report functioning and health, users need to be able to map the world of measures to the ICF. The qualitative mapping of measurement instruments to the ICF relies on linkage rules (5, 7). The quantitative mapping relies on transformations using the Rasch model (8).

Qualitative mapping is applied for the content comparison of measurement instruments, e.g., when studying their comparative content validity. The ICF-based comparison of measurement instruments can therefore assist researchers and clinicians to identify and select a most suited measurement instrument for a specified purpose. ICF-based comparisons also enable researchers to ensure that all ICF categories of an applicable ICF Core Set representing an international standard for a specific health condition or health service context are covered by candidate measurement instruments and hence to report functioning according to international standards (35). **Table 2** lists studies that have compared most widely used measurement instruments for specified health conditions as well as a comparison of generic health status measures.

Table 2 - Mapping of measurement instruments to the ICF.

Context	Health Condition	Reference	Measurements/Instruments
Early post-acute Context	Neurological conditions Musculoskeletal conditions Cardiopulmonary conditions Geriatric patients	[1]	Functional Independence Measure (FIM), Functional Assessment Measure (FAM); Barthel Index (BI)
Long-term context	Obesity	[2]	Bariatric Analysis and Reporting Outcome System (BAROS); Bariatric Quality of Life Index (BQL); Lite, Impact of Weight on Quality of Life Questionnaire (IWQOL); LEWIN-TAG Questionnaire (LEWIN-TAG); Obesity Adjustment Survey-Short Form (OAS-SF); Obesity-Related Coping (OCQ); Obesity-Related Distress Questionnaire (ODQ); Obesity Eating Problems Scale (OE); Obesity-Related Problems Scale (OP); Obesity-Related Well-being Questionnaire (ORWELL); Short-Specific Quality of Life Scale (OSQOL); Obesity and Weight-Loss Quality of Life (OWLQOL); Weight-Related Symptom Measure (WRSM)
	Osteoarthritis	[3]	Health Assessment Questionnaire (HAQ); Australian/Canadian Osteoarthritis Hand Index (AUSCAN); Cochin scale; Functional Index of Hand OA (FIHOA); Score for Assessment and Qualification of Chronic Rheumatoid Affections of the Hands questionnaire (SACRAH); Arthritis Impact Measurement 2 Short Form questionnaire (AIMS2-SF)
	Osteoarthritis	[4]	Western Ontario and McMaster Universities (WOMAC) and Lequesne-Algofunctional Indices
	Low back pain	[5]	North American Spine Society Lumbar Spine Outcome Assessment Instrument (NASS); Oswestry Low Back Disability Questionnaire (ODI); Roland-Morris Disability Questionnaire (RMQ)

Context	Health Condition	Reference	Measurements/Instruments
	Osteoporosis	[6]	Quality of Life Questionnaire of the European Foundation for Osteoporosis (QUALEFFO-41); Osteoporosis Assessment Questionnaire (OPAQ 2.0); Osteoporosis Assessment Questionnaire Short Version (OPAQ-SV)
	Stroke	[7]	Stroke Impact Scale (SIS); Stroke-Specific Quality of Life Scale (SSQOL); Stroke and Aphasia Quality of Life Scale (SAQOL-39); Quality of Life Index - Stroke Version (QLI-SV); Stroke-Adapted Sickness Impact Profile-30 (SA-SIP30); Burden of Stroke Scale (BOSS); Quality of Life Instrument for Young Hemorrhagic Stroke Patients (HS-Quale)
	Ankylosing spondylitis	[8]	Bath Ankylosing Functional Index (BAS-FI); Dougados Functional Index (DFI); Health Assessment Questionnaire modified for the spondylarthropathies HAQ-S); Revised Leeds Disability Questionnaire (RLDQ)
	Chronic obstructive pulmonary diseases	[9]	St. George's Respiratory Questionnaire (SGRQ); Chronic Respiratory Questionnaire, Standardized Version (CRQ-SAS); Pulmonary Functional Status & Dyspnea Questionnaire, Modified Version (PFS-DQM); Pulmonary Functional Status Scale (PFSS); Breathing Problems Questionnaire (BPQ); Seattle Obstructive Lung Disease Questionnaire (SOLDQ); Quality of Life for Respiratory Illness Questionnaire (QOLRIQ); Airway Questionnaires 20 (AQ20); London Chest Activity of Daily Living Scale (LCADL); Maugeri Foundation Respiratory Failure Questionnaire (MRF28); Clinical COPD Questionnaire (CCQ)
Generic	Different conditions	[10]	Medical Outcomes Study 36-Item Short-Form Health Survey (SF-36); Nottingham Health Profile (NHP); Quality of Life Index (QLI); World Health Organization Quality of Life Scale (WHOQOL-BREF); World Health Organisation Disability Assessment Schedule II (WHODASII); European Quality of Life Instrument (EQ-5D)

Context	Health Condition	Reference	Measurements/Instruments
	Different conditions	[7]	Medical Outcomes Study 36-Item Short-Form Health Survey (SF-36); Reintegration to Normal Living Index (RNL); Sickness Impact Profile (SIP); European Quality of Life Instrument (EQ-5D); LHS London Handicap Scale (LHS); Nottingham Health Profile (NHP); Dartmouth COOP Charts (COOP); 15-Dimensional Measure of Health Related Quality of Life Test (15-D); Assessment of Life Habits (LIFE-H); Assessment of Quality of Life (AQoL); Craig Handicap Assessment and Reporting Technique (CHART); Health Utilities Index Mark II (HUI II); Health Status Questionnaire (HSQ); Lancashire Quality of Life Profile (LQLP); Quality of Life Index (QLI); World Health Organization Quality of Life Scale (WHOQOL)
Occupational context	Different conditions	[11]	Canadian Occupational Performance Measure (COPM); Assessment of Motor and Process Skills (AMPS); Sequential Occupational Dexterity Assessment (SODA); Jebsen Taylor Hand Function Test (JT-HF); Moberg Picking Up Test (MPUT); Button Test (Button); Functional Dexterity Test (FDT)

Source: (44)

1. Grill E, Stucki G, Scheuringer M, Melvin J (2006) Validation of International Classification of Functioning, Disability, and Health (ICF) Core Sets for early postacute rehabilitation facilities: comparisons with three other functional measures. Am J Phys Med Rehabil 85:640-649

2. Stucki A, Borchers M, Stucki G, *et al.* (2006) Content comparison of health status measures for obesity based on the international classification of functioning, disability and health. Int J Obes (Lond) 30:1791-1799

3. Stamm T, Geyh S, Cieza A, *et al.* (2006) Measuring functioning in patients with hand osteoarthritis-content comparison of questionnaires based on the International Classification of Functioning, Disability and Health (ICF). Rheumatology (Oxford) 45:1534-1541

4. Weigl M, Cieza A, Harder M, *et al.* (2003) Linking osteoarthritis-specific health-status measures to the international classification of functioning, disability, and health (ICF). Osteoarthritis Cartilage 11:519-523

5. Sigl T, Cieza A, Brockow T, *et al.* (2006) Content comparison of low back pain-specific measures based on the International Classification of Functioning, Disability and Health (ICF). J Clin Pain 22:147-153

6. Borchers M, Cieza A, Sigl T, *et al.* (2005) Content comparison of osteoporosis-targeted health status measures in relation to the International Classification of Functioning, Disability and Health (ICF). Clin Rheumatol 24:139-144

7. Geyh S, Cieza A, Kollerits B, *et al.* (2007) Content comparison of health-related quality of life measures used in stroke based on the international classification of functioning, disability and health (ICF): a systematic review. Qual Life Res 16:833-851

8. Sigl T, Cieza A, van der Heijde D, Stucki G (2005) ICF-based comparison of disease-specific instruments measuring physical functional ability for ankylosing spondylitis. Ann Rheum Dis 64:1576-1581

9. Stucki A, Stucki G, Cieza A, *et al.* (2007) Content comparison of health-related quality of life instruments for COPD. Respir Med 101:1113-1122

10. Cieza A, Stucki G (2005) Content comparison of health related quality of life instruments based on the ICF. Qual Life Res 14:1225-1237
11. Stamm TA, Cieza A, Machold KP, *et al.* (2004) Content comparison of occupation-based instruments in adult rheumatology and musculoskeletal rehabilitation based on the International Classification of Functioning, Disability and Health. Arthritis Rheum 51:917-924

Qualitative mapping in combination with quantitative mapping is used for the identification of measurement items addressing the construct covered by a specified ICF category and the construction of Rasch scales to estimate the level of functioning for this category. An example of qualitative mapping combined with quantitative mapping is the transformation of information from electronic records (25).

ICF-based measurement of functioning

Measuring a single ICF category

In principle, there are two approaches to measure a specified ICF category, i.e., to quantify the extent of variation therein. The first is the direct coding of the ICF Qualifier used as rating scale ranging from 0 to 4 (**Table 3**). Coding therefore is a form of measurement since it involves the assignment of numbers to attributes of ICF categories. The second is to use information obtained with a clinical test or a patient-oriented instrument and to transform this information into the ICF Qualifier used as a reference scale.

Table 3 - Direct coding of the *ICF Qualifier* used as *rating scale* ranging from 0 to 4.

ICF Qualifier*		Percentage of Problem
Body functions, body structures, activity, and participation		
0 – NO problem (none, absent, negligible, ...)		0-4%
1 – MILD problem (slight, low, ...)		5-24%
2 – MODERATE problem (medium, fair, ...)		25-49%
3 – SEVERE problem (high, extreme, ...)		50-95%
4 – COMPLETE problem (total, ...)		96-100%
Environmental factors		
0 – NO barrier	+0 – No facilitator	0-4%
1 – MILD barrier	+1 – MILD facilitator	5-24%
2 – MODERATE barrier	+2 – MODERATE facilitator	25-49%
3 – SEVERE barrier	+3 – SEVERE facilitator	50-95%
4 – COMPLETE barrier	+4 – Complete facilitator	96-100%

* "Having a problem may mean an impairment, a limitation, a restriction, or a barrier, depending on the construct," i.e., depending on whether we are classifying body functions and structures (impairments), activity and participation (limitations or restrictions), or environmental factors (barriers or facilitators).

With the direct coding of the ICF Qualifier, a physician or health professional integrates all accessible and suitable information from the patient's history and clinical and technical exams to code a specified category according to established coding guidelines

(31). To ensure quality in a specific setting, it is advisable to regularly assess the reliability of coding (18). The rating of certain ICF categories may be facilitated by complementary instructions provided in addition to the descriptions of the ICF categories as provided in the ICF reference material. Complementary instructions have been, for example, developed by the American Psychological Association (1).

When transforming information obtained with a clinical test or a patient-oriented instrument, the ICF Qualifier serves as a reference scale. The results from a clinical test or a patient-oriented measurement instrument are transformed into the ICF Qualifier using the linking methodology (8).

For many ICF categories, there are suitable clinical tests that include standardized expert and technical examinations or patient-oriented measurement instruments that include patient and proxy-reported, self-administered, or interview-administered questionnaires, which are routinely used in clinical practice or for research purposes. In this case, information already available can be transformed to report the results with respect to a relevant ICF category in the standard language of the ICF.

In the case where there are no readily available clinical tests or patient-oriented instruments with interval-scale properties that can be used to assess a specified ICF category, one may consider the construction of an ICF category interval scale using parts of clinical test batteries or selected measurement items of patient-oriented measurement instruments that cover a specified ICF category (8). The obtained raw scores on the ICF category scale can then be transformed into the ICF Qualifier, which serves as a reference scale. A major advantage of the second approach is that the original format of the items used to construct the ICF category interval scale remains unchanged. Thus, it is possible to use the information provided by items within the context of their original instruments and, at the same time, within the context of the ICF. This application can be extremely useful, given the increasing use of the ICF and the ICF Qualifier as references when documenting and reporting functioning and disability (22, 45).

Measuring across ICF categories

Based on the ICF, it is possible to develop self-reported measurement instruments. The WHO has developed the WHODAS II (29, 54), a generic self-administered questionnaire used in adults >18 years of age, which covers the ICF components activity and participation. It includes six domains: *understanding and communicating, getting around, self-care, getting along with others, household and work activities*, and *participation in society*. It has been developed cross-culturally and is applicable across the spectrum of cultural and educational backgrounds. In addition to self-report, an interviewer and proxy version is available. The time to complete the questionnaire for the 12-item version is approximately 5 minutes, and for the 36-item version, it is 20 minutes.

For specific conditions and/or settings, one may want to use a specific measurement instrument. A suitable starting point for the development for such measurement instruments are the ICF Core Sets. The ICF Research Branch of the WHO FIC CC Germany at the University of Munich is thus cooperating with and supporting research groups in the process to develop self-reported questionnaires based on the ICF Core Sets (www.icf-research-branch.org).

The ICF can also serve as the basis for the development of ICF-based clinical measurement instruments. Clinicians' ratings of the ICF Qualifier across a number of ICF categories, e.g., across the categories of an ICF Core Set, can be reported in the form of a categorical profile. A categorical profile across a valid set of ICF categories such as an ICF Core Set provides an estimation of a person's *functioning state*. The functioning state is the central information for clinicians when planning and reporting the results of a health care intervention. **Figure 5** shows an example of the functioning states at the start and the end of a rehabilitation program.

The aggregation of information obtained from a categorical profile using the Rasch model results in a summary score (10, 19). In the case of aggregation of information across a valid set of categories such as ICF Core Set, the summary score provides an estimation of a person's functioning status. If using an electronic clinical chart, the creation of a score from a categorical profile created based on an ICF Core Set does not require additional work. Functioning status information provides clinicians with an intuitive, overall understanding of a patient's general level of functioning. It can be used by clinicians, service program providers, and payers, e.g., for the assignment of patients to suitable rehabilitation service programs, to monitor and manage persons functioning along the continuum of care and across service program providers, to evaluate service programs, to predict resources and hence costs, and to derive payment schemes.

The principle of how to develop one- or multi-dimensional clinical measurement instruments based on clinicians' ratings of the ICF Core Sets has been recently demonstrated (9, 10, 19). It could also be demonstrated how to apply such scores across countries by adjusting for differential item function. It is thus possible to compare functioning status information across countries and world regions.

The ICF, a unifying model for PRM

ICF-based conceptualization of the public health strategy rehabilitation and the medical specialty (PRM)

Rehabilitation can be understood as the public health strategy that focuses on functioning and that complements the preventive, curative, and supportive strategy (**Table 4**) (39). As a universally shared concept of functioning, the ICF can therefore serve as a framework and taxonomy for conceptual descriptions and definitions of rehabilitation (39) and accordingly of PRM and the rehabilitation professions.

Table 4 - Rehabilitation in the context of four health strategies.

	Preventive Strategy	Curative Strategy	Rehabilitative Strategy	Supportive Strategy
Primary goal	Prevent health conditions (e.g., vaccination to prevent polio)	Cure health conditions (e.g., tuberculosis)	Restore functioning (e.g., rehabilitation after hip replacement)	Optimize quality of life (e.g., pain control in cancer)
Alternative goals	Reduce incidence of conditions (e.g., tobacco control to reduce incidence of lung cancer)	Remission (e.g., chemotherapy for cancer) Disease control (e.g., biologics in rheumatoid arthritis) Damage control in injury	Optimize functioning (e.g., rehabilitation in chronic conditions, such as, multiple sclerosis; in ageing; in acute conditions with sequelae such as spinal cord injury or stroke)	Preserve autonomy (e.g., assistance to preserve independence)
Key outcomes	Health Survival	Survival Functioning	Functioning Quality of Life	Quality of life Health
Related outcomes	Functioning and disability Quality of life	Quality of Life Health	Health Survival	Survival Functioning
Sector	Health	Health	Health (reference or root sector) Education Labor Social	Health (reference or root sector) Social

Source: (6)

Initiated by the professional affairs committee of the PRM section of the European Union of Medical Specialists (UEMS) and in cooperation with the *Journal of Rehabilitation Medicine* (JRM), the official journal of ISPRM, a process toward universally agreed conceptual descriptions of rehabilitation (39), PRM, and the rehabilitation professions (45) has been started in 2007. A brief version of the proposed conceptual description describes rehabilitation as the "health strategy applied by PRM and professionals in the health sector and across other sectors that aim to enable people with *health conditions* experiencing or likely to experience *disability*, to achieve and maintain optimal *functioning* in interaction with the *environment*" (39). A brief version of the conceptual description for PRM describes it accordingly as "the medical specialty that, based on the assessment of *functioning* and including the diagnosis and treatment of *health conditions* performs, applies and coordinates biomedical and engineering and a wide range of other interventions with the goal of optimizing *functioning* of people experiencing or likely to experience *disability*" (45).

ICF-based conceptual descriptions of rehabilitation as a health strategy (39) and of PRM may contribute to the development of a common understanding of rehabilitation across professional and scientific disciplines and an enhanced recognition of rehabilitation through stakeholders, funding agencies, and policymakers.

ICF-based organization of "human functioning and rehabilitation research"

The meaningful structuring of research areas requires the delineation of distinct scientific fields. Distinct scientific fields are pivotal for the fruitful division of labor, the advancement of innovations, and the development of a common identity among researchers. A possible approach for the structuring of a putative research area called human functioning and rehabilitation is the general distinction in basic, applied, and professional sciences applicable to research in general, and the rehabilitation relevant distinction between the comprehensive perspective based on the ICF as the WHO's integrative model of human functioning and the more focused perspective of the biomedical aspects of functioning (**Fig. 1**). Human functioning and rehabilitation can accordingly be structured in five distinct scientific fields ranging "from the cell to society" (20, 43, 46, 47). At the core of the proposed organization of human functioning and rehabilitation research is the suggestion to establish the human functioning sciences and integrative rehabilitation sciences as basic and applied sciences for rehabilitation from the comprehensive perspective (8, 10, 41). They complement the biosciences and biomedical rehabilitation sciences and engineering, which focus on the biomedical aspects of functioning and the professional rehabilitation sciences to which PRM belongs. **Figure 2** shows a graphical depiction and short descriptions of the five proposed distinct scientific fields (43, 47). **Table V** (46) lists research domains of the distinct fields.

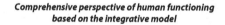

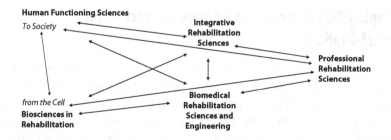

Fig. 2 - Graphical depiction and short descriptions of the five proposed distinct scientific fields (37, 43).

Table 5 - Domains of research in the five distinct scientific fields of human functioning and rehabilitation research.

Human functioning sciences – Theory and models of functioning – Classification and measurement of functioning – Functioning epidemiology – Functioning impact assessment

Integrative rehabilitation sciences
– Rehabilitation services research
    including health policy and law, rehabilitation economics and community-based parti-
    cipatory research
– Rehabilitation intervention research
    including rehabilitation intervention program research; rehabilitation technology as-
    sessment in clinical and community settings, technology transfer; and applying research
    designs ranging from randomized controlled trials to observational studies
– Rehabilitation administration and management
    including the development of integrated care and service concepts and ICF-based case
    management programs as well as the design of other structures and processes in rehabi-
    litation institutions

Biosciences in rehabilitation (examples) – Tissue injury and repair – Plasticity – Homeostatic mechanisms of muscle contraction
Biomedical rehabilitation sciences and engineering – Research in relation to organ systems, e.g., cardiopulmonary, musculoskeletal or neurologi- cal rehabilitation research – Research in relation to intervention principles, e.g., rehabilitation engineering, occupational therapy and physiotherapy research, drug trials
Professional rehabilitation sciences – Standards and guidelines for the provision of best care – Rehabilitation quality management – Scientific education and training of professionals in rehabilitation – Development and evaluation of the rehabilitation team

Source: Modified from Stucki *et al.* (39).

Developing PRM in the context of "human functioning and rehabilitation"

The building of research capacity in the distinct scientific fields of human functioning and rehabilitation can importantly contribute to the development of PRM. Similar to other medical specialties that have greatly benefited from the development of biomedicine with a close interaction between medicine and the biosciences, PRM may benefit from the interaction between the emerging human functioning sciences and integrative rehabilitation sciences and an increased interaction between the established biomedical rehabilitation sciences and engineering.

As a research area, human functioning and rehabilitation complements established themes from the biomedical perspective (**Fig. 1**). In the context of life sciences, it can be seen as an extension of biosciences toward a comprehensive understanding of human life, including human interaction and communication, against the background of the natural and social environment. Based on a better understanding of human functioning and disability, there is a wide range of largely unexplored possibilities to optimize populations' functioning and minimize persons' experience of disability in the presence of a health condition. PRM is uniquely positioned to integrate and translate scientific advances into benefits for people and the society.

With the increasing recognition of the need for interdisciplinary research, there is the opportunity to initiate the building of interdisciplinary research centers for human functioning and rehabilitation at universities and regional or national collaboration networks (37). Comprehensively understood human functioning and rehabilitation research is ideally positioned to gather scholars from different disciplines around a common theme. Its strong focus on the translation of research into benefits for people's lives also bears an enormous potential for the collaboration of researchers, stakeholders, industries, and services with a common goal.

Human functioning and rehabilitation research from the comprehensive perspective can thus become a catalyst of interdisciplinary research that crosses the boundaries of natural sciences and engineering research, human and behavioral sciences, social sciences, and a wide range of related scientific areas. Rehabilitation research is also uniquely positioned to cross the boundaries of medicine and the health sector at large, and to translate knowledge across sectors including education, labor, and social affairs.

The successful development of human functioning and rehabilitation depends on the successful development of a respective workforce. Currently, education and training of human functioning and rehabilitation researchers based on the integrative model of functioning are hardly available. It is thus time to introduce innovative educational concepts and training programs as suggested in a recent paper (36).

The ICF in rehabilitation management

The ICF has the potential to have significant contribution to the quality of rehabilitation service and care delivery. It can serve as a starting point to structure clinical assessment and rehabilitation management (11, 35, 38, 40). A structured rehabilitation management generally involves the four steps of the Rehab-Cycle: assessment, assignment, intervention, and evaluation (41). The ICF framework is useful in all of these steps because it facilitates the organization of the collection and documentation of relevant information regarding functioning. To facilitate the implementation of the ICF in rehabilitation management, ICF-based documentation tools have been developed for use in clinical practice (30). The so-called ICF Assessment Sheet, ICF Categorical Profile, ICF Intervention Table, and ICF Evaluation Display will be presented in the following case example of a 35-year-old woman who suffered traumatic spinal cord injury AIS (Asia Impairment Scale) A (complete paralysis) at T8-level 4 months ago.

Assessment

Generally, assessment as the first step in the Rehab-Cycle involves three substeps: [1] the description of a patient's problems and needs, [2] the setting of mutually agreed goals, and [3] the determination of intervention targets. In the context of a case management situation, the assessment step includes the identification of patients' problems and needs and the definition of *global goals* and the *service program goals* of an anticipated rehabilitation program that is further specified in the assignment and intervention step.

In the context of care provided in a rehabilitation service program, the assessment includes the identification of patients' problems and needs, the review and potential modification of the assigned service program goal, the definition and modeling of the *cycle goals* and the determination of intervention targets. Intervention targets are defined to be aspects of functioning that have an impact on a cycle goal. Furthermore, intervention targets have to be modifiable through treatment and relevant for the improvement of a patient's functioning state in the actual situation of the rehabilitation process.

Patients' problems can be assessed in a nonsystematic or systematic way using an appropriate ICF Core Set. To use a systematic approach using an ICF Core Set either alone or in addition to a nonsystematic approach is advisable to ensure that all potentially relevant problems have been addressed. The systematic approach is particularly useful when training members of the rehabilitation team. The systematic approach also has the advantage that different team members can take primary responsibility for defined ICF categories. Information from the patient, clinical examinations, technical investigations, or observations may be used to assess the amount of problems in the specific ICF categories. To use a systematic way for appraising the amount of a problem in the different aspects of functioning, each ICF category is rated within the ICF Qualifiers (**Table 3**) based on the results of the gathered information.

The ICF Assessment Sheet and the ICF Categorical Profile have been developed to illustrate the results of the assessment. In the case example here, the ICF Core Set for spinal cord injury for early post-acute situation (24) served as the basis for the assessment. The ICF Assessment Sheet (**Fig. 3**) illustrates a comprehensive overview of the patient's functioning from the perspectives of both the patient and the health professionals (34). To describe the problems in functioning, the patient's words are used in the upper section of the sheet (patient's perspective). ICF codes, composed of an ICF category from the ICF Core Set and the generic ICF Qualifier (e.g., b152.3 = severe problems in emotional functions), were used in the lower section (health professional's perspective).

The ICF Categorical Profile (**Fig. 4**) is based on the list of ICF categories taken from a health condition-specific ICF Core Set. If no ICF Core Set exists for a particular health condition, those ICF categories that are relevant for the description of the actual state of the patient are identified by the rehabilitation team. A list of categories is then composed. The profile illustrates the functioning state of a patient individual at the time of assessment.

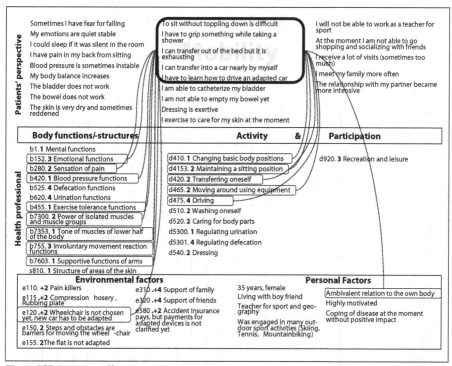

Fig. 3 - ICF Assessment Sheet.

Both the ICF Assessment Sheet and the ICF Categorical Profile provide relevant information for the definition of mutually agreed goals. Moreover, both tools allow the documentation of goals and intervention targets. In the ICF Assessment Sheet, cycle goals are highlighted in the patient's perspective section, "mobility" for example in our case. The intervention targets are illustrated within the connecting lines to the ICF categories in the health professional's section. For example, "b152.3 Emotional functions" (fear of falling), "b455.2 Exercise tolerance functions," "d420.2 Transferring oneself," and "e120.+2 Wheelchair" were determined to be intervention targets to improve the cycle goal "mobility." For each cycle goal, a separate ICF Assessment Sheet may be created.

In the ICF Categorical Profile, rehabilitation goals (global, service program, and cycle goals) are entered above the list of ICF categories. Intervention targets are chosen from the list of ICF categories and are marked by entering an abbreviation that demonstrates the relation to the according cycle goal in the respective column. For example, to improve the cycle goal "Self-care," "s810.1 Structures of areas of the skin," "d420.2 Transferring oneself," and "d540.2 Dressing" were determined to be intervention targets. For each intervention target, a goal value highlighting the expected improvement was defined based on an ICF Qualifier and entered in the respective column. For example, the goal would be to reduce the amount of the problem in the intervention target "b280 Sensation of pain" from ICF Qualifier to 2 to 0.

Fig. 4 - CF Categorical Profile (Extraction).

Assessment Four Months Post-trauma

Global goal: community integration
Service program goal: independence in daily living
Cycle goal 1: self-care
Cycle goal 2: mobility
Cycle goal 3: recreation and leisure

		Goal Relation	Goal Value
Global goal			0
Service program goal			0
Cycle goal 1			0
Cycle goal 2			0
Cycle goal 3			1

ICF Categories		ICF Qualifier* (Problem 0 1 2 3 4)	Goal Relation	Goal Value
b130	Energy and drive functions			
b134	Sleep function			
b152	Emotional functions		CG2	1
b260	Proprioceptive functions⁺			
b265	Touch functions⁺			
b270	Sensory functions related to temperature and other⁺			
b280	Sensation of pain		CG2	0
b410	Heart functions			
b415	Blood vessel functions			
b420	Blood pressure functions		CG2	0
b440	Respiration functions			
b445	Respiratory muscle functions			
b455	Exercise tolerance functions		CG3	0
b525	Defecation functions			
b530	Weight maintenance functions			
b550	Thermoregulation functions			
b620	Urination functions			
b640	Sexual functions			
b710	Mobility of joint functions		CG2	0

Fig. 4 - CF Categorical Profile (Extraction).

b715	Stability of joint functions			
b7300	Power of isolated muscles and muscle groups		CG2, 3	1
b7303	Power of muscles in lower half of the body			
b7353	Tone of muscles of lower half of the body		CG2, 3	1
b740	Muscle endurance functions[+]		CG 3	0
b750	Motor reflex functions[+]			
b755	Involuntary movement reaction functions[+]			
b760	Control of voluntary movements[+]			
b7603	Supportive functions of arms		CG2	0
b810	Protective functions of the skin			
s120	Spinal cord and related structures			
s610	Structure of the urinary system			
s810	Structure of areas of skin		CG1	0
d230	Carrying out daily routine			
d240	Handling stress and other psychological demands			
d410	Changing basic body positions		CG2	0
d4106	Shifting the body's centre of gravity		CG2	1
d4153	Maintaining a sitting position		CG2, 3	0
d420	Transferring oneself		CG1, 2	0
d430	Lifting and carrying objects			
d445	Hand and arm use			
d450	Walking			
d4600	Moving around within the home		CG2	0
d4602	Moving around outside the home or other buildings		CG2	0
d465	Moving around using equipment		CG2	0
d470	Using transportation		SPG	0
d475	Driving		CG2	0
d510	Washing oneself		CG1	0

Fig. 4 - CF Categorical Profile (Extraction).

Code	Description	Facilitator / Barrier		
d520	Caring for body parts		CG1	0
d5300	Regulating urination		CG1	0
d5301	Regulating defecation		CG1	0
d540	Dressing		CG1	0
d570	Looking after one's health		GG	0
d850	Remunerative employment		GG	0
d920	Recreation and leisure		CG2	1
e110	Products or substances for personal consumption		CG2	+3
e1151	Assistive products for personal use in daily living		SPG	+4
e1201	Assistive products for personal ... mobility ...		CG2	+4
e140	Products and techn for culture, recreation, and sport		CG3	+1
e150	Design, construction ... of buildings for public use			
e155	Design, construction ... of buildings for private use		SPG	+4
e310	Immediate family			
e320	Friends			
e355	Health professionals			
e410	Individual attitudes of immediate family members			
e420	Individual attitudes of friends			
e555	Associations and organizational services, systems...			
e580	Health services, systems, and policies			

Facilitator: 4+ 3+ 2+ 1+ 0   Barrier: 0 1 2 3 4

Influence of Personal Factors

Code	Description	Positive	Neutral	Negative		
pf	Sportive person					
pf	Motivation					
pf	Relation to the own body				CG2, 3	+
pf	Coping of disease				SPG	+

Assignment and intervention

After the determination of goals and intervention targets, the assignment step refers to the assignment of the intervention targets to health professionals and intervention principles accordingly. The intervention step refers to the specification of the intervention techniques, indicator measures, and target values that are to be achieved in a predefined period. Monitoring of the intervention is also considered. To document the assignment and the implementation of intervention techniques, the ICF Intervention Table was developed (**Table 6**). In the ICF Intervention Table, those ICF categories determined to be intervention targets and marked in the ICF Assessment Sheet and/or ICF Categorical Profile are transferred to the left column. For each intervention target, the responsible health professionals are marked and intervention principles assigned to each profession based on the ICF category. It is not uncommon that for some intervention targets, different intervention principles were assigned to the same health profession (e.g., "b152 Emotional functions" being treated by a psychologist with psychological counseling and Feldenkrais therapy). In other cases, different health professionals might aim to satisfy the same intervention principle toward a common therapeutic goal. For example, the nurse, physiotherapist, and occupational therapist implement transfer training procedures in various settings to improve "d420 Transferring oneself."

The ICF Intervention Table serves as a comprehensive overview of the complete rehabilitative interventions and the involvement of each member of the rehabilitation team. Specific intervention techniques will be defined and implemented by the team members in the entire Rehab-Cycle and modified if necessary. Information about the intervention techniques and results of test and examinations over the course of the Rehab-Cycle will be documented by the team members elsewhere and may be reported in team meetings. Shortly before the end of the Rehab-Cycle, an evaluation or reevaluation of the rehabilitation program will take place. In our case example, the (re)evaluation took place three months after the assessment period.

Evaluation

The evaluation step refers to the evaluation of goal achievement with respect to cycle goals and intervention targets that were determined beforehand. Each intervention target will be evaluated by the responsible team member using the same instruments as they did during the assessment. The results of the evaluation will be placed in the ICF Evaluation Display (**Fig. 5**).

Table 6 - ICF Intervention Table.

	Intervention Target	Intervention Principles	Phys	Nurse	PT	Spo	OT	Psy	SW	First Value*	Goal Value*	Final Value*
b152	Emotional functions	Psychological counseling						X				
		Feldenkrais therapy						X		3	1	2
b280	Sensation of pain	Medication	X									
		Detonization of muscle stiffness			X					2	0	2
b420	Blood pressure functions	Compression hosery	?	X	?	?	?	?	?	1	0	0
b455	Exercise tolerance functions	Swimming, Fitness training	?	?	?	X?	?	?	?	2	1	1
b7300	Power of isolated muscles and muscle groups	Circuit training	?	?	X	?	?	?	?	2	1	1
b7353	Tone of muscles of the lower half of the body	Sauna	?	?	X?	?	?	?	?	2	1	2
		Hippotherapy			X							
		Medication	X									
b740	Muscle endurance functions	Circuit training, Fitness training	?	?	?	?X	?	?	?	2	0	1
b755	Involuntary movement reaction functions	Body balance training	?	?	?X	?	?	?	?	3	1	1
b7603	Supportive functions of arms	Circuit training	?	?	?	X?	?	?	?	2	0	1
		Prop up training	?	?	X	?	?	?	?			
s810	Structure of areas of skin at risk	Daily skin control	?	X	?	?	?	?	?	1	0	0

Body function/structure

	Intervention Target	Intervention Principles	Phys	Nurse	PT	Spo	OT	Psy	SW	First Value*	Goal Value*	Final Value*
d410	Changing basic body positions	Repetitive training	?	?X	X	?	?	?	?	2	0	1
d4153	Maintaining a sitting position	Body balance training	?	?	X	?	?	?	?	2	0	0
d420	Transferring oneself	Repetitive training of transfers	?	?X	X	?	X	?	?	2	0	1
d4602	Moving around outside the home or other buildings	Outdoor training	?	?	?	?	X	?	?	2	0	0
d465	Moving around using equipment	Wheelchair training	?	?	X?	X	?	?	?	2	0	0
d475	Driving	Instruction and training	?	?	?	?	X?	?	?	4	0	1
d510	Washing oneself	Assistance and instruction	?	X	?	?	?	?	?	2	0	0
d520	Caring for body parts	Assistance and instruction	?	X	?	?	?	?	?	2	0	0
d5300	Regulating urination	Assistance and instruction	?	X	?	?	?	?	?	1	0	0
d5301	Regulating defecation	Assistance and instruction	?	X	?	?	?	?	?	4	0	0
d540	Dressing	Assistance and instruction	?	X	?	?	X	?	?	2	0	0
d850	Remunerative employment	Vocational counseling				?		X	?	2	0	1
d920	Recreation and leisure	Sport activities	?	?		X	?	?	?	3	1	1

Activity/Participation

	Code	Intervention Target	Intervention Principles	Phys	Nurse	PT	Spo	OT	Psy	SW	First Value*	Goal Value*	Final Value*
Environmental factors	e110	Products or substances for personal consumption	Medication	X	?	?	?	?	?	?	+2	+3	+2
	e1151	Assistive products for personal use in daily living	Choice/adaptation of required devices	?	?	?	?	X	?	?	+2	+4	+4
	e1201	Assistive products for personal ... mobility ...	Clarification, counselling and order	?	?	?	?	X	?	?	+2	+4	+4
	e140	Products and techn. for culture, recreation, sport	Choice and adaption of sport equipment				X				0	+1	+4
	e155	Design, construction...of buildings for private use	Clarification and organization	?	?	?	?	X	?	X	2	+4	+4
Personal factors	pf	Coping of disease	Psychological counseling	?	?	?	?	?	X	?	0	+	+
	pf	Relation to the own body	Feldenkrais therapy	?	?	?	?	?	X	?	0	+	+

Phys: physician, PT: physiotherapist, Spo: sport therapist, OT: occupational therapist, Psy: psychologist, SW: social worker.
* The values are rated within the use of the generic ICF Qualifiers.

Fig. 5 - ICF Categorical Profile (Extraction).

	ICF Qualifier (Problem)	Goal Relation	Goal Value	ICF Qualifier (Problem / Not Evaluated Yet)	Goal Achievement
Global goal: community integration			0		–
Service programme goal: independence in daily living			0		✓
Cycle goal 1: self-care			0		–
Cycle goal 2: mobility			0		✓
Cycle goal 3: recreation and leisure			1		✓

ICF Categories	ICF Qualifier (Problem 0–4)	Goal Relation	Goal Value	ICF Qualifier (Problem 0–4 / Not Evaluated Yet)	Goal Achievement
b152 Emotional functions		CG2	1		–
b280 Sensation of pain		CG2	0		–
b420 Blood pressure functions		CG2	0		✓
b455 Exercise tolerance functions		CG3	1		✓
b710 Mobility of joint functions		CG2	0		✓
b7303 Power of isolated muscles and muscle groups		CG2, 3	1		✓
b7353 Tone of muscles of lower half of the body		CG2, 3	1		–
b740 Muscle endurance functions		CG 3	0		–
b755 Involuntary movement reaction functions		CG1,2,3	1		✓
b7603 Supportive functions of arms		CG2	0		–

Fig. 5 - ICF Categorical Profile (Extraction).

Code		Facilitator					Barrier						
		4+	3+	2+	1+	0	1	2	3	4			
s810	Structure of areas of skin										CG1	0	✓
d410	Changing basic body positions										CG2	0	-
d4106	Shifting the body's centre of gravity										CG2	1	✓
d4153	Maintaining a sitting position										CG2, 3	0	✓
d420	Transferring oneself										CG1, 2	0	-
d4602	Moving around outside the home or other buildings										CG2	0	✓
d465	Moving around using equipment										CG2	0	✓
d470	Using transportation										SPG	0	✓
d475	Driving										CG2	0	-
d510	Washing oneself										CG1	0	✓
d520	Caring for body parts										CG1	0	✓
d5300	Regulating urination										CG1	0	✓
d5301	Regulating defecation										CG1	0	✓
d540	Dressing										CG1	0	✓
d850	Remunerative employment										GG	0	-
d920	Sport										CG2	1	✓
e110	Products or substances for personal consumption										CG2	3+	-

Fig. 5 - ICF Categorical Profile (Extraction).

		Influence of Personal Factors					Influence of Personal Factors			
		Positive	Neutral	Negative			Positive	Neutral	Negative	
e1151	Assistive products for personal use in daily living				SPG	4+				✓
e1201	Assistive products for personal … mobility …				CG2	4+				✓
e140	Products and techn. for culture, recreation, and sport				CG3	1+				✓
e155	Design, construction … of buildings for private use				SPG	4+				✓
pf	Coping of disease				SPG	+				✓
pf	Body awareness				CG2	+				✓

The ICF Evaluation Display is based on the ICF Categorical Profile, and only those ICF categories that were defined to become intervention targets are listed. A column is added to illustrate the results of the evaluation. This procedure facilitates the comparison of the assessment value, the goal value, and the evaluation value. This comparison provides an insight into whether or not a goal has been achieved, e.g., the aim of reducing the problem on "b280 Sensation of pain" from ICF Qualifier 2 to 0 (i.e., moderate to no problem). The evaluation profile shows that the problem was still rated as 2 (based on the ICF Qualifier) in the end. Hence, the set goal was not achieved. In contrast, the goal to reduce the problem on 'd465 Moving around using equipment' from 2 to 0 was achieved.

The above discussion presents the importance of the ICF Evaluation Display. First, it illustrated the changes in functioning state after one Rehab-Cycle with consideration to treating and managing each aspect of functioning. Second, it provides important information regarding the decision-making process on future rehabilitative programs.

Training materials for the implementation of the ICF in practice are provided on the Internet by the Swiss Paraplegic Research, which uses the example of spinal cord injury (http://www.icf-casestudies.org).

Conclusion

The ICF has the potential to become the universally shared model for PRM, the "medicine of functioning." The adoption of the ICF as a unifying model for PRM can contribute to the urgently needed development of research capacity in the area of human functioning and rehabilitation. The ICF can serve as reference for the reporting of functioning across a wide range of measurement instruments and as a starting point for the development of universally applicable international standards and practical tools, as well as clinical and self-reported measures the ICF. The application of the ICF may thus also contribute to the worldwide harmonization of classification and measurement instruments relevant for PRM. The use of the ICF in rehabilitation management may enhance a structured approach and may enhance the communication within the team with respect to problems, goals, intervention targets, and interventions concerning a patient individual. It could improve the communication between health care settings and insurers or case managers. An ICF-based rehabilitation management approach is useful within the context of clinical quality management and assurance, research and evidence-based rehabilitation, training, and best practice, and in the formulation, implementation, and evaluation of guidelines. Within the context of disability evaluation, the ICF provides a comprehensive framework for assessment and modeling of the determinants of disability.

In agreement with the editor of *PM&R* and the editor of the *Journal of Rehabilitation Medicine*, the readers of *PM&R* are invited to write letters to these journals commenting on the suggestions made in this chapter regarding the use of the ICF as a unifying model for PRM. It is hoped that this discussion, facilitated by the *Journal of Rehabilitation Medicine* and *PM&R*, will contribute to the development of human functioning and rehabilitation research and the development of PRM.

Acknowledgments

The authors would like to thank Gisela Immich for assistance with the preparation of the manuscript, Dr. Reuben Escorpizo for reviewing this chapter, and Drs. Alarcos Cieza, Jan Reinhardt, John Melvin, Gunnar Grimby, Nenad Kostansjek, Bedirhan Üstün, and Susanne Stucki for their invaluable contributions to the ideas presented in this chapter.

References

1. American Psychological Association (2000) Procedural manual and guide for standardized application of the International Classification of Functioning, Disability and Health (ICF). Field trial version [cited May 24, 2008]; available from: http://icf.apa.org/
2. Bickenbach JE, Chatterji S, Badley EM, Ustun TB (1999) Models of disablement, universalism and the international classification of impairments, disabilities and handicaps. Soc Sci Med 48:1173-1187
3. Brandt EN, Pope AM, Institute of Medicine (eds) (1997) Enabling America: assessing the role of rehabilitation science and engineering. National Academy Press, Washington, DC
4. Chamie M (1995) What does morbidity have to do with disability? Disabil Rehabil 17:323-337
5. Cieza A, Brockow T, Ewert T, *et al.* (2002) Linking health-status measurements to the international classification of functioning, disability and health. J Rehabil Med 34:205-210
6. Cieza A, Ewert T, Ustun TB, *et al.* (2004) Development of ICF Core Sets for patients with chronic conditions. J Rehabil Med 44:9-11
7. Cieza A, Geyh S, Chatterji S, *et al.* (2005) ICF linking rules: an update based on lessons learned. J Rehabil Med 37:212-218
8. Cieza A, Hilfiker R, Boonen A, *et al.* (2009) Items from patient-oriented instruments can be integrated into interval scales to operationalize categories of the International Classification of Functioning, Disability and Health. J Clin Epidemiol 62:912-921, 921 e911-913
9. Cieza A, Hilfiker R, Boonen A, *et al.* (2009) Towards an ICF-based clinical measure of functioning in people with ankylosing spondylitis: a methodological exploration. Disabil Rehabil 31:528-537
10. Cieza A, Hilfiker R, Chatterji S, (2009) The International Classification of Functioning, Disability, and Health could be used to measure functioning. J Clin Epidemiol 62:899-911

11. Cieza A, Stucki G (2006) The International Classification of Functioning, Disability and Health (ICF): a basis for mulitdisciplinary clinical practice. In: Bartlett SJ, Bingham CO, Maricic MJ, *et al.* (eds) Clinical care in Rheumatic Disease Association of rheumatology health professionals, 3rd ed. Division of ACR, Atlanta, pp. 79-87

12. Cieza A, Stucki G (2008) The International Classification of Functioning Disability and Health: its development process and content validity. Eur J Phys Rehabil Med 44:303-313

13. Dewey J (1925) Experience and nature. Dover Publications, New York

14. Epping-Jordan J, Ustun B (2000) The WHODASII leveling the playing field for all disorders. WHO Bull Ment Health 6:5-6

15. Ewert T, Fuessl M, Cieza A, et al. (2004) Identification of the most common patient problems in patients with chronic conditions using the ICF checklist. J Rehabil Med 22-29

16. Geyh S, Cieza A, Kollerits B, *et al.* (2007) Content comparison of health-related quality of life measures used in stroke based on the international classification of functioning, disability and health (ICF): a systematic review. Qual Life Res 16:833-851

17. Grill E, Ewert T, Chatterji S, *et al.* (2005) ICF Core Sets development for the acute hospital and early post-acute rehabilitation facilities. Disabil Rehabil 27:361-366

18. Grill E, Mansmann U, Cieza A, Stucki G (2007) Assessing observer agreement when describing and classifying functioning with the International Classification of Functioning, Disability and Health. J Rehabil Med 39:71-76

19. Grill E, Stucki G (2009) Scales could be developed based on simple clinical ratings of International Classification of Functioning, Disability and Health Core Set categories. J Clin Epidemiol 62:891-898

20. Grimby G, Melvin J, Stucki G (2007) The ICF: a unifying model for the conceptualization, organization and development of human functioning and rehabilitation research. Foreword. J Rehabil Med 39:277-278

21. Imrie R (2004) Demystifying disability: a review of the International Classification of Functioning, Disability and Health. Sociol Health Illn 26:287-305

22. Jette AM (2006) Toward a common language for function, disability, and health. Phys Ther 86:726-734

23. Kirchberger I, Stamm T, Cieza A, Stucki G (2007) Does the Comprehensive ICF Core Set for rheumatoid arthritis capture occupational therapy practice? A content-validity study. Can J Occup Ther 74:267-280

24. Kirchberger I, Cieza A, Biering Sørenser F, *et al.* (2010) ICF Core Sets for individuals with spiral cord injury in the early post-acute context, Spiral Cord. 48(4):305-12

25. Mayo NE, Poissant L, Ahmed S, *et al.* (2004) Incorporating the International Classification of Functioning, Disability, and Health (ICF) into an electronic health record to create indicators of function: proof of concept using the SF-12. J Am Med Inform Assoc 11:514-522

26. Nagi SZ (1965) Some conceptual issues in disability and rehabilitation. In: Sussmann MB (ed) Sociology and rehabilitation. American Sociological Association, Washington, DC

27. Nagi SZ (1976) An epidemiology of disability among adults in the United States. Milbank Mem Fund Q 6:439-467

28. Pope AM, Tarlov AR, (eds) (1991) Disability in America: toward a national agenda for prevention. National Academies Press, Washington, DC

29. Posl M, Cieza A, Stucki G (2007) Psychometric properties of the WHODASII in rehabilitation patients. Qual Life Res 16:1521-1531

30. Rauch A, Cieza A, Stucki G (2008) How to apply the International Classification of Functioning, Disability and Health (ICF) for rehabilitation management in clinical practice. Eur J Phys Rehabil Med 44:329-342

31. Reed GM, Lux JB, Bufka LF, et al. (2005) Operationalizing the International Classifcation of Functioning, Disability and Health (ICF) in clinical settings. Rehabil Psychol 50:22-31

32. Stamm TA, Cieza A, Machold K, et al. (2005) Exploration of the link between conceptual occupational therapy models and the International Classification of Functioning, Disability and Health. Austr Occup Ther J 53:9-17

33. Stamm TA, Cieza A, Stucki G (2005) Exploration of the link between occupational therapy models and the International Classification of Functioning, Disability and Health: A response from colleagues in Norway. Austr Occup Ther J 53:143-144

34. Steiner WA, Ryser L, Huber E, et al. (2002) Use of the ICF model as a clinical problem-solving tool in physical therapy and rehabilitation medicine. Phys Ther 82:1098-1107

35. Stucki G (2005) International Classification of Functioning, Disability, and Health (ICF): a promising framework and classification for rehabilitation medicine. Am J Phys Med Rehabil 84:733-740

36. Stucki G (2007) Developing human functioning and rehabilitation research. Part I: Academic training programs. J Rehabil Med 39:323-333

37. Stucki G, Celio M (2007) Developing human functioning and rehabilitation research. Part II: Interdisciplinary university centers and national and regional collaboration networks. J Rehabil Med 39:334-342

38. Stucki G, Cieza A (2004) The International Classification of Functioning, Disability and Health (ICF) Core Sets for rheumatoid arthritis: a way to specify functioning. Ann Rheum Dis 63:ii40-ii45

39. Stucki G, Cieza A, Melvin J (2007) The International Classification of Functioning, Disability and Health (ICF): a unifying model for the conceptual description of the rehabilitation strategy. J Rehabil Med 39:279-285

40. Stucki G, Ewert T (2005) How to assess the impact of arthritis on the individual patient: the WHO ICF. Ann Rheum Dis 64:664-668

41. Stucki G, Ewert T, Cieza A (2002) Value and application of the ICF in rehabilitation medicine. Disabil Rehabil 24:932-938

42. Stucki G, Grimby G (2004) Foreword. Applying the ICF in medicine. J Rehabil Med 44:5-6

43. Stucki G, Grimby G (2007) Organizing human functioning and rehabilitation research into distinct scientific fields. Part I: Developing a comprehensive structure from the cell to society. J Rehabil Med 39:293-298

44. Stucki G, Kostanjsek N, Ustun B, Cieza A (2008) ICF-based classification and measurement of functioning. Eur J Phys Rehabil Med 44:315-328

45. Stucki G, Melvin J (2007) The International Classification of Functioning, Disability and Health: a unifying model for the conceptual description of physical and rehabilitation medicine. J Rehabil Med 39:286-292

46. Stucki G, Reinhardt JD, Grimby G (2007) Organizing human functioning and rehabilitation research into distinct scientific fields. Part II: Conceptual descriptions and domains for research. J Rehabil Med 39:299-307
47. Stucki G, Reinhardt JD, Grimby G, Melvin J (2007) Developing "Human Functioning and Rehabilitation Research" from the comprehensive perspective. J Rehabil Med 39:665-671
48. Stucki G, Ustun TB, Melvin J (2005) Applying the ICF for the acute hospital and early post-acute rehabilitation facilities. Disabil Rehabil 27:349-352
49. United Nations General Assembly (2006) Convention on the rights of persons with disabilities. Resolution 61/106 [cited May 29, 2008]; available from: www.un.org/esa/socdev/enable/conventioninfo.htm
50. Ustun B, Chatterji S, Kostanjsek N (2004) Comments from WHO for the Journal of Rehabilitation Medicine Special Supplement on ICF Core Sets. J Rehabil Med 7-8
51. WHA (2005) Disability, including prevention, management and rehabilitation. Report No. WHA 58.23. World Health Assembly, Geneva
52. WHO (1992) International statistical classification of diseases and related health problems. 10th revision. World Health Organization, Geneva
53. WHO (2001) International Classification of Functioning, Disability and Health (ICF). WHO Publishing, Geneva
54. WHO (2001) World Health Organization Disability Assessment Schedule II (WHODAS II) [cited May 24, 2008]; available from: http://www.who.int/icidh/whodas/index.html
55. WHO (2003) ICF Checklist. Version 2.1a, Clinician Form for International Classification, of Functioning, Disability and Health [cited May 24, 2008]; available from: http://www.who.int/classifications/icf/training/icfchecklist.pdf
56. Zola IK (1989) Toward the necessary universalizing of a disability policy. Milbank Q 67:401-428

Rehabilitation and norms

J.-M. Mouillie, V. Saoût and I. Richard

Medical practice aims at creating a norm; as such it is both normalizing and standard-izing. It implies evaluations that draw a distinction between what is "normal" and what is pathological: this traditionally defines both its goals and its field of practice. Rehabil-itation medicine is both on the margin and at the very heart of this founding distinction, and therefore also of the concepts or representations that underlie the definition of the norm and the actions triggered when a deviation from this norm is observed.

At first sight, the question of what is "normal" may seem peripheral because from the outset, the clinical situations in which physical and rehabilitation medicine (PRM) first developed, whether traumatic amputations or the poliomyelitis epidemic, made it necessary to renounce the imaginary goal of a cure, defined as restoration to a previous condition, and replaced it with the objective of helping patients accept and adapt to their altered living conditions. But a closer look reveals that the "norm" is actually quite central to the practice of PRM and involves a number of specific, related issues.

When H. Rusk, in 1951, associated "rehabilitation" with "physical medicine," he presented it as a "global concept" involving all the various aspects of the patient's situ-ation that are affected by the handicap. "Rehabilitation (is) neither a purely psychiatric concept nor a purely physical medicine concept; it (is) a total concept to meet the total needs of a disabled person" (36, p. 188). In its various fields of practice, from functional rehabilitation to long-term follow-up care within the community, the practice of PRM is at the junction between medicine and society at large. Its field of analysis and inter-vention is therefore shifted from compensating for an impairment or restoring a func-tion to adapting to a given set of social situations, with the risk that it will rely on, or even contribute to define, a set of "normal" social roles and situations. Historical shifts in the uses of the word "rehabilitation," occasionally in combination with "camp," are a reminder – assuming one was needed – of the conceptual pitfalls involved, such as the fact that adaptation to the patient's social environment is never in itself a "normal" sign of health, in the sense that it is "desirable."

We will therefore start with definitions of the principal meanings of the word "nor-mal" and their possible use in the context of PRM. We will then analyze how, histori-cally, the "abnormality" of disabled individuals has been closely linked to the process of their exclusion and, in more complex ways, to strategies aiming at their so-called integration. Finally, we will examine how shifting the goal, or goals, from restoring normality to restoring normativity, defined as the possibility for patients to define their own norms, can perhaps contribute to bring about a therapeutic process that is both respectful toward patients and coherent with the creation of a social model of disability.

Meanings of the word "normal"

The word "normal" is used in a variety of senses that can lead to confusions in actual usage. It is therefore necessary to distinguish between these meanings, although our intention here is not so much to review available meanings as to set about clarifying the concepts we will be referring to.

Like any other standard, the word "normal" originally implies a judgment that defines or determines a criterion for comparison, a threshold, a boundary, or a dividing line. This element of comparison can be either quantitative or qualitative in nature. The word "normal" thus refers to a numerically dominant, statistical norm; conversely, "abnormal" refers to a statistical minority. "Normal" and "abnormal" also imply value judgments. Thus defined, "abnormality" can be both numerically dominant and negatively valued.

We can therefore distinguish between at least five different meanings to the word "normal."

In a statistical sense, within the context of a measured observation, "normal" refers to a value or a frequency recorded in most, but not all, cases observed for a given phenomenon, under comparable observation conditions. Under this definition, "normality" refers to an observable fact defined by a numerical value above which appears a deviation (be it a pathological risk, an intolerance, or a sign of morbidity). This quantitatively defined normality refers to an art of measured observation that is an integral part of the elaboration of science. Biology and physiology thus contribute to sketch a picture of "man in general" (3), an epistemological fiction that needs to be questioned in terms of its conformity with the actual human being, which is never quite the average human being, within a framework of critical reflection bearing on the logic that underpins this type of knowledge.

This first meaning is an extension of the assessment often expressed in everyday life where "normal" refers to a frequency subjectively perceived or experienced. In this empirical, psychological sense, "normal" refers to what remains unexamined/unquestioned by ordinary experience because it is taken for granted or explained away. Saying something is "normal," in this sense, means "I understand that this is how things are, ordinarily." In a more general sense, what is "normal" is whatever fulfills my expectations in terms of ordinary experience: it will seem normal that, under a given latitude, the sun should rise once in every 24 hours; that nights should be devoted to sleep; or that an acquaintance should greet me when we meet. These are "regular" events that would not take place if I lived in a very small, isolated group in the middle of a polar night. The word "normal," in this sense, refers to the customary setting of the subject's everyday life, to the set of living habits that one is often not aware of until they are suspended or disrupted. This descriptive sense, referring to an empirical observation, is therefore linked to psychological experience, where the concept of "normality" is not entirely independent from an implied value judgment.

In a third sense, the word "normal" implies a value judgment relatively to an individual, social, or cultural subjective variability. Here, we have shifted from a descriptively defined type of normality (cognitively or empirically based) to a prescriptively defined one: I will describe as "normal" whatever is coherent with my preconceived values and prejudices. This is what is made tangible by a disruption in my habits or points of reference. What is not "normal" refers to whatever disturbs the "natural" order of things, the permanent character of which, or a desire for which, is the basis for the subject's feeling that things should be just so rather than otherwise. The word "normal" thus describes what is perceived to be good, desirable, or appropriate; what complies with a rule or standard perceived as the only one valid or as preferable to others; or what is in a state perceived as desirable by a given group or individual. Health, perceived as the normal condition of a living being, is in this sense a concept that discriminates against illness. Even more so than in the statistical sense, the exception and the norm are inseparable to the extent that each creates the other, and upholders of moral norms tend to disparage the deviations that they themselves have contributed to create. The word "normal," in this sense, refers to what complies with positively valued standards. This qualitatively defined normality often includes a denial of its nature as a social construct, based on an evaluation, and is often claimed to be "natural." It is associated with an ideal understood as a maximum life potential. It is fairly common that "health" in its modern sense combines both these meanings, i.e., "normal" and "ideal." In any case, in all of these uses, normality, identified with what is good, fair, or harmonious, is a moral, aesthetic (7), ideological, and metaphysical concept. In this third sense, the word "normal" implies a positive value judgement, while "abnormal" refers to what is condemned or deviant, regardless of its statistical frequency. What is "normal" is what ought to exist.

The word "normal" can also refer to a mode of being defined by a living being for his or her own life. The norm is thus understood as a regulation aimed at preserving an organic individual and as an open attitude, ready to adapt to the unexpected in a given situation. "Normativity" thus refers to the work of living, which can never be reduced to the mere forms it establishes except in the case of illness, and this is precisely how illness is defined: as the experience of a restriction to this normativity. G. Canguilhem, in his works, insists on this normative capacity in living beings, in which normality is identified with the individual being's lack of subordination to his or her natural or social environment, whereas abnormality is defined as a dependency on the environment that threatens the individual's viability (7). The individual subject is therefore a reference for normativity: in other words, the subjects themselves become their own standard for self-assessment. In this sense, the concept of "normality" is both objective and specific to the individual; it is not a value judgment or a law of nature but rather a trait specific to the individual. In the same line of thought, Canguilhem has developed the idea of a biological normativity, understood as an adaptive plasticity to the natural or artificial environment (7). To underline the necessity of shifting from the perspective of "nature" and its essential constants to processes of adaptation and reconfiguration, Canguilhem precisely refers to normativity rather than norms or normality. To be normal is to be normative, i.e., to be able to modify one's own norms.[1] The normativity inherent to normality is therefore defined not in terms of frequency but as the possibility of adapting to the environment, subjectively assessed by the individual in a given situation.

In a final sense, the word "normal" can generally refer to a standard, a consensus, or in other words what is agreed on as the norm, in the sense of an authority or a reference, implicit or explicit, prevalent within a community: its habitus, shared references, common ethos, or whatever is coherent with the dominant paradigm. Within this category of normality, it is necessary to draw a distinction between the conventionally normative institution (intentional and consciously decreed) and the original normative institution, not consciously thought, such as symbolic institutions. Normality understood in this sense is first and foremost the norm established as the reference, deviations from which will variously be categorized as abnormal, eccentric, illegal, heretical, or immoral (in a sense that is not necessarily pejorative, and therefore more neutral than meaning number 3).

The word "normal" therefore refers to a norm, and the question is how this is defined: with reference to the statistical calculation of a frequency (meaning 1), to the psychological experience of a habit and a quality of what is logical (meaning 2), to a value judgment as to what is legitimate (meaning 3), to a mode of being, specific to a subject who defines his or her own living norms (meaning 4), or to a dominant community institution (meaning 5). Particular care should be taken to distinguish the descriptive sense of the word (which is specific to the first two meanings) and its prescriptive sense (specific to meaning 3) from normality as a standard, which is not always simple (particularly with meanings 4 and 5). Drawing a distinction between these two interpretations of normality is a necessary prerequisite to an ethical and epistemological reconsideration of the goals of medical practice and therapeutic intervention.

It is crucial that this distinction be maintained in order to ensure that science is not used to support a particular ideology and that its proponents do not let the patient-carer relationship, which should be liberating, be replaced with a power relationship, and thus a threat to the patient's liberty.

---

1. "Being healthy means being not only normal in a given situation but also normative in this and other eventual situations. What characterizes health is the possibility of transcending the norm, which defines the momentary normal, the possibility of tolerating infractions of the habitual norm and instituting new norms in new situations" (7, pp. 196-197)

The "abnormal other": a long history of discrimination

There is no question that describing individuals as "handicapped" questions his or her normality. First, being impaired excludes them from statistical "normality," in the first of the senses defined above. Second, in their own perception as well as in others', their impairment – when it is acquired rather than innate – forces them to modify their living habits and makes it difficult to adapt to new situations, with the effect that previous living norms are seriously disrupted. Neither of these two meanings is in itself sufficient to trigger the process of discrimination, which is based neither on deviation from the statistical norm nor on the subject's own perception of a disruption.

A handicap, in the pejorative sense, is the way disability leaves the patient's body or mind affected with an essential disadvantage (18, 34). Individuals, once they are identified to their handicap, are thereby sorted into a category of "essentially" diminished beings. "We tend to impute a wide range of imperfections on the basis of the original one" (18, pp. 15-16). This marking and sorting into categories provide a structure for the process of discrimination against individuals, which are both reduced to a single characteristic and contaminated in their entire being by the "negativity" associated with this particular trait. Discrimination on the grounds of handicap is "ontological," in the sense that it discriminates against the subject's very being, rather than against the circumstances that reveal the subject's handicap.

Here, normality functions as a binary criterion, according to which the category of humanness is assigned or denied by stigmatizing those who do not measure up to an ideal: on the one hand are normal, authentic, true human beings, whereas all other "different" individuals are, in a sense, "inferior" human beings.

Historical accounts provide damning evidence of such stigmatization. An emblematic illustration of the traditional practice of physically or symbolically eliminating individuals that were considered morphologically or physiologically undesirable, because they were weak, deformed, of inferior birth, or considered useless burdens, is provided by the practice allegedly prevalent in ancient Sparta, where every family was required to bring newborns to a tribunal that decided on the child's right to live and become a citizen and progenitor. The existence of the medieval court of miracles can in no way be interpreted as confirmation for the imagined ideals of tolerance that are occasionally depicted in popular films and literature. Not until the late nineteenth century did the category of physical monsters, ranging from errors of nature to the esthetically grotesque and demonic outrages, cease to be taken for granted; it is survived only by the category of the moral monster. The canonically ideal body represented statutorily and the cruel depiction of physical imperfection bear witness to a centuries-old practice of sorting both bodies and individuals.

The practice of focusing on disabilities in order to alleviate them may be far from recent, but until recently it remained exceptional. Dominant practices amounted to a loosely conceived form of eugenics, until the nineteenth century, when Darwinian theories were interpreted as an excuse to turn this into a system, in the form of a scientific, health-oriented, moral, and political ideology. This evolution reached an apex with the criminal Third-Reich National Socialist process of physically eliminating any individuals that were considered as embodiments of evil (4).

Disability, examined in the light of history, reveals a long-suffering history of abuse. Contemporary efforts to move beyond exclusion are calling into question fundamental representations of human identity. Most of these are unthought and belong to the realm of the imagination. Disabled individuals embody a particular category of outcasts, in the sense that they force us to come face to face with our own vulnerability (38). The uncanny strangeness of the "abnormal" other is fascinating to the observer and holds up a cruel mirror to one's narcissism, a shattered image of one's illusions, that revives the infantile anxiety and the hidden insecurities that are inherent to one's identity (26).

Such was the backdrop against which disability care was to appear. Its very existence contributes to integrating the "abnormal" other, potentially excluded from humanity, back into the fold of potential recipients of medical attention, now focused on reaffirming solidarity between fellow human beings.

PRM: an alternate construction of the normal-abnormal contrast

PRM developed as a consequence of a number of major historical changes that contributed to turn the cripple, formerly a bearer of essential stigmata attributable to nature, fatality, or a curse, into a disabled person who has been injured or mutilated and for whom society is directly or indirectly accountable. The two main salient historical facts here are the industrial revolution and the increasing numbers of war veterans disabled in the Napoleonic wars and, even more massively so, during the First World War. The industrial revolution created a whole new category of patients: victims of work-related injuries. The change was a social one rather than epidemiological. Also the development of a structured labor movement, particularly in the mining industry, had the effect that disability ceased to be explained by mere fate and was instead attributed to third-party liability, which paved the way for a system where compensation, whether symbolic or financial, was expected. The other decisive event was the First World War, killing thousands and leaving thousands more either disabled or disfigured by severe facial injuries (known in French as "gueules cassées," literally "shattered faces"). The perception of these new categories of disabled persons as fellow workers or war heroes went against the historical tendency to consider them as abnormal; their sheer number, during and after the war, dramatically changed the way they were usually perceived and of raising the question of their inclusion in society.

The poliomyelitis epidemic and the development of resuscitation techniques that made it possible for patients to live with major motor deficits contributed to the completion of this paradigm shift. A handicap was no longer a consequence of congenital defects or accidental mishaps; it became the habitual consequence of a number of pathologies otherwise included within the field of remedial medicine. Rehabilitation medicine, born of war surgery and of workers' demands, thus came to be included in the larger field of general medicine, a phenomenon that only increased throughout the twentieth century, as chronic diseases and the aging of the population became major public health issues, at least in Western societies (6, 12, 16, 32, 33, 37, 38, 44).

The paradigm shift from disability to handicap and the development of PRM have to some extent undermined the process of excluding "abnormal" individuals, but the rehabilitation process was still closely linked to the quest for normality. Rehabilitation was structured around the necessity of replacing or regaining a function or a previous situation: limbs that had been lost to war, or to a workplace injury, had to be restored, and crooked limbs were to be straightened (43).

As for rehabilitation, it was understood, first and foremost, as rehabilitating patients for work. Michel Foucault, insisting on social normativity as coercion, has shown how the normalization process relied on authoritarian structures, the aim of which was to subdue and to produce subjects who in turn became instruments of normalization. He places medical authority at the heart of this process, as the seat of a knowledge that discriminates between what is normal, i.e., desirable, and the pathological, either curable or to be disposed of. Rehabilitation by and for work, which is both a means and an end, was consistent with the logic of a system prevalent from the nineteenth century on, aimed at producing machine-men, men that were productive tools (13). Rehabilitation could be seen as the central, emblematic embodiment of this general process, the end of which was to conform, correct, discipline, rectify, train, and exploit. Working on the body made it ready for work. Subjects were made to incorporate prostheses, techniques, and postures that made them viable for productive work. Physical rehabilitation, as voluntarist intervention, embodied a general process of turning the body into an instrument controlled by social norms.

This integration is part of a framework of social normalization, where the worker – average, gauged, and fit for all purposes – was the exemplary figure of normality (10). The legal obligation to employ "disabled workers," which dates from the 1950s (10), did not go hand in hand with equal treatment between workers: disabled workers were granted lesser status than able-bodied fellow workers, both in terms of salary and in terms of the responsibilities they are entrusted with.

This sometimes-unformulated relationship to work as a social norm remains predominant in institutional practices and in international literature. Resuming employment, remaining in employment, and adapted work are to this day accepted as criteria for assessing an individual's participation in society and as goals – usually explicit and positively valued – of the rehabilitation process. No doubt work can be an essential element in the patient's social integration, but it seems problematic that integration should look no further.

This attention given to function and to social roles was to be theorized in a model introduced by Wood in 1981. The United Nations (UN) proclaimed 1981 the International Year of Disabled Persons; this was followed by the Decade of Disabled Persons (1983-1992), proclaimed by the General Assembly of the UN. The International Classification of Impairments, Disabilities and Handicaps (ICIDH) (46), developed by the World Health Organization (WHO), was published in 1980. Its stated purpose was to complement the International Classification of Diseases with a classification of their disabling consequences. According to these definitions, an impairment is "any loss or abnormality of psychological, physiological, or anatomical structure or function." A disability is defined as "any restriction or lack (resulting from an impairment) of ability to perform an activity in the manner or within the range considered normal for a human being." A handicap is "a disadvantage for a given individual, resulting from an impairment or a disability, that limits or prevents the fulfilment of a role that is normal (depending on age, sex, and social and cultural factors) for that individual." The reference to "normal" abilities appears in all three definitions and is neither called into question nor clarified.

Within this model, PRM therefore remains a process aimed at normalization, which can be interpreted in three broad senses:

- Similarity to the majority, whether this is defined as a statistical average or as an imaginary representation. The rehabilitation process aims at reaching a norm or standard that is predefined or perceived as dominant and that tends to set an ideal goal, such as resuming employment;
- Integration, which consists of fusing a novel situation back into a synthetic unity of the individual patient's life. Rehabilitation is therefore understood as the restoration of a continuum in self-perception, beyond the traumatic event, and of perception by patients of their condition as "normal for me";
- Adaptation, i.e., integrating the patient back into the community, in conformity with social norms.

The social model of disability: how the issue of normality shifted from the individual to the environment

The publication of the ICIDH was undeniably a turning point in the definition of disability, but the concept is still structured around the individual, in a medical perspective, and leaves little room to factors in the environment. It implies a linear, chronological succession from one concept to the next (from impairment to disability and on to handicap), which is not always the case. It describes situations in terms that are negative and carry stigma for the individuals concerned. Confronted with this model that explicitly referred to a standard of normality, a logic that entailed labeling disabled people, collectively, as "abnormal," other teams have developed concepts that make it possible to phrase the issue of difference in alternate terms (22, 31). In the 1990s, Patrick Fougeyrollas stressed the importance of environmental factors and suggested the alternate model known as the disability creation process (DCP), which focuses on disability not as a characteristic but as a *situation*, a restriction of life habits, and created the International Network on the Disability Creation Process (INDCP) (14, 15, 25, 30). Disability is thus perceived as a "situational state," brought about by interaction between personal factors and environmental factors, which can be facilitators or obstacles, and unlike the ICIDH, the DCP has the effect of redefining disability as a dynamic process clearly dissociated from any characteristics inherent to the individual who is subjected to discrimination.

Once the limits of the ICIDH were made clear, it was revised; in 2001 the WHO approved the International Classification of Functioning, Disability and Health (ICF) (19, 45). Where the ICIDH was clearly biomedical in its perspective, the ICF is written in a frame of mind that is more focused on the environment. The vocabulary it uses is positive, whereas the ICIDH used a negatively valued terminology. The definition of disability is no longer centered on the individual, in a strictly medical perspective, but it has become a social concept. The ICF provides a classification of "health components," whereas the ICIDH focused only on classifying the "effects" of disability on health.

More recently, after several years of negotiations with representatives of persons with disabilities and with other nongovernmental organizations, on December 13, 2006, the UN General Assembly adopted the Convention on the Rights of Persons with Disabilities, which came into force on May 3, 2008 (41). The preamble to the convention states that "disability is an evolving concept and (that) disability results from the interaction between persons with impairments and attitudinal and environmental barriers that hinder their full and effective participation in society on an equal basis with others." The convention advocates the elimination of discrimination against persons with disabilities and requires that they enjoy independence, equal opportunities, and "full participation and inclusion in society."

This shifting of the norm, from a definition centered on the individual (where it is up to the individual to adapt to society, according to his or her specific impairments) to one where it is up to society to implement policies designed to adapt the environment to the individual's (according to their expectations, needs, and choices), has largely been brought about by a protest movement known as the Disabled Peoples' International (DPI), which was founded in 1982 and is particularly active internationally (8), by the Independent Living Movement (24), which arose in the United States in the 1970s, and by the academic disability studies networks. In Europe was created in 1996 the European Disability Forum, which is a nongovernmental organization (11). Like the DPI motto ("Nothing about us without us"), they advocate that "no decisions concerning disabled people are taken without disabled people."

One of the major consequences of this revised perception of disability has been to affect social choices regarding the accessibility of locations and activities. This has meant not only adapting existing venues to make them accessible but even more also dramatically altering building standards and urban design rules in order to allow access for and integration of persons with every kind of disability. This has led to creating new standards for buildings and for spatial arrangements: the social "treatment" of disability has again led to setting norms and standards, with the difference that these norms apply on a larger scale than norms applying to individuals; instead, they have become constraints on society as a whole.

One example of how this new paradigm translates into national legislation is the French law «pour l'égalité des droits et des chances, la participation et la citoyenneté des personnes handicapées» (28). This law makes it clear that the plan focuses on the individual and advocates nondiscrimination, respect, and the expression of life choices and accessibility (in the broader sense of the word), in order to help patients be active as citizens and as participants in social life. The law offers individuals the possibility of expressing a "life project." This is defined as "an expression of the individual's self-projection into the future and the expression of his or her wishes and choices." The law calls for implementing policies that would "make up for the effects of disability" (such as human or technical assistance, adapting the disabled person's home or car, animal assistance) according to what is outlined in the individual's "life project" (5).

Is it possible to reconcile medical practice and the social model of disability?

The social model of disability and the ICF have been slow to replace Wood's model in the field of PRM. This may well be due to real obstacles as well as to the need for development of new concepts (20). Medical practice, including that focused on rehabilitation, necessarily remains focused on the individual patient. Clinical analysis cannot dispense with an assessment of impairments and activities or with a reference to normality. For this reason, it can be difficult to design therapeutic strategies where the stated purpose of the process is not, or not only, defining "normalization" as bringing about the greatest possible similarity to the majority and conformity to social norms. It is no doubt necessary to deal with these issues before one can find a final, alternate possibility for "normalisation," in the fourth of the senses defined above.

If normality is first and foremost defined as normativity, as non-subordination of living beings to their environment, then adaptation and creativity can be reconciled within the therapeutic process, thus allowing every patient to design, reveal, or recreate their own standard of "normality" (2).

So, ultimately, what the concept of rehabilitation must be based on is the idea of restoring creativity, and not – as we made it clear from the start – on a *restitutio ad integrum* to a previous condition: normality is less a matter of conforming to a given norm than it is the ability to switch to a different norm according to the requirements of the one's environment, situations, needs, wishes, or motivations. This is what Goldstein refers to as "responsivity" (*responsivität*) and Canguilhem as "normative" ability. «Thus, being well means to be capable of ordered behavior that may prevail in spite of the impossibility of certain performances that were formerly possible. But the new state of health is not the same as the old one» (17, p. 332). Whether rehabilitation is understood as resigning to a functional deficit or resisting it, its main goal should be to enable patients to acquire structured behaviors that allow them to live a life adapted to the requirements of their environment.

The "normalization" inherent to rehabilitation thus takes on an entirely different meaning: its orientation is now defined by the patient rather than designed around predetermined goals and activities. Both the aim and the orientation of the rehabilitation process (such as the choice of this or that particular prosthetic device, surgical procedure, or social role) remain open, and all that needs to be adapted is the care provided to the patient. The concept of "normalization" would then be restricted in its application to the possibility for patients to freely determine their lifestyle, within a given environment and a set range of possibilities, as for anyone else. Professional practitioners would keep a neutral perspective, and the process would be limited to offering new life standards and then taking the patient's point of view into account when choosing among the solutions available (29).

Implementing such a change of references in actual practice would require thinking about how it can be articulated to our current habits and with other constraints such as assessment of therapeutic strategies and evidence-based medical practice (9, 35).

Since the publication of Wood's model, the assessment of therapeutic strategies has mainly been centered on assessing disabilities – or activities in the terms used by the ICF. These tools are often inadequate in terms of respecting individual normativity. However, some progress has been made in this direction, for instance, by introducing into the Functional Independence Measure a possibility of scoring for "otherwise normal" performance, e.g., the possibility of performing a given task with technical assistance (21). The assessment of patient participation is difficult to ascertain (9, 35), probably because the normalization that underlies the design of this sort of scale would nowadays be considered unacceptable.

The most promising tools, in this perspective, seem to fall into two categories: on the one hand are quality-of-life (QOL) assessments (1, 39) and on the other, methodological tools that allow individualization of rehabilitation (27, 40).

Specific focus on the patients' quality of life reflects both a social perspective (since a person's quality of life is closely related to the quality of life of others and to their interactions with their social environment) and an eminently individual-centric attitude. Quality of life, in order to be assessed, has to be broken down into a number of components. These are chosen when the scale is designed (e.g., a sensation of tiredness, difficulty walking, or mood swings), depending on the goals that are to be achieved when the scale is used.

The use of specific or generic health-related quality-of-life scales in the practice of PRM can however be made relevant if, in agreement with the modern perception of disability, they shift away from quantifying impairments and function and focus on the patient's involvement. Health-related quality of life cannot be assessed by a third-party observer; it must be analyzed by patients themselves and this is what qualifies them as a means of including the patient's choices into the assessment process.

Of all the stages in the therapeutic process, defining the goals of a readaptation program may well be the one during which the conscious or unconscious temptation and attempts to strive for normality are strongest. In the patient's life history, at least in acquired pathologies such as a vascular accident or a traumatic medullary lesion, the process begins at a time when the emotional shock experienced by the patient as an effect of a traumatic event can make it difficult for him or her to exercise freedom of choice.

The wish, which can be legitimate, to admit evidence-based medicine as a key deciding factor in the choice of therapeutic gestures will increase the carer's influence in a given choice. Also such decisions as the choice of a micturition mode, or the date when the patient can spend his or her first weekend back at home, will be made for an average patient, which is necessarily different from the actual patient.

Tools are now being developed that may help fight this rampant tendency toward forced normalization. One example of these is goal attainment scaling based on individualizing goals (23). They tend to be developed in the form of goal attainment scales in a number of fields of rehabilitation and make it possible to reconcile individualized goals, treatment assessment, and data analysis on a large scale (40). Another example could be the use of the Canadian Occupational Performance Measure (COPM) (27) in which patients choose from a suggested list of goals that matter most to them. These goals are then the basis for assessment as to the success or failure of the procedure.

Another possibility that needs to be examined would be to weight the various items measuring the patient's activity level and quality of life by a factor set by the patient in order to reflect where the patient's priorities lie. Further research remains necessary to assess the metrological effectiveness of this kind of scales. But, beyond the issue of what kind of tool should be used, what remains absolutely necessary is to listen to what patients have to say, or to what their friends and family can convey, when it comes to defining what matters to them.

Once goals are defined, the rehabilitation process will involve multiple stages of learning, the prerequisites and conditions of which will be developed at length in the later chapters of this book. In rehabilitation, as in any kind of training, motivation appears to be one of the key factors toward effective learning.

The determining factors for this motivation can be external, and in a paradigm that differs little from what continues to prevail in education, the carer is the one who knows what needs to be learned, defines the stages in the learning process, and offers positive or negative feedback, thus reinforcing motivation and keeping discouragement at bay. We have seen how most of the senses of the word "normal" lead practitioners of PRM to precisely this attitude.

Recent trends in education have made it clear that external motivation is shaky and best replaced with internal motivation and processes in which the student is an active learner, defining his or her own learning goals (42). The issues at stake in the rehabilitation process could well be the same as in education, which implies that the therapist's role should be to facilitate a learning process.

Conclusion

What is advocated here is therefore a form of rehabilitation where the medical process of restoring normality goes hand in hand with restoring the patient's self-normativity rather than with the promotion of a particular ideal of health or performance, determined "externally." Only in its perfect adequacy to the individual patient's life, experienced in natural, intimate, and social situations, can the therapeutic process be shown to be relevant and therefore justified.

Putting such principles into practice entails reexamining every stage in the rehabilitation process. Assessing the various components of a patient's situation both is absolutely necessary and inherently implies a reference to an external standard. It will therefore be useful to keep developing metrology tools that make it possible to collectively analyse data, the collection of which remains tailored to the individual. The aim and the risk-to-benefit ratio, of a routine clinical use of metrology tools developed for research purposes, still need to be closely examined.

Determining the goals of the process is a crucial stage, during which the subject's choices may or may not be solicited, heard, and taken into account. In a real-life environment, where the development of standard procedures can contaminate the entire carer-patient relationship, the question arises whether monitoring the patient's degree of involvement in setting these goals will become a necessary evil, along with providing risk information. Particular issues can arise when the patient's actual ability to exercise their freedom of choice is affected by impaired consciousness or cognitive functions, or the emotional shock caused by a traumatic event.

The process of learning new gestures and new ways of living therefore becomes central to the therapeutic process. Depending on whether goals and references will have been set by the patient within the framework of a process of normativity or defined externally, the patient will be able to call on his or her own motivational resources or depend on the feedback provided by the therapist.

References

1. Andresen EM, Meyers AR (2000) Health-related quality of life outcomes measures. Arch Phys Med Rehabil 81(suppl 2):S30-S45
2. Barrier P (2008) The self-normativity of chronical patient: an innovatory concept for medical relationship and therapeutic education. Alter Eur J Disabil Res 2:271-291
3. Bernard C (1865) Introduction à l'étude de la médecine expérimentale, First ed. J.-B. Baillère, Paris. (1927) An introduction to the study of experimental medicine, Dover Publications Inc.
4. Binding K, Hoche A (1920) Die Freigabe der Vernichtung lebensunwerten Lebens, ihr Maß und ihre Form. Felix Meiner Verlag, Leipzig
5. Bracq-Meeschaert S (2007) L'influence de la loi de 2005 sur les organisations de santé. Réflexions sur un processus qui pourrait permettre de dépasser la simple logique de soin dans l'appréhension du handicap. J Readapt Med 27(2-3):81-83

6. Braddock DL, Parish SL (2001) An institutional history of disability, pp. 11-68. In: Albrecht GL, Seelman KD, Bury M (eds) Handbook of disability studies. Sage Publications, London

7. Canguilhem G (1966) Le Normal et le Pathologique. Presses Universitaires de France, Paris. (1991) The normal and the pathological. Zone Books, New York

8. Disabled Peoples' International: http://v1.dpi.org/lang-en/

9. Djikers M, Whiteneck G, El-Jaroudi R (2000) Measures of social outcomes in disability research. Arch Phys Med Rehabil 81(12, suppl 2):S63-S80

10. Doriguzzi P (1994) L'histoire politique du handicap. L'Harmattan, Paris

11. European Disability Forum: http://www.edf-feph.org/

12. Folz TJ, Opitz JL, Peters DJ, Gelfman R (1997) The history of physical medicine and rehabilitation as recorded in the diary of Dr Frank Krusen: Part 2. Forging ahead (1943-1947). Arch Phys Med Rehabil 78(4):446-450

13. Foucault M (1977) Surveiller et Punir, Naissance de la prison, Gallimard, Paris, 1975. Discipline and punish: the birth of the prison. Pantheon Books, 1st American edition, New-York

14. Fougeyrollas P, Cloutier R, Bergeron H, et al. (1998) The Quebec classification: disability creation process. International Network on Disability Creation Process, Canadian Society for the International Classification of Impairments, Disabilities and Handicaps, Lac St-Charles, Quebec, Canada

15. Fougeyrollas P, Noreau L, Bergeron H, et al. (1998) Social consequences of long term impairments and disabilities: conceptual approach and assessment of handicap. Int J Rehabil Res 21:127-141

16. Gelfman R, Peters DJ, Opitz JL, Folz TJ (1997) The history of physical medicine and rehabilitation as recorded in the diary of Dr Frank Krusen: Part 3. Consolidating the position (1948-1953). Arch Phys Med Rehabil 78(5):556-561. Erratum in: Arch Phys Med Rehabil 1998; 79(1):116

17. Goldstein K (1934) Der Aufbau des Organismus. Nijhoff, The Hague. (1939) The organism, First ed. American Books Co., New York. (1995) Zone Books, New York

18. Goffman E (2006) Stigma: notes on the management of spoiled identity, First ed 1963. Penguin Books,

19. Gray DB, Hendershot GE (2000) The ICIDH-2: developments for a new era of outcomes research. Arch Phys Med Rehabil 81(12, suppl 2):S10-S14

20. Gzil F, Lefève C, Cammelli M, et al. (2007) Why is rehabilitation not yet fully person-centred and should it be more person-centred? Disabil Rehabil 29(20-21):1616-1624

21. Hamilton BB, Granger CV, Sherwin FS, et al. (1987) A uniform national data system for medical rehabilitation. In: Fuhrer M (ed) Rehabilitation outcomes: analysis and measurement. Brookes, Baltimore, pp. 137-147

22. Hamonet C, Magalhaes T (2003) The concept of handicap. Ann Readapt Med Phys 46(8):521-524

23. Hurn J, Kneebone I, Cropley M (2006) Goal setting as an outcome measure: a systematic review. Clin Rehabil 20(9):756-772

24. Independent Living Movement: http://www.independentliving.org/

25. International Network on the Disability Creation Process: http://www.ripph.qc.ca/?rub2=0&rub=nouvelles&lang=en

26. Korff-Sausse S (2001) D'Œdipe à Frankenstein, figures du handicap. Desclée de Brouwer, Paris

27. Law M, Baptiste S, McColl M (1990) The Canadian Occupational Performance Measure: an outcome measure for occupational therapy. Can J Occup Ther 57(2):82-87

28. Law «pour l'égalité des droits et des chances, la participation et la citoyenneté des personnes handicapées», n 2005-102, February 11, 2005, available at http://www.legifrance.gouv.fr/affichTexte.do;jsessionid=B9C5C4B212D3C7217116D72AF3C EF945.tpdjo17v_1?cidTexte=LEGITEXT000006051257&dateTexte=20090808

29. Leplège A, Gzil F, Cammeli M, et al. (2007) Person-centredness: conceptual and historical perspectives. Disabil Rehabil 29(20-21):1555-1565

30. Levasseur M, Desrosiers J, Saint Cyr TD (2007) Comparing the disability creation process and International Classification of Functioning, Disability and Health models. Can J Occup Ther 74(special no):233-242

31. Minaire P (1992) Disease, illness and health: theoretical models of the disablement process, Bull World Health Organ 70(3):373-379

32. Opitz JL, Folz TJ, Gelfman R, Peters DJ (1997) The history of physical medicine and rehabilitation as recorded in the diary of Dr Frank Krusen: Part 1. Gathering momentum (the years before 1942). Arch Phys Med Rehabil 78(4):442-445

33. Peters DJ, Gelfman R, Folz TJ, Opitz JL (1997) The history of physical medicine and rehabilitation as recorded in the diary of Dr Frank Krusen: Part 4. Triumph over adversity (1954-1969). Arch Phys Med Rehabil 78(5):562-565

34. Ravaud JF, Stiker HJ (2001) Inclusion/exclusion: an analysis of historical and cultural meanings, pp. 490-512. In: Albrecht GL, Seelman KD, Bury M (eds) Handbook of disability studies. Sage Publications, London

35. Resnik L, Plow MA (2009) Measuring participation as defined by the International Classification of Functioning, Disability and Health: an evaluation of existing measures. Arch Phys Med Rehabil 90(5):856-866

36. Rusk HA (1972) A world to care for. Random House, New York

37. Rusk HA (2008) A world to care for. 1972. Am J Public health 98(2):254-255

38. Stiker HJ (1982) Corps infirmes et sociétés, Essais d'anthropologie historique. Aubier-Montaigne, Paris. (1999) A history of disability. The University of Michigan Press, Ann Arbor

39. The WHOQOL Group (1998) The World Health Organization Quality of Life Assessment (WHOQOL): development and general psychometric properties. Soc Sci Med 46:1569-1585

40. Turner-Stokes L (2009) Goal attainment scaling (GAS) in rehabilitation: a practical guide. Clin Rehabil 23:362-370

41. United Nations (2006) Convention on the rights of persons with disabilities, December 13, 2006, available at http://www.un.org/disabilities/documents/convention/convoptprot-e.pdf

42. Viau R (1998) La motivation en contexte scolaire. Ed De Boeck, Bruxelles

43. Vigarello G (2004) Le corps redressé, First ed 1978. Armand Colin, Paris

44. Wirotius JM (1999) Histoire de la rééducation. Encycl Med Chir (Elsevier, Paris), Kinésithérapie-Médecine physique-Réadaptation, 26-005-A-10, 25 pp

45. World Health Organization (2001) International classification of functioning, disability and health. WHO, Geneva
46. World Health Organization (1980) International classification of impairments, disabilities and handicap. WHO, Geneva

PART II

IMPLICIT LEARNING: A BASIC LEARNING PROCESS

A historical perspective on learning: the legacy and actuality of I. M. Pavlov and N. A. Bernstein

A. Roby-Brami and R. Goasdoué

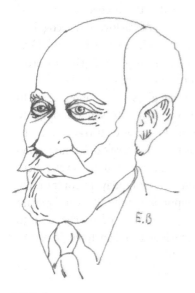

I.P. Pavlov

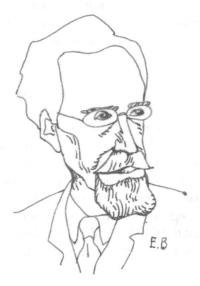

N.A. Bernstein

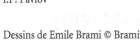

Dessins de Emile Brami © Brami

Introduction

The aim of the present chapter is to examine the mechanism of learning at the level of sensorimotor functions rather than at a higher cognitive level. Indeed, although the mechanisms subserving motor control and learning are still disputed, it is generally admitted that the control of even the simplest gesture such as pointing or grasping implies initial learning during development as a child and continuous adaptation to the context of action.

Learning is defined as a relatively permanent modification of the organism's activity resulting from its interactions with the external environment. There are two theoretical streams: the main stream that we may call very schematically computo-representational neurosciences, which aims to improve understanding of the physiology of the nervous system, and various alternative approaches that share a more systemic or dynamical point of view, with strong references to psychology and a common aim to understand human activity. These two approaches differ on some important points, particularly on the question of the mechanisms of learning. This debate would necessitate an extensive and detailed review of the experimental, theoretical, and modeling evidences supporting or refuting both approaches, which are well beyond the scope of this chapter. We chose to tackle the question *from a historical point of view*, through the controversy that occurred between Pavlov and Bernstein during the1930s.

Pavlov, a Nobel Prize winner, is universally recognized as the discoverer of classical conditioning (46). Bernstein was a younger contemporary of Pavlov, now recognized as an important pioneer in the field of motor control. In 1936, he wrote the book *Contemporary Issues on the Physiology of the Central Nervous System*, expressing his disagreement with Pavlov's views on motor learning, which remained unpublished until 2003 (8). Beyond the hard historical context, this controversy gives us the opportunity to review the scientific and epistemic lineage of these two great scientists. In our opinion, their controversy personalizes the still current confrontation between two key concepts: "reflexes" and "activity," to apprehend the multiple aspects and levels of learning nowadays. The ideas of Pavlov and the concept of reflexes have structured the development of research both in psychology and neuroscience right up until today. In contrast, the ideas of Bernstein were forgotten until their recent reappraisal in the 1970s and remain less recognized outside the specific field of motor control. The aim of this chapter is to suggest that the ideas he developed should be better considered and analyzed, in particular their potential applications for education and rehabilitation.

Biographies and historical context of the controversy between Pavlov and Bernstein

Biography of Ivan Petrovich Pavlov

Pavlov was a Russian physiologist, psychologist, and physician who is universally known for his work on conditioned reflexes. He is considered as a pioneer in many fields such as psychology, integrated physiology, and neuroscience.

Pavlov was born on September 14, 1849 at Ryazan, where his father was a village priest. He was educated at the theological seminary at Ryazan. Pavlov decided to devote his life to natural science. During his brilliant academic career, he directed the Department of Physiology at the Institute of Experimental Medicine from 1890 to the end of his life (45 years). This center became one of the most important for physiological research.

Pavlov was mainly inspired by the progressive ideas of I. M. Sechenov, the father of Russian physiology, who investigated the physiological basis of mental processes and postulated that the mnesic trace of past sensations could be recalled by the evocation of any of its parts (nowadays called cued recall). In the 1890s, Pavlov investigated the neural control of digestion in dogs by externalizing a salivary gland, so he could collect, measure, and analyze the saliva and its responses to food under different conditions. He noticed that the dogs tended to salivate before food was actually delivered to their mouths and set out to investigate this "psychic secretion," as he called it after Sechenov. He then carried out a long series of experiments in which he manipulated the stimuli occurring before the presentation of food. He determined several basic laws for the establishment and extinction of what he called "conditioned reflexes" that are the basis of the theory he developed until the end of his life (45, reviewed in 57).

Pavlov's experiments on digestion earned him the 1904 Nobel Prize in Physiology and Medicine (47). In 1907, he was elected as an academician of the Russian Academy of Sciences and received in the following years many honorary memberships abroad.

After the October Revolution, a special government decree signed by Lenin on January 24, 1921, noted «the outstanding scientific services of academician I. P. Pavlov, which are of enormous significance to the working class of the whole world». Pavlov and his collaborators were given unlimited scope for scientific research and received continuous government support despite Pavlov's critical opinions of the soviet regime (50).

The 15th International Physiological Congress, consecrating his work, was held in Leningrad and Moscow in 1935. Pavlov nurtured a great school of physiologists, which produced many pupils who continued to develop his ideas along with a host of followers all over the world. I. M. Pavlov died in Leningrad on February 27, 1936.

Conditioned reflexes and Pavlov's theory

Pavlov described conditioned reflexes in detail and used his observations to theorize upon the functioning of the brain and mental activity (46). Conditioned reflexes are based on the stimulus-response paradigm. Any external agent (the conditional stimulus) can, by coinciding in time with an ordinary reflex (e.g., food, which is the unconditional stimulus of salivation), become the signal for the formation of a new artificial conditioned reflex. Thus, conditioning creates a new link between the conditional stimulus and the response. Pavlov emphasized the importance of repetition for the formation of this new link. He paid particular attention to the experimental conditions, especially timing and selectivity of the stimuli. To this purpose, he built a laboratory some years later in St. Petersburg with a complicated system of acoustic insulation necessary for the experiments, the so-called "Tower of Silence" (57).

Pavlov's objective was to study all psychic activity objectively, instead of resorting to subjective methods and to experimentally investigate the most complex interrelations between an organism and its external environment. "A conditioned reflex should be regarded as an elementary psychological phenomenon, which at the same time is a physiological one. It followed from this that the conditioned reflex was a clue to the mechanism of the most highly developed forms of reaction in animals and humans to their environment and it made an objective study of their psychic activity possible" (45). Thus Pavlov rejected the subjective interpretation of «*psychic*» salivary secretion. More generally, for him all psychic activity was of a reflex nature – though not a permanent but a temporary or conditioned reflex. He was also interested in language that he called the second system of signalization (the external or internal stimulations being the first system of signalization), and this field was further developed by his followers. His objectivism was very innovative at that time by reference to contemporary psychophysics. Pavlov's work largely developed and popularized the stimulus-response paradigm, which dominated experimental psychology until the 1960s.

The method of conditioned reflexes allowed Pavlov to analyze the mechanism of "higher nervous function" in the cerebral cortex (46). He considered learning as a formation of connections among cortical centers parallel to the formation of associations at the psychological level. Although he was inspired by his contemporary C. S. Sherrington (1857-1952), who investigated the neuronal bases of spinal reflexes, Pavlov did not directly investigate the neuronal bases of behavior.[1] His findings on brain physiology were based on the demonstration of active inhibitory processes and the analysis of the complex interplay between excitation and inhibition during conditioning and not through lesional experiments that he used very little himself. "… conditioning is accompanied by excitatory and inhibitory processes extending over the hemispheres according to a variety of laws" (16).

Classical conditioning is recognized as a precursor of learning theory. However, Pavlov distinguished two mechanisms of association leading to modification of activity: adaptation through conditioning and learning through "trial and error" (developed later by Skinner in behaviorism). Pavlov thought that conditioned reflexes were at the basis of rapid adaptation to the environment and reserved the term of learning to the acquisition of knowledge resulting from trial and error. He thought that, unlike associations due to conditioned reflexes that could easily be extinguished, associations learned by trial and error were more stable and long lasting (69).

In the late part of his life, Pavlov worked on conditioning animals to pain and described the organism's response to overwhelming stimuli, what he called transmarginal inhibition.

Biography of Nicolaï Alexandrovitch Bernstein

Although much less universally known than Pavlov, Bernstein is recognized by the scientific community, even by his detractors, as a pioneer in the knowledge of action and movement control both in psychology and neurosciences and as a founder of cybernetics.

---

1. In contrast, Pavlov's ambition to understand psychological phenomenon by using objective physiological method departs from the Sherrington's views (13).

N. A. Bernstein was born in Moscow in 1896; his father was a well-known psychiatrist and his uncle a famous mathematician. After finishing his medical studies, he served as a medical doctor in the Red Army (1919-1921) then worked as a neuropsychologist. In 1922 he was recruited by the laboratory of biomechanics in the central institute of work in Moscow. In 1930-1941 he headed the laboratory of biomechanics in the central scientific institute of physical activity and set up biomechanics laboratories in other institutions. His method (kymocyclography) directly stems from Marey's chronophotography (Marey 1830-1904) with some technical improvement such as 3-D recordings and mathematical signal processing. Bernstein was particularly interested in the details of human movements and their variability with the double purpose of improving working conditions and understanding the underlying neuropsychological mechanisms.

Bernstein's observation of movement variability brought him to propose his theory on hierarchical control of action and movement coordination. He was influenced by the theory of dynamical systems investigated by the mathematicians Lyapunov (1857-1918) and Andronov (1901-1952), and he adapted these ideas on the organization of autonomous systems to the physiology of the motor system. He was also particularly interested and influenced by the neurophysiological works of Charles S. Sherrington (1857-1952) and Alfred Fessard (1900-1982). He deepened his theoretical thinking along with the ideas of the psychologist L. Vygotski (1896-1934) on the role of the material and social environment for development (56). He proposed a general theory of activity of the living organism that he named "physiology of activity" as a tribute to Vygotski, who proposed "psychology of activity."

Bernstein focused on action and the achievement of goals and not to a chaining of reflexes. This brought him to criticize Pavlov's theory in the book *Contemporary Studies on the Physiology of Nervous System*, written during the 1930s (7). This text is not so much a critique of the works of Pavlov himself but of the application of his theory to mental action and language by his pupil A. G. Ivanov-Smolenski. Mainly, it was an opportunity for Bernstein to present his own vision of cerebral function and particularly to transpose the paradigm of activity to physiology. The book was ready for publication, and the proofs were signed, when Pavlov died in 1936. Bernstein then refused the publication since he considered he should not argue against an opponent who could not answer.[2]

Bernstein spent the period of the war in Tashkent. Back in Moscow, he received recognition for the practical applications of his works (in sport, for bracing in rehabilitation, and for the training of cosmonauts). In 1947 he received the Stalin prize for his major book *The Construction of Movement* (2), which has never been integrally translated in English. In 1949, Bernstein was accused, during the anti-Semite campaign of

---

2. His student Pr Iosif Moiseevitch Feigenberg kept the proofs until now and directed the publication in 2003 in Moscow. This book is unfortunately still not translated despite its importance for the history of science.

"violating the principles of the party and the historical perspective." In 1950 a session of the Academy of Science proclaimed that Pavlov's doctrine was the official doctrine of the communist party. Considered as a public enemy, Bernstein was fired and his laboratory closed. Never disowning his convictions, shut in his home, he devoted his next years to writing. In particular, he wrote the pedagogical book "on dexterity and its development," which remained unpublished until 1991 (9).

Bernstein was rehabilitated after Stalin's death in 1953 and worked in the Institute of Neurology until his death in 1956, where he participated in a multidisciplinary seminar devoted to cybernetics (see below). Since Bernstein's death in 1966, the Institute of Higher Nervous Activity has been continuing his work on motor coordination, keeping his archives, and promoting his thinking.

The psychology of activity

The concept of activity was developed by Soviet psychologists in the 1930s, in particular the "Troïka": Vygotski (1896-1934), Leontiev (1903-1979), and Luria (1902-1977) (56), and transposed into physiology by Bernstein. This concept is at the heart of the controversy between Bernstein and Pavlov.

The concept of activity is a genuine paradigm shift mainly proposed as an alternative for the classic "stimulus-response" scheme. Leontiev suggested that the development of research in psychology needs to get beyond this debate, which began in XIXth psychophysics (39). This dualism leads the subject to be considered as passively receiving stimulations from his environment. Yet, the work by Soviet psychologists and Bernstein showed that perception is active since it implies exploration. In addition, studying only responses conceals the processes that determine the response. Vygotski qualified the responses as *«fossilized behavior»* since they are only traces of activity. The definition by Leontiev *«Activity is the non additive, molar unit of life for the material corporeal subject»* clearly shows the paradigm shift: the unit for analysis is no longer response but activity as a whole.

In the following section, we present the general properties of "psychology of activity" (reviewed in 39) and show how they were continued and adapted by Bernstein for his "physiology of activity."

Goal-directed activity and levels of description

The active dimension of activity is given the principal place, and much of this work focuses on the motives of activity. Every activity is goal directed, and the motive needs to be considered in order to understand its organization. The following example illustrates this principle and the structure of activity in three levels: to feed his family (motive), a person can go hunting (action), but the tools and techniques will not be the same depending on the hunted quarry (operations) (39). Bernstein follows the principle of a hierarchical description but more precisely focused at the level of operations. The highest level for Bernstein corresponds to Leontiev's "actions" and describes the goal as a *«representation of what will later occur»* (5, 6). Three lower levels detail the functioning of the operation level (the lowest level is that of tonus) consistent with the description of the central nervous system by Hughlings Jackson (16) and Luria (40) (reviewed in 24, 56). The descriptions by Bernstein (2, 9, 10) are on the border between activity and neurophysiological description. He links these domains, which are usually, but wrongly, considered as separate.

A developmental approach

One of the main aims of the theory of activity is to apprehend the processes of development in the most general sense. The idea of using development to understand activity was at first very much linked to the principles of dialectical materialism. According to P. P. Blonsky (1921, quoted in 67), "Behavior can be understood only as history of behavior." The history of behavior is considered at multiple timescales from phylogenesis to microgenesis, which are the short-term changes observed during learning. This preoccupation is present in Bernstein's works, in particular in his synthetic book on dexterity that presents considerations on phylogenesis, child development, and learning.

Interaction, mediation, internalization

These three notions, which are intricately related, are essential features of the theory of activity. Interactions, whether social or with the physical environment, are often mediated by tools. Language and symbolic gestures are considered by Vygotski as tools for social interactions (66). For example, pointing gestures, which are from a developmental point of view unfinished prehension gestures, become expressive means to designate objects and thus are tools for social interactions. This idea led to new interpretations of inner speech in children. Vygotski largely developed these concepts in his studies of the development of disabled children in the framework of defectology (65). He considers handicap as a sociocultural developmental phenomenon where compensation comes from socialization and culture (23). He introduced the concepts of "primary defects" (organic impairment) and "secondary defects" (distortions of higher psychological functions due to social factors), and in his search for alternative tests for handicapped students, he introduced the notion of the "zone of proximal development."

According to the Marxist perspective, the followers of the theory of activity underline the dialectic nature of tools since the potential they offer allows the individual to develop as well as give himself or herself a means to act on the world. This conception led to the concept of psychological instruments developed by Vygotski: the tools and in general the systems of signs are means for instrumentation. V. V. Ivanov (1977, quoted in 67) extends the notion of mediation and considers that behavior cannot be controlled otherwise than through intermediates (tools belonging to systems of signs). "Man cannot govern his own behavior directly and creates signs in order to control it indirectly." The concept of internalization is complementary to those of interaction and mediation. It describes the transition between the external plane of activity, from interaction with the environment, and the internal mental plane. This process supports transformations (generalizations, and so on) that will make internalized processes more general, more efficient, and able to anticipate future adaptations. This shift from external to internal, which is fundamental for the understanding of learning, allows the constitution of a "model of the future" in order to extrapolate in a statistical manner and anticipate «*the course of events in the environment*» (5, 10 reviewed in 11).

The role of social interactions is of minor importance in the work of Bernstein, but the interactions with the environment are critical. Bernstein showed on multiple occasions the importance of interactions with the environment for the organization of movement and for the exploratory strategies used for learning. He rejected the mechanicist interpretation of the control of the biomechanical parameters of locomotion. For Bernstein, motility results from an interaction between all the structures of the central nervous system and external factors, and evolves over time, the cerebral structures being able to modify themselves as a consequence of experience. What is important is the active search of a motor solution within the variability of the infinite number of possible solutions. Movement coordination according to Bernstein is a much more flexible system than conditioned reflexes and cannot be based on one particular neuronal mechanism but on the organization of the whole common activity.

The idea that we do not command behavior directly is similar to the hierarchical description of control proposed by Bernstein and to his idea that we do not directly control movement in all its details. The concept of tools, ubiquitous in the theory of activity, is also very significant in Bernstein's work since he dedicated a large part of his experimental work to the use of very varied tools from the hammer to the piano (4, 5).

The Bernstein-Pavlov controversy

The early work of Bernstein in the 1930s led to the question of the relationship between function and its neuronal substrate (i.e., the question of cerebral localization) and that of plastic changes in the central nervous system. Bernstein blamed Pavlov for considering the conditioned reflex as an isolated pathway (two central points, linked together by a synchronous association link) not generalized and separated from the rest of the personality.[3] This debate meets another debate: that between holism and atomism.

Bernstein was particularly interested in child development and posits that development cannot be reduced to the mechanical result of external influences. By opposition, he claims that learning is also determined by the history of the organism and of its species, and the long-lasting traces it has left, in keeping with the concept of activity. For him memory is a huge architecture of facts, is historically constructed, and is the support of consciousness as a matter organized in a specific way. In contrast to Pavlov, who insisted on the importance of repetition for the rooting of combinations of reflexes, Bernstein claimed in a very modern way that repetition does not exist since it can never

---

3. This criticism is shared by Luria (56).

be repetition of the same. The situation is always variable from one occurrence to another; the observer has to consider the whole situation, including the context, the observer himself, and the existing memory traces. So repetition induces qualitative and not only quantitative changes (7). For Bernstein, repetition is a primitive way of learning, useful only in the highly simplified and artificial context of the laboratory (the "tower of silence"), in contrast to the rich context of usual human or animal life. Consistently and in a complementary way, Bernstein claimed that perception is an active search process. Individuals are never passive, according to the concept of activity. "Those aspects of the remaining variability that have no reactive adaptive value can justifiably be looked upon as search-variability, in which the active exploration of the environment, its gradients, the optimal way to act, et cetera, come to the fore" (10, reviewed in 43).

Later, Bernstein suggested that the basis of motor control by the central nervous system is not muscular contractions but synergies that allow the control of the incredible complexity of the human body. He challenged the idea that commands for movements are directly issued by the brain. He posited that performance of any kind of movement results from an infinite variety of possible combinations, or degrees of freedom, of neuromuscular and skeletal elements. The system should, therefore, be considered as self-organizing, with body elements coordinated, or assembled, in response to specific tasks. Bernstein presented a hierarchical organization of the motor system in keeping with the concept of activity, putting in parallel the structure of the CNS according to the neurologist Hughlings Jackson and the phylogenetic description of animal movements. This topology of motor acts also influenced his contemporary A. R. Luria (56). The functional hierarchical organization is arranged within levels and between levels (the principle of minimal interaction proposed in 22). Bernstein proposed that motor development was dependent not only on brain maturation but also on adaptations to body constraints (changes in the growing infant's body mass and proportions) and to exogenous conditions (gravity, surface, specific tasks to be performed). He coined the term biomechanics, describing the application of mechanical principles and methods to biological systems. Many of the key issues in modern-day movement coordination were formulated by Bernstein, including the anticipation of the goal, the degrees of freedom problem, motor equivalence, and non-univocality of motor commands, and peripheral effects.

Legacy

Despite the political separation by the Iron Curtain, the theories of Pavlov developed largely in the West, particularly through behaviorism formulated and developed by Watson and then Skinner. The main works by Skinner in the United States during 1950s to 1960s coincided with the revival of Pavlovian studies in the USSR. Conversely, the applications of cybernetics were well developed in the USSR. Bernstein formulated in the 1930s some key concepts similar to those formulated as cybernetics by Wiener and, in the late part of his life, led a seminar devoted to the theoretical implications of cybernetics.

Pavlov and Behaviorism

Expansion of behaviorism in the United States

Since his Nobel Prize in 1904, Pavlov became universally recognized and celebrated as a major scientist in physiology. His legacy in psychology, based on his later works on conditioning, was developed by American psychologists, particularly through the writings of John B. Watson (1878-1958), who founded behaviorism, and E. Thorndike (1874-1949). This direction differed from Pavlov's general purpose since he noted "that the practical American mind found it more important to know the external behavior of a man, than to guess about his internal state" (42).

Behaviorism became popular in its radical form mainly through the contribution of B. H. Skinner (1904-1990), who was an influential American psychologist and founded his own school of experimental research psychology and radical behaviorism, and recognized his dept toward Pavlov (17). The key concept is operant conditioning, sometimes called instrumental conditioning or instrumental learning. Operant conditioning uses the consequences of voluntary behavior or response to modify the occurrence and form of behavior. This was demonstrated through systematic experiments in the operant conditioning chamber invented by Skinner. The chamber contained feeding mechanisms, activated by key or lever presses, that enabled measurement of the rate of response. Successful responses producing satisfying consequences (reinforcement) are imprinted and thus will occur more frequently. Unsuccessful responses producing undesirable consequences (punishment) will subsequently occur less frequently. Operant behavior functions within the environment and is maintained by its consequences, while classical conditioning is obtained by modifications of preceding conditions and is not maintained by consequences. Reinforcement, punishment, and extinction, which are the main tools of operant conditioning, are either positive (delivered following a response) or negative (withdrawn following a response). The power of conditioning relies on particular schedules over time with fixed or variable intervals and ratios of reinforcement or punishment as a function of behavioral responses. Extinction is the lack of any consequence following a behavior.

In contrast to classical conditioning in which the unconditioned stimulus (e.g., food) occurs shortly after the conditioning stimulus (e.g., sound), a prior stimulus is not necessary for operant conditioning (although the context of response may be considered as a stimulus). Another difference is that classical conditioning establishes associations between stimuli while operant conditioning establishes associations between response and stimulus.

This behavioral approach has proven to be successful in many areas; in particular, it has largely contributed to the development of a psychotherapeutic approach (cognitive behavioral therapy) that aims to influence problematic and dysfunctional emotions, behaviors, and cognitions through a goal-oriented, systematic procedure.

Therapy for posttraumatic shock (51) is also based on the work of Pavlov on conditioning to pain and transmarginal inhibition. This is also the case for methods of extreme mental conditioning procedures or brain washing exerted by several organizations such as military camps.

Hebb and adaptation in formal neural networks

Pavlov directly influenced the works by D. O. Hebb (1904-1985), a Canadian psychologist who is considered as the father of neuropsychology and neural networks. In particular, he proposed a theory, inspired by classical conditioning at the neuronal level, which became known as Hebbian learning. This method of learning is best expressed by the following quote from his book *The Organization of Behavior* (30): "When an axon of cell A is near enough to excite cell B and repeatedly or persistently takes part in firing it, some growth process or metabolic change takes place in one or both cells such that A's efficiency, as one of the cells firing B, is increased." This is often paraphrased as "Neurons that fire together wire together." The mechanism of Hebbian learning was a source of the development of learning in artificial neural networks. Creation of some modern artificial neural networks is still based on the transmission of signals via electrical impulses and Hebbian synapses.

Hebbian learning and cerebellar physiology

The Hebbian theory also had great impact in neuroscience in the field of cerebellar physiology (29). The convergence of parallel fibers and climbing fibers on Purkinje cells was initially proposed as being a Hebbian synapse. Later, Ito confirmed experimentally the phenomenon of long-term depression (LTD), i.e., the decrease in transmission between parallel fibers and Purkinje cells after conjunctive stimulation of the parallel fibers and climbing fibers. It is now largely admitted that the microcomplex of the cerebellar networks and LTD could be the basis of an adaptive mechanism in the brain and the acquisition of adaptive models[4] (see below).

Bernstein and Russian Cybernetics

Conversely to behaviorism, cybernetics was born in the United States but was developed particularly in the USSR, both on the applied and fundamental sides. Bernstein is also considered as a pioneer in the theoretical branch of Eastern cybernetics.

---

4. "Initially all parallel-fiber synapses on Purkinje cells may be functional, so that Purkinje cell are fully activated by a mossy fiber input and in turn inhibit nuclear neurons that otherwise might be activated by the mossy fiber input. If the consequent silence of nuclear neurons results in errors, climbing-fiber signals are generated to depress the parallel fiber-Purkinje cell transmission, thereby releasing nuclear neurons from Purkinje cells inhibition and generating output from the microcomplex. This will lead to improvement of the overall system performance with reduced errors" (29).

Cybernetics, the science of the control of regulated systems, is based on a modeling of exchanges and information and principles of interaction. It relates more to the functioning of the whole system than to the analysis of the components. It was later designed as the science of mastered analogies between organisms and machines.

Cybernetics began in the United States as an interdisciplinary science in the 1940s during the Macy conferences for which mathematicians, logicians, anthropologists, psychologists, and economists who aimed to build a general science on mind functioning all gathered. This was formalized by the mathematician Norbert Wiener (1894-1964) in his book *Cybernetics, or Control and Communication in the Animal and the Machine*, which was published in 1948 (68). The "first cybernetics" was later divided into three branches: cognitive sciences, artificial intelligence, and a movement known as second-order cybernetics (reviewed in 18). Second-order cybernetics is a theory of auto-organizing systems formalized in the 1950s by Heinz von Foerster (1911-2002), an Austrian-American physician and philosopher. In the field of biology, this trend initiated by Maturana and Varela (41, 64) and Atlan (1) was particularly fertile in France.

Wiener's book was published in the USSR in 1958 and became very popular. At the end of the 1950s and the beginning of the 1960s, there was a cybernetics boom in the USSR. In contrast to the few academic cybernetics departments in the United States, many cybernetics departments were created in universities and scientific institutions of the USSR. Most of these organizations had a practical technical purpose for engineering.

Bernstein did not participate in the founding of cybernetics in the 1940s. However, he is recognized for his contribution to the description of neuromuscular feedback, a key concept of cybernetics, and for proposing its strict mathematical definition in differential equations (62). Bernstein's idea largely influenced the thinking in the USSR with regard to the biological basis of cybernetics. After their meeting with Bernstein, the famous mathematician I. M. Gelfand (1913-2009) and the theoretical physicist M. L. Tsetlin created a laboratory in the Institute of Information Transmission, where they initiated a multidisciplinary seminar with the biologist V. S. Gurfinkel. Their contribution was mainly related to the stream of second-order cybernetics. Bernstein and his colleagues in the multidisciplinary seminar contributed largely to the influence of fundamental research on control in the USSR, and this was largely disseminated in the world from the end of the 1960s. People participating in this seminar became the relay for Bernstein's thinking, particularly on movement sciences.

The works of Bernstein were little known in the West until the translation and publication in 1967 of a book written in 1935 (5), *The Coordination and Regulation of Movement*. After that, his influence grew as demonstrated by the exponential curve of quotations. He was recognized as a pioneer and quoted even by scientists who defended ideas far from his own. His direct disciples (Berkenblit, I. M. Feigenberg, A. G. Feldman, L. P. Latash, M. L. Latash, G. N. Orlovsky, G. L. Shik, ...), many of whom emigrated to the West after 1990, developed his scientific legacy. A scientific society exists with the aim of developing Bernstein's legacy,[5] and regular international meetings are organized. In France, collaboration between French and Russian scientists renewed the tradition elicited by E. J. Marey on the physiology of sensorimotor activity.

Presence and impact on motor control and sensorimotor learning today

Pavlov and Bernstein had very different personal destinies. During the 1930s Pavlov was a universally respected Nobel Prize winner and Bernstein a younger physician and scientist working in a difficult historical context. Both were great scientists whose legacy extends well beyond their own work. Their dialog is materialized by the book *Contemporary Issues on the Physiology of the Central Nervous System* (7), which testifies the theoretical, experimental, and historical richness of their controversy particularly on the mechanism of learning. Now, more than 70 years later, after complicated streams of scientific influence in new disciplines such as behaviorism and cybernetics, as well as complicated exchanges between Eastern and Western scientific traditions, an echo of their controversy remains. Despite an exponential growth of knowledge on learning, brain function, and sensorimotor control, the controversy between two "types" of theories corresponding to two "types" of learning mechanisms remains vivid. On the one hand, we largely recognize the wide legacy of Pavlov in the mainstream view on motor control and learning. On the other hand, several scattered theoretical alternatives (dynamical systems approach, ecological psychology, motor control) defend minority ideas close to those defended by Bernstein and his direct followers.

Motor control: problems to solve in the control of movement

This opposition in ideas can be illustrated on the question of motor control, i.e., on the mechanisms by which the central nervous system commands and controls the complex mechanical structure of the body. Bernstein is especially famous for evidencing the theoretical questions related to motor control (6). Indeed, the apparent ease with which we move and smoothly execute simple goal-directed gestures contrasts deeply with the complexity of the problem. The first aspect is that of multilevel redundancy. In general, the human body has at its disposal a larger number of degrees of freedom (DoF) that is necessary for the task. This is true at the anatomical level of the joints: for example, to reach an object in 3-D space, 6 DoFs are needed (to position and orientate the hand relative to the object). However, the human arm has at least 7 DoFs (3 rotations in the glenohumeral shoulder joint, 2 in the elbow, and 2 in the wrist, without mentioning the trunk, scapula, and hand). This redundancy is still greater if we consider muscles (in general, several muscles can activate one rotation, many mus-

---

5. International Society for motor control. http://www.i-s-m-c.org

cles are bi-articular, and so forth), or even motor units. So redundancy affords multiple ways to execute a movement. The second aspect is linked to Newtonian laws of mechanics that work on our body. All movements are performed within the field of gravity. In addition, the body is structured as a multilink effector, so any movement of one segment has consequences on the neighboring segments, due to action-reaction effects, and finally on the whole body chain until the postural support; therefore, the dynamical interactions of rotating segments are mathematically very complex. These interactions are prone to induce an important perturbation of the movement. Therefore, any movement involves not only the control of the joints that had to be moved but also the stability of the other joints and generally the simultaneous control of posture and equilibrium. This postural control is anticipatory since it is generated before the onset of movement (12).

Actions are generally goal directed so that movement involves a representation of the future as underlined by Bernstein according to the theory of activity. Goal-directed action opens the question of anticipation for motor control (32).

In addition, the environment within which the movement is performed may itself induce external perturbations; some can be anticipated and predicted (i.e., obstacles or interactions with objects), and others may cause unexpected perturbations or cannot be exactly predicted due to some variability and noise.

So, human or, more generally, biological motion implies the mastering of a complicated mechanical movement in the field of gravity. However, movements are characterized by a smooth execution and by a great regularity evidenced by well-known kinematic invariants. For example, the movement of the finger for a goal-directed task such as pointing has a linear trajectory and a smooth velocity profile, both showing that the constraints of motor control are anticipated by the central nervous system before the onset of movement (32). The mechanism of anticipated control is disputed, but all the theories concur to the idea that those mechanisms have to be acquired during the development and continuously updated during life, by a continuous adaptation process.

Acquisition of internal models and programs: role of reinforcement learning

The concept of motor programs means that the details of the movement are generated by an anticipatory mechanism before the onset of movement itself. Theoretical work on motor programs stem from both a psychological and a neurophysiological context.

Schmidt and generalized motor programs

The most classical view on motor anticipation is the idea of motor program or schemata as proposed by Schmidt (52). For him, the motor programs were generalized for a same action, and each movement instance was influenced by the parameter as a function of sensory information. The idea of generalized programs avoided the need for extensive memory storage. For him, the schema was "a rule developed by practice and experience across a lifetime, which described a relationship between the outcomes achieved on past attempts at running a program and the parameters chosen on those attempts" (52). Schmidt distinguished between recall schemata (relationships between the parameters of the program and the outcome) and recognition schemata (relationship between the past sensory consequences generated by the program and the outcome of the program), and he described the role of feedback for the permanent tuning and adaptation of the parameters of these schemata constituting the generalized motor program. He also formalized the distinction between several kinds of feedback information [knowledge of results (KR) and knowledge of performance (KP); see Robertson *et al.* this volume] that both act as reinforcement. The theory of generalized motor programs is not behaviorist but keeps the emphasis on repetition in order to evoke the "correct movement" and the idea that that the perceptual trace in memory is an increasing function of the number of repetitions ["law of exercise," initially proposed by Thorndike (60)]. Recent experiments with augmented feedback did not always obey the predictions of the theory (reviewed in 55), perhaps because the generalized motor program theory explains the improvement of motor execution, but not the acquisition of the program, when evidence suggests that KR may act more on the acquisition of the skill itself than on the tuning of the parameters. This theory does not explain, for example, motor learning by mental practice, and it is suggested that all the repetitions of the task are not equivalent and that cognitive effort could weigh the effect of each repetition (55).

Brain control of movement

A great number of studies in neuroscience have investigated the neuronal mechanisms of motor control and learning. Classically, motor control is assumed to be hierarchical with relatively sequential but overlapping steps: planning as a function of task requirement in the prefrontal cortex (34); coordination as a function of initial condition and context in a network between premotor and parietal associative areas (15); and then execution in the primary motor area with activation of the pyramidal neurons.

In this context, the acquisition of motor behavior is related to the adaptation and plasticity of brain structures, the cerebral and cerebellar cortices, and basal ganglia.

Adaptive motor learning and internal models in the cerebellum

Many studies devoted to the control of smooth movement and its adaptation to changing conditions of execution focused on the cerebellum, following the description by Ito of the properties of the cerebellar microcomplex (see above). Indeed, the structure of the cerebellum could be the neuronal basis of internal models. Models of adaptive learning based on cerebellar wiring diagrams have been used to understand how the central nervous system adapts itself to control the complex mechanics of the body. The cerebellum can form "an internal model mimicking the motor plant that is controlled by the motor cortex" (29).[6] Such a forward internal model predicts the consequences of actions and can be used to overcome time delays associated with feedback control. Later, Kawato proposed that the cerebellum also used inverse models that can provide the neural command necessary to achieve some desired trajectory (33). A more recent model of cerebellar function includes multiple paired forward and inverse models. This arrangement could explain both motor learning and control (70). The progressive learning within the cerebellar forward and inverse models is tuned to progressively reduce errors in order to obtain one optimal solution minimizing the cost of the movements and the noise in the command (reviewed in 61). Optimization, as a result of the adaptation of internal models, is therefore able to provide a solution for the "ill-posed[7]" problem of redundancy (26). Learning in such a circuit is supervised since the objective is given by the task, and the mechanisms operate to converge on a reduction of the errors given by the feedback.

The cerebellum is now viewed as the stocking structure of multiple models of the environment or tools mediating the movements. The choice of a particular model would occur as a result of the dense reciprocal relationships between the cerebral associative areas and the cerebellum. These models are backed up by experimental evidence with motor learning and adaptation paradigms and brain imaging studies (27, 28). In a recent review, based on studies in patients with lesions of the central nervous system, Shadmehr and Krakauer (54) map the functional aspect of such an integrated model of motor control between the cerebellum, cortical brain areas, and the basal ganglia. Theories based on motor programs do not exclude corrective online control of movement that is now largely demonstrated (48).

Although these theories are far from behaviorism since their aim is to "open the black box" and investigate the neuronal basis of motor control, they still rely heavily on Pavlov's view on leaning. First, the historical lineage relayed by Hebb is clear; second, the experimental paradigms share a surprising common basis, which is the role of feedback for supervision and reinforcement, the great number of movement trials, the goal of optimization, the objective to reduce the variability, the emphasis on repetition, and the mechanism by the formation of a neuronal trace whose strength increases with repetition. The kinematic invariants are in general viewed as optimal solutions that are what needs to be specifically learnt.

A dynamical view on motor control in Bernstein's tradition

Besides these mainstream theories on motor control, based on the idea of motor programs and internal models, several concurrent theoretical approaches have been developed. These approaches are quite diverse but share common principles based on systemic models rooted in the action perception cycle with a common reference to Bernstein.

---

6. Forward and inverse models are terms stemming from engineering and robotics that can be put together with recall and recognition schemata respectively.

7. The coordination of a redundant system is an "ill-posed" problem since it has no unique solution.

Synergies and the use of variability

Learning is the result of activity and of spontaneous exploration of the possible actions depending on the context. The focus is put on variability of the different instances of movements instead of repetition of the same, on the importance of varied and rich sensory information in a natural context, on sudden success, and on the long-lasting remaining skill. For example, in order to learn to ride a bike, a child has to make many attempts, but the exact conditions and the sensorimotor context, including the help of adults, vary from one attempt to another and are far from being repetitions of the same movement. Then, the child finally succeeds in the mastering of the very complex dynamical interactions between his movements, the forward progression of the bike, and the complex dynamical equilibrium of the cyclist and bike pair. This sudden understanding is what Bernstein called with humor the "aha" effect (9). Once somebody has learned to ride a bike, he can improve velocity or other parameters, but the skill itself is never forgotten, in contrast to the gradual extinction of Pavlovian conditioned reflexes.

As Bernstein showed, the full mastering of professional, artistic, or sports skills (hammering, playing piano, …), needs many repetitions of intensive practice in variable conditions of execution. Joint coordination is always different, despite the kinematic regularity of the part of the limb, which is most important for the task, the working point (36). Bernstein's followers, along with Gelfand, demonstrated how variability is positive, since it allows accommodation of the trial-to-trial variations of the context. Gelfand and Latash (21) proposed the replacement of the word "redundancy" by the word "abundance."[8] In this framework, the redundancy of the motor system is not an "ill-posed problem" but a fundamental characteristic of motor control, allowing fluidity, flexibility, and adaptability of motor acts as well as their automatic resistance to perturbation. Movement in the different degrees of freedom is organized is such a way as to maintain the important variables for the task, while releasing the variability in the other degrees of freedom (53, 63, reviewed in 38). According to this hypothesis, synergies are organized according to two complementary properties: (i) covariation in several DoFs, which can be combined additively in order to reduce the dimensionality of the control and (ii) automatic compensation from one DoF to another, in case of perturbation or random fluctuation of execution. This latter property corresponds to motor equivalence (25).

Mass-spring models and equilibrium point control

Complementary to Bernstein's work, A. G. Feldman has been developing since the 1960s the theory of equilibrium point control in which the limbs are modeled as a mass-spring mobile (reviewed in 19). This theory can be generalized to a redundant system: in this case the command specifies a referent configuration corresponding to a set of thresholds for the recruitment of motorneurons. The final configuration of the limb reaches its final state according to the central command (referent configuration) and to

---

8. The Russian word for redundancy may have both meanings.

the mechanical constraints in the environment (i.e., the command moves the limb if it is free or increases the force in an isometric situation). Thus, the force is not directly specified by the central nervous system but results from the dynamical interactions between the command and the biomechanics of the limb and of the environment, including gravity (44). Therefore, the equilibrium point theory avoids the need for an internal model of the limbs and the environment, since the necessary adaptation to changing conditions occurs through tuning of the command from trial to trial (20).

Dynamical systems for learning and development

Another influential stream of research is based on the concept of dynamical systems. The common basis of this thinking is inspired by the physical models of nonlinear dynamical systems, an area of applied mathematics used to describe the behavior of complex interactions usually by employing differential equations. Models of coupled oscillators have been applied with success on rhythmic movements, which have been largely studied by this school, for example, juggling (3) in line with Bernstein's early study on the dynamics of piano playing (4). These theories oppose the theories of motor programs and internal models. Here the focus is put on the interactions between the subject and his or her environment and the auto-organization of the behavior rather than on supervised learning. The priority in this line of thinking is not to investigate the neuronal basis but to understand the construction of behavior and cognition resulting from the action perception cycle in a constructionist way. This view is in agreement with that of Gibson, the founder of ecological psychology, who argued that animals and humans form a "system" with the environment such that, to fully explain some behavior, it is necessary to study the environment in which this behavior took place. The environment affords opportunities for actions, the "affordances" that critically depend on the individual body of the person (or animal!) acting. The arrangement of the environmental context of action as a field of promoted actions is a means for adults or experts to encourage the discovery and learning of new skills in the developmental or academic context (14, 49). The concepts of affordance and the "field of promoted actions" allow the bridging of the gap between recent advances in psychophysiology of action and perception and the sociocultural theories for the dynamical construction of behavior during development and learning, initiated by Vygotski in the 1930s (66).

In most cases, dynamical models of interactions are not explicitly modeled but rather used as a metaphor. Dynamical systems theory deals with long-term qualitative behavior and uses the concepts of physics: self-organization (the spontaneous creation of coherent forms), emergent properties, limit cycle, ... Experimentally, the focus is put on (i) long-term observation of a small number of individuals, taking into account their own bodily characteristics (e.g., respiratory, circulatory, nervous, musculoskeletal, perceptual), (ii) the characteristics of the environment (perceptual, mechanical, ...), and (iii) the aim being to investigate the determinants of the transitions between behaviors. An influential theorist in this field is E. Thelen (58, 59), who studied the motor development of children. She showed that the onset of behavior depended on many intricate factors involving not only the maturation of the central nervous system but also the characteristics of the body, or its state, and of the environment. For example, she showed that infant stepping, which is present after birth, can be elicited before the acquisition of locomotion in a pool, suggesting that it is masked by biomechanical factors, and can be released when the constraints of gravity are lessened by water. Similar analysis aims to understand the particular construction of behavior of individuals whatever their condition. Latash and Anson (37) proposed that the movement patterns observed in pathological conditions should not be considered as pathological but "atypical" since they may represent the best motor solution for a person taking into account his or her impairment and life context. However, this position is contested; "atypical" movements may have detrimental consequences or may limit rehabilitation and finally lead to a poorer outcome.

In opposition to the reductionist approach of mental activity on neuroscience, these approaches share the ambition to develop nonreductionist materialistic theories of human activity (10).

Conclusion

In summary, the impressive legacy of Pavlov has fertilized very different fields in psychology, neuroscience, and formal neurons. It is commonly accepted in the community and very largely applied for learning, teaching, and therapy with unquestionable efficiency. It remains nowadays the mainstream paradigm for learning and adaptation and has received much evidence from basic and integrated neuroscience.

Although quite varied, the approaches in Bernstein's tradition share common principles that differ markedly from the tradition of conditioning inherited from Pavlov. The drive for learning is action itself and not stimuli. The focus is put on dynamical processes and not on representation (called traces by Pavlov) and on the sensorimotor history of each individual. All the elements of interaction are considered, including the characteristics of the body structure, and the multiple facets of the physical, social, and cultural environment. The theories of reference are more related to physical models of auto-organization and autopoiesis than to neuronal models developed by computational neuroscience. In addition, the concept of activity allows dualist positions to be rejected as Leontiev suggests: "We must analyze the system of objective activity in general. This includes the corporal subject – the brain and the perceptual and motor organs" (39).

However, rather than being alternative, these two streams of research should be presented as complementary approaches since they do not really share the same object of research. Skinner claimed "neuroscientists need science of behavior; without it, they would not know what to look for in the nervous system and therefore might look for things they would never find" (quoted in 17). An analysis of activity in the physical and sociocultural context (and not only of behavior) should precede and complement research on brain activity. For both scientific and sociological reasons, a synthesis is still to come. The hazards of life and history in a particularly troubled period meant that the physiology of activity proposed by Bernstein as a new paradigm (35) remained of minority interest and did not evoke a generally accepted shift in scientific thinking.

However, the authors hope that the readers of the present text will share their fascination for the destiny of these two eminent people, both as men and as researchers, who so brilliantly personify the ongoing hot debate on learning.

Acknowledgments

The authors are indebted to Nicolas Balzamo for the translation in French of a chapter of Bernstein (1936/2003). The translation was supported by the Federative Institute for Research on Disability (IFR 25). We thank Johanna Robertson for reviewing the English. A. Roby-Brami is supported by the INSERM. Original pictures of I. P. Pavlov and N. A. Bernstein by Emile Brami, copyright Emile Brami.

References

1. Atlan H (1979) Entre le cristal et la fume. Seuil, Paris
2. Bassin PV, Bernstein NA, Latash LP (1966) (English translation 1999) On the problem of the relation between structure and function in the brain from a contemporary viewpoint. In: Latash LP, Latash ML, Meijer OG (eds) Part I. Motor Control (1999) 3:329-332, 342-345. Part II. Motor Control (2000) 4:125-149
3. Beek PJ, Turvey MT (1992) Temporal patterning in cascade juggling. J Exp Psychol Hum Percept Perform 18:934-947
4. Bernstein NA, Popova (1930) Studies on the biodynamics of the piano strike (English translation 2003). In: Kay BA, Turvey MT, Meijer OM (eds) (2003) An early oscillator model. Studies on the biodynamics of the piano strike. Motor Control 7:1-45
5. Bernstein NA (1935) (English translation 1967) The coordination and regulation of movements. Pergamon Press, Oxford
6. Bernstein NA (1945) (English translation 1998) The current problem of modern Neurophysiology. In: Sporns O, Edelman GM (eds) Bernstein dynamic view of the brain: the current problem of modern neurophysiology. Motor Control (1998) 2:283-305
7. Bernstein NA (1936-2003) Contemporary issues on the physiology of the central nervous system (in Russian). Smysl, Moscow
8. Bernstein (1947) The construction of movement (in Russian). Medzig, Moscow
9. Bernstein NA (1947-1991) (English translation 1996) Dexterity and its development. In: Latash ML, Turvey MT (eds) Dexterity and its development (1996). Lawrence Erlbaum, New Jersey, pp. 1-235
10. Bernstein NA (1965) (English translation 2000) On the road towards a biology of activity. In: Bongaardt R, Pickenhain L, Meijer OG (eds) Bernstein's anti-reductionistic materialism: on the road towards a biology of activity. Motor control (2000) 4:377-406

11. Bongaardt R, Meijer OG (2000) Bernstein's theory of movement behavior: historical development and contemporary relevance. J Mot Behav 32:57-71

12. Bouisset S, Do MC (2008) Posture, dynamic stability, and voluntary movement. Neurophysiol Clin 38:345-362

13. Brazier M (1977) La neurobiologie du vitalisme au matérialisme. La recherche 83:965-972

14. Bril B (2002) Apprentissage et context. Intellectica 35: 251-268

15. Burnod Y, Baraduc P, Battaglia-Mayer A, et al. (1999) Parieto-frontal coding of reaching: an integrated framework. Exp Brain Res 129:325-346

16. Buser P (2006) Slowly forgetting the Pavlovian adventure? C R Biol 329:398-405

17. Catania C, Laties VG (1999) Pavlov and Skinner: two lives in science (an introduction to BF Skinner's "Some responses to the stimulus 'Pavlov'", J Exp Anal Behav 72:455-461

18. Dupuy JP (1994) Aux origines des sciences cognitive. La Découverte, Paris

19. Feldman AG, Goussev V, Sangole A, Levin MF (2007) Threshold position control and the principle of minimal interaction in motor actions. Prog Brain Res 165:267-281

20. Foisy M, Feldman AG (2006) Threshold control of arm posture and movement adaptation to load. Exp Brain Res 175:726-744

21. Gelfand I, Latash ML (1998) On the problem of adequate language in motor control. Motor Control 2:306-313

22. Gelfand IM, Tsetlin ML (1966) On mathematical modelling of the mechanisms of the central nervous system. In: Gelfand IM, Gurfinkel VS, Fomin SV, Tsetlin ML (eds) Models of the structural-functional organisation of certain biological systems. Nauka, Moscow, pp. 9-26 (English translation: 1971. MIT Press, Cambridge).

23. Gindis B (1995) Viewing the disabled child in the sociocultural milieu. Vygotsky's quest. School Psychol Int 16:155-166

24. Glozman JM (2007) A. R. Luria and the history of Russian neuropsychology. J Hist Neurosci 16(1):168-180

25. Gracco GL, Abbs JH (1986) Variant and invariant characteristics of speech movements. Exp Brain Res 65:156-166

26. Guigon E, Baraduc P, Desmurget M (2007) Computational motor control: redundancy and invariance. J Neurophysiol 97:331-347

27. ImamizuH, Kuroda T, et al. (2003) Modular organization of internal models of tools in the human cerebellum. Proc Natl Acad Sci U S A 100(9):5461-5466

28. Imamizu H, Kuroda T, Miyauchi S, Yoshioka T, Kawato M (2003) Modular organization of internal models of tools in the human cerebellum. Proc Natl Acad Sci U S A 100:5461-5466

29. Ito M (2002) Historical review of the significance of the cerebellum and the role of Purkinje cells in motor learning. Ann N Y Acad Sci 978:273-288

30. Hebb DO (1949) The organization of behavior: A neuropsychological theory. Wiley, New York

31. Hughlings Jackson J (1889) On the comparative study of disease of the nervous system. Br Med J 2:355-362

32. Jeannerod M (1988) The neural and behavioral organization of goal-directed movements. Clarendon Press, Oxford

33. Kawato M, Furukawa K, Suzuki R (1987) A hierarchical neural-network model for control and learning of voluntary movement. Bio Cybern 57:169-185

34. Koechlin E, Ody C, Kouneiher F (2003) The architecture of cognitive control in the human prefrontal cortex. Science 302:1181-1185

35. Kuhn TS (1962) The structure of scientific revolutions. University of Chicago Press, Chicago

36. Latash ML (1996) The Bernstein problem: how does the central nervous system make its choices? In: Latash ML, Turvey MT (eds) Dexterity and its development. Lawrence Erlbaum, New Jersey, pp. 277-303

37. Latash M.L., Anson G. (1996) What are "normal movements" in atypical populations. Behav Brain Sci 19:55-106

38. Latash ML, Scholz JP, Schöner G (2007) Toward a new theory of motor synergies. Motor Control 11:276-308
    experience. MIT Press, Cambridge, MA

39. Leontiev AN (1972) (English translation 1981) The problem of activity in psychology. In: Wertsch J (ed) The concept of activity in soviet psychology (1981). Armonk, New York: M.E. Sharpe, Inc., pp. 37-71

40. Luria AR (1969) (French translation 1978) Les fonctions corticales supérieures de l'homme (1978). PUF, Paris

41. Maturana H, Varela F, (1980) Autopoiesis and cognition: the realization of the living. In: Cohen RS, Wartofsky MW (eds), vol. 42, Boston Studies in the Philosophy of Science. Reidel Publishing, Dordecht

42. Medvedeva TA (2008) Cybernetics and the Russian intellectual tradition. Conference Cybernetic Heritage in the Social and Human Sciences and Beyond, Centre for Baltic and East European Studies (CBEES). Södertörn University, Stockholm

43. Meijer OG, Bruijn SM (2007) The loyal dissident: N. A. Bernstein and the double-edged sword of Stalinism. J Hist Neurosci 16:206-224

44. Ostry DJ, Feldman AG (2003) A critical evaluation of the force control hypothesis in motor control. Exp Brain Res 153:275-288

45. Pavlov IP (1903) The experimental psychology and psychopathology of animals. 14th International Medical Congress in Madrid, Spain

46. Pavlov IP (1927) Conditioned reflexes: an investigation of the physiological activity of the cerebral cortex. http://psychclassics.yorku.ca/Pavlov/index.htm

47. Pavlov IP (1904) Autobiography/biography. In: Nobel lectures, physiology or medicine 1901-1921 (1967). Elsevier Publishing Company, Amsterdam. http://nobelprize.org/nobel_prizes/medicine/laureates/1904/pavlov-bio.html

48. Prablanc C, Desmurget M, Gréa H (2003) Neural control of on-line guidance of hand reaching movements. Prog Brain Res 142:155-170

49. Reed E, Bril B (1996) The primacy of action in development. A commentary of N. Bernstein. In: Latash ML, Turvey MT (eds) Dexterity and its development. Lawrence Erlbaum, New Jersey, pp. 431-451

50. Samoilov VO (2007) Ivan Petrovich Pavlov (1849-1936). J Hist Neurosci 16:74-89

51. Sargeant W (1957) Battle for the mind: A physiology of conversion and brain-washing. Malor Books, Cambridge, MA

52. Schmidt RA (2003) Motor schema theory after 27 years: reflections and implications for a new theory. Res Q Exerc Sport 74(4):366-75. Review

53. Scholz JP, Schöner G, Latash ML (2000) Identifying the control structure of multijoint coordination during pistol shooting. Exp Brain Res 135:382-404

54. Shadmehr R, Krakauer JW. (2008) A computational neuroanatomy for motor control. Exp Brain Res 185:359-381. Schmidt RA (1975) A schema theory of discrete motor skill learning. Psychol Rev 82:225-260

55. Sherwood DE, Lee TD (2003) Schema theory: critical review and implications for the role of cognition in a new theory of motor learning. Res Q Exerc Sport 74:376-382

56. Siksou M, (2008) Les psychologues de la Troïka et la notion de fonction. In: Parot F (ed) Les Fonctions en psychologie. Wavre, Mardaga, pp. 161-185

57. Smith GP (2000) Pavlov and integrative physiology. Am J Physiol Regul Integr Comp Physiol 279:743-755

58. Thelen E, Corbetta D, Kamm K, et al. (1993) The transition to reaching: mapping intention and intrinsic dynamics. Child Dev 64:1058-1098

59. Thelen E, Smith LB (1994) A dynamic systems approach to the development of cognition and action. A Bradford Book, MIT Press, Cambridge

60. Thorndike E (1932) The fundamentals of learning. Teachers College Press, New York

61. Todorov E (2004) Optimality principles in sensorimotor control. Nat Neurosci 7:907-915

62. Trogemann G, Nitussov AY, Ernst W (2001) Computing in Russia: the history of computer devices and information technology revealed. VIEVEG (Bertelsmann, Springer), Wiesbaden

63. Tseng Y, Scholz JP, Schöner G, Hotchkiss L (2003) Effect of accuracy constraint on joint coordination during pointing movements. Exp Brain Res 149:276-288

64. Varela F, Thompson E, Rosch E (1991) The embodied mind: cognitive science and human

65. Vygotski LS (1928) (French translation 1994) Textes choisis. In: Barisnikov K, Petitpierre G, (eds) Vygotski: Défectologie et déficience mentale. Delachaux et Niestlé, Neuchâtel, 258 pp

66. Vygotski LS (1934) (French translation 1997) Pensée et Langage, 1997. La Dispute, Paris

67. Wertsch JV (1979) The concept of activity in soviet psychology. An introduction. In: Wertsch J (ed) The concept of activity in soviet psychology. Sharpe, New York

68. Wiener N (1948) Cybernetics: Or the control and communication in the animal and the machine. Librairie Hermann & Cie, Paris, France

69. Windholz G (1992) Pavlov's conceptualization of learning. Am J Psychol 105(3):459-469

70. Wolpert DM, Miall RC, Kawato M (1998) Internal models in the cerebellum. Trends Cogn Sci 2:338-347

Introducing implicit learning: from the laboratory to the real life

E. Bigand and C. Delbé

Introduction

The dissociation between implicit and explicit cognition has a long history in psychology. As early as 1920, Clark Hull (25) investigated the learning of Chinese ideographs and identified the process of concept formation by abstraction of common elements, a process that occurs without explicit knowledge from the subjects of these regularities. Perceptual learning is another example of those processes that take place largely in the absence of awareness of the rules that govern the stimulations of the environment. Helmholtz (24) was one of the first to refer to *implicit inference* made by the perceptual system and to *perceptual learning*. Some years later, the distinction between implicit and explicit cognition contributed to mark the end of the behaviourism psychology. At this time, Tolman (74) reported an experiment that was difficult to account for in the framework of conditioning theories of Skinner (69). In this experiment, rats were put in a complex labyrinth and had to learn to get food at the exit. Not surprisingly, the rats receiving positive reinforcement learned faster than a control group of rats that never received food at the exit. The interesting new point of Tolman's study was to define a third group of rats, for which no food was available at the exit during the first part of the experiment. According to the behaviourist school, this group was not supposed to learn anything and was actually shown to behave exactly as the control group. In the second part of the experiment, this third group started to receive food at the exit. It was expected that learning would begin with this trial, and that rats of the third group would start improving their performance in the same way as rats of the first experimental. The new discovery of Tolman was that the performance of these rats increased much faster than those of the first experimental group. This difference led Tolman to conclude that the rats of the third group have implicitly learned the structure of the labyrinth during the first part of the study, and that this learning was externalized during the second part, when food was introduced at the exit. This implicit leaning account raised a lot of theoretical problems for the behaviourist school, since it assumed that some internal representations of the labyrinth was elaborated in the rats, a concept that was not compatible with the stimulus response theory of Skinner (69).

In the middle of the twentieth century, the concepts of learning without awareness and incidental learning became central for several psychologists. For example, Francès (19) was one of the first French psychologists to apply this concept to music perception and to argue that Western listeners, similarly to the rats in their labyrinth, had actually internalized the rules by which tones and chords are combined in Western music. In contrast with musicians, who received an explicit training in music, nonmusician listeners do not know the name of the musical organization and structures they have learned, but they have developed an implicit representation of these structures. As for Tolman's rats, this implicit knowledge may be evidenced by appropriate experiments. As was shown later, this implicit learning process reaches a surprising level of sophistication, such that it allows nonmusician listeners to respond to musical structures in a way that weakly differs from highly trained musicians (for a review, see 7).

Both examples illustrate a basic principle in cognitive psychology: "We know more than we can tell" (44). Other most striking examples of the dissociation between implicit and explicit cognition were then provided by neuropsychology. For example, amnesic patients of Schacter (67) were bad at explicit memory tests compared to matched control participants but performed as good as the control group when implicit memory tasks were used. Examples of this sort are numerous and may be found for a large variety of pathologies, such as unilateral spatial neglect, apraxia, and aphasia (32). For example, in a typical Stroop experiment, participants are required to give the name of the color of the ink of words appearing on a computer screen. When the word itself designates a color, interfering effect occurs in normal subject when the ink does not fit with the meaning of the road (e.g., red ink used to display the word "green"). In such a case, identifying the ink takes more time because the participant cannot avoid to read the word and to activate its meaning. This process occurs automatically in an implicit way in normal people. Interestingly, a Stroop effect can be replicated in aphasic patients (61). This suggests that implicit access to mental lexicon is preserved in aphasia.

Peretz, Gagnon, and Bouchard (47) reported a similar case with a brain damage patient, IR, who suffers from a severe loss of music recognition and expressive abilities, as first evidenced by Peretz, Belleville, and Fontaine (46). To illustrate her musical deficit, IR was unable to recognize very famous tunes such as "Happy Birthday," while it was easy to identify the tune on the basis of its words. When performing a same-different comparison task between two musical excerpts, she complained about the difficulty of the task and about its considerable cognitive load, even when the two musical excerpts corresponded to two different pieces of Mozart, for example. Obviously, IR was strictly unable to report subtle changes in musical structure, such as a change from major (c, d, e, f, g, a, b) to minor (c, r, eb, f, g, ab, b) mode. The interesting point is that such a change in mode is always experienced by normal listeners as a modulation of the emotional expressivity of music, with minor mode being more sad (15). The critical point of Peretz, Gagnon, and Bouchard' study (47) was to show that IR managed to differentiate major and minor versions of a given musical excerpt, without any difference with matched controls, only when she was simply asked to evaluate whether the music was sad or happy. Moreover, IR behaved as did match controls even when the duration of the excerpts was drastically reduced below 1 s. Finally, in a further experiment, Tillmann, Peretz, Bigand, and Gosselin (73) demonstrated that, using an implicit task (i.e., a so-called priming paradigm), IR managed to respond to very subtle changes in the musical function of chords, a finding that stands at the opposite of what we may have anticipated on the basis of her responses to the explicit test (73).

Examples of such dissociations between explicit and implicit cognition are numerous in neuropsychology (14). They are consistent with the conventional cognitive framework that rests on the existence of a powerful cognitive unconscious that stores, manipulates, and transforms representations in an implicit way, so doing by using algorithms that are incompatible with the constraints of the conscious thought. Although this model was recently questioned (50), it still remains dominant in current cognitive psychology and neurosciences. Explicit cognition is usually viewed as the external part of an iceberg, the largest immerged part defining implicit cognition. It was also argued that conscious though is a passive spectator of the job made by implicit cognition. As quoted by Baars (4), "a classic metaphor for consciousness has been a 'bright spot' cast by a spotlight in the stage of a dark theatre." The overall function of consciousness is to provide very widespread access to brain regions, implementing unconscious processes. Documenting the strength of implicit cognition, notably implicit learning, has a lot of implications for education and rehabilitation, both activities being essentially dominated by explicit training and explicit cognition. As will be seen in the present book (see Chapters 6, 7, and 10), implicit cognition offers new strategies for education and rehabilitation, without supplementing them. Of course, the purpose is not to promote a dichotomy between what Cleeremans and Jiménez (13) designates as Commander Data (all cognitive processes are explicit) and Zombies (all processes are implicit). Explicit representations are indispensable in a numerous situations. For example, we need explicit semantic knowledge about rules and facts of the external environment (Paris is the capital of France, 3 + 4 = 7, and so on). We also need explicit episodic memory ("I met him last Monday at the theater"). However, implicit cognition confers numerous advantages for interacting with the external environment. For example, procedural skills, such as driving or playing piano (for a professional performer), have to be internalized in an implicit way. Learning implicitly complex structures of the environment could also provide adaptive advantages for both healthy and abnormal subjects. In the present chapter, we will focus on the basic characteristics of these implicit learning processes by addressing the following three questions: what are the characteristics of implicit learning? In which situation do human learn implicitly? What is the nature of the knowledge acquired through implicit learning?

What are the characteristics of implicit learning?

Implicit learning refers to the fact that "abstract information about any stimulus in the environment may be acquired largely independently of the subjects' awareness of either the process of acquisition or the knowledge base ultimately acquired" (58, p. 16). As quoted by Reber, the discovery of implicit learning conflicted with the idea that humans are rational and logical, and make decisions on coherent patterns of reflection and analysis. Such an explicitly based rational behavior, which was metaphorically referred as Commander Data strategy by Cleeremans and Jiménez (13) contrasts with the fact that, in most situations, humans solve problems, reach conclusions, and appropriately behave without this conscious and rational process they were assumed to use. This second attitude, referred to as the "Zombie" strategy by Cleeremans and Jiménez (13), was shown to occur even with statisticians making decision that violates the Bayesian principles (which they were knowing explicitly) or physicians making inappropriate choice in a triage-type setting (26). The importance of implicit cognition in everyday life was also emphasized by social psychology. In situations where people appeared to act according to explicit and consciously developed inferences, they were in fact drawing on implicit knowledge systems (76). Lewicki and collaborators notably demonstrated how social behavior rests on statistical regularities between personality traits and external features (such as the length or the type of hair) that are internalized implicitly (35). In one famous study (36), psychology students were presented with pictures of several workers of a clinical institution, pictures that they were supposed to work with during several days. Personality traits were artificially paired with external body features (e.g., the length of the hair); for example, people with long hair were said to have some specific personality traits (e.g., perseverance) and people with short hairs another trait (e.g., helpfulness). For another group, this pairing was reversed. It was assumed that psychology students would implicitly internalize these associations during the presentation of these pictures, and that this implicit knowledge would then influence their response to a subsequent test involving pictures already presented as well as new workers. The data confirmed that students tended to responded according to this implicit knowledge. The previous examples already quoted, going from perceptual learning to social psychology, illustrated one of the first characteristics of implicit learning processes: their *generality*.

A second characteristic of implicit learning is its *automaticity*. In order to illustrate this point, let us consider the numbers presented in **Table 1**. Look carefully to the numbers of the leftmost column and then look those of both right columns. If you were asked to indicate which of these two right columns fits best with the left one, you would probably choose the columns opening with the number 38,247. If this was actually the case, you will encounter huge difficulties to explain why. Moreover, once knowledge is implicitly acquired, it applies in an automatic and irrepressible way. Music cognition offers several examples of the automaticity of implicit processes. As already mentioned above, Western listeners implicitly internalized the regularities of Western music (72).

This implicit knowledge was shown to influence their perceptual expectancy about musical events in a very fast acting way (8). More importantly, this implicitly acquired musical knowledge was found to automatically influence the processing of linguistic information in sung music. That is to say, even when the experimental task recommended participants to explicitly process either phoneme information (9) or semantic information (54), without paying attention to music, the musical rules influenced their linguistic processing. This automaticity of implicit knowledge was observed for both musically untrained listeners and highly trained participants. This emphasizes that explicit training cannot influence the activation of this implicit knowledge.

Table 1 - Which of the two right columns fits better with the left column?[1]

14,356	38,247	69,245
63,498	12,538	17,529
91,243	72,301	56,140
35,042	64,823	42,185

Neuropsychological studies have evidenced one of the most compelling aspects of implicit learning: its *robustness*. Implicit learning is preserved in neurological and psychological injuries that otherwise compromise conscious explicit though. Korsakoff (29) and Clarapède (12) provided the first striking demonstrations of preserved implicit memory in the absence of explicit memory. Claparède shook the hand of an amnesic patient with a pin inside the hand. The patient never explicitly reported a memory of this suffering experience; nevertheless, he refused Claparède's hand after this date. The robustness of implicit process is not only preserved in memory disorder (for a survey, see Chapter "Implicit learning and implicit memory in moderate to severe memory disorders") but was also observed with prosopagnosia, Parkinson disease (70), aphasia and dyslexia (77), brain-damaged amusia (46), and several other cognitive disorders. Implicit learning ability was also reported in case of personality disorders such as psychosis, chronic alcoholics, and depressive subjects (1). Implicit learning was also found to be less dependent of IQ than explicit learning. Standardized tests of intelligence, actually, mostly investigate explicit cognitive functions but not intelligent behaviors that rest on implicit cognition. Reber, Walkenfeld, and Hernstadt (59) correlated the performance of a group of participants differing by their IQ, in explicit and implicit learning tasks. A quite-high correlation was found between IQ and explicit performance ($r = .69$), and a low one with implicit performance ($r = .25$, *ns*). This suggests that intelligent behaviors could rest on implicit cognition, despite a low IQ. Finally, the robustness of implicit learning in healthy subject is also demonstrated by the long-living trace of information learned implicitly. Many implicit learning tasks show remarkable retention by subjects over weeks and even years, during which concomitant explicit knowledge has faded (53, 71).

---

1. The solution is given at the end of the present chapter.

A further interesting and related feature of implicit learning is that it is weakly affected by personality differences and moreover by *age differences*. Implicit learning of highly sophisticated information was notably observed in very young infants (20). Several studies by Saffran and collaborators remarkably illustrated this ability in the auditory learning domain (for a review, see 63). In these experiments, participants were presented with a synthesized speech stream generated by concatenating six multisyllabic nonsense words (e.g., "bupada") in a random order. The only cue that makes learning the artificial words possible was a statistical one: the transitional probabilities relating the syllables were higher for those occurring inside a word compared to those occurring at the border of words. Few minutes of exposure to these stimuli suffices for eight-month-old infants, first-grade children, and adults (3, 65) to be able to differentiate words from nonwords, even when both latter groups were not encouraged to pay attention to the speech stream (66). Moreover, it is worth noting that the same learning abilities have been observed for nonhuman primates (23). Overall, this emphasizes the robustness of the learning process involved and suggests that this process is unlikely to occur at an explicit level of consciousness (but see 50 for a debate). Recent studies extended this finding to visual (27) and nonverbal auditory stimuli (64), suggesting that implicit learning may occur for a large variety of stimulations, such as artistic ones. Finally, other researchers have investigated the influence of age on both explicit and implicit learning (for a review, see 40).

In sum, implicit learning differs from explicit learning, along several features of interest: this is a phenomenon of considerable generality that occurs automatically, that resists to cognitive and neurophysiologic injuries, that is weakly affected by personality differences and disorders, and that may occurs with a similar efficiency between people of different ages. These features underline the adaptive advantage of implicit learning and raise the question of its evolutionary origin. Although evolutionary psychology remains a rather new issue (for an introductory approach, see 75), the adaptive function of implicit learning was addressed as early as 1976 by Rozin (62). Cognitive abilities are supposed to be organized in different encapsulated modules, each of which had evolved its own restricted programs for its particular functions (see 18 and 52). Over evolutionary time, the modular units become more and more accessible to each other, resulting ultimately in the emergence of consciousness. Reber (58) suggested a similar evolution for implicit learning mechanisms. Implicit learning is likely to have occurred prior to explicit learning though in phylogenesis. The primacy of implicit learning in phylogenesis is related to its robustness. According to Jackson's principle (see 17), the degree of resistance of a mental function to disease or natural deterioration is directly related to the evolutionary antiquity of that function in the species. Recently evolved functions are lost first, and those of greater evolutionary ages are lost later. A similar evolution is recapitulated in ontogenesis. Implicit learning occurs before explicit learning in infants, and the former is shown to resist more to aging than the latter. The main adaptive advantage of implicit learning would be to allow humans to learn the highly complex structure of their environment, an issue that could not be addressed by explicit though only.

Implicit learning strategies are typically supposed to occur as soon as our explicit learning, though, is overloaded by the numerous interrelationships that should be taken into account to solve a given problem. Learning a foreign language was sometimes taken as an example of such a too complex structure. Although one explicit strategy, developed in schools, consists in learning explicitly all the rules of the grammar of the language, another efficient strategy consists in traveling to the foreign country in order to be intensively exposed to its language.

In which situation do humans learn implicitly?

Implicit learning in the laboratory

Implicit learning may be addressed in experimental settings, with artificial stimuli that mimic the complexity of the natural environment. Of course, the complexity of these stimuli is reduced compared to the real life, but the time to learn this complexity is also considered shortened in the used experimental settings. As such, we can consider that experimental psychology reproduced in miniature the implicit learning processes that occur during life in the natural environment. A large set of experimental settings have been used to investigate implicit learning abilities. The most famous procedure will be presented here.

One of the most common paradigms in this field involves the learning of an **artificial finite-state grammar** (55, 57, 58; see **Fig. 1**, *left*). During an initial phase, subjects have to memorize sequences of letters that conform to the rules of the grammar. During a second phase, the subjects are asked to judge the grammaticality of new sequences of letters, half of which are nongrammatical (**Fig. 1**, *right*). Participants usually perform better than chance, with accuracy varying between 60% and 80%, yet they are slightly successful in describing the rules used to generate the letters. According to Reber (55, 57), these participants have acquired an implicit knowledge of the abstract rules of the grammar.

Another famous procedure is the serial reaction time (SRT) task (45), in which a target appears in different locations on a screen and, for each presentation, participants are required to press a button on the keyboard corresponding to the position of the target as quickly as possible. The participants are not informed that a specific sequence of locations is repeated. Over time, participants respond faster, indicating simple practice effects. However, when a random pattern is suddenly presented instead of the old one, reaction times increase, thus demonstrating that participants learned the sequence despite little conscious access to this knowledge. This leads to the typical pattern of learning curve shown **Fig. 2**.

Other procedures tap into different cognitive processes. For example, in a dynamic control task, participants interact with a simulated system, e.g., a sugar production factory (5). On each trial, they are required to vary the number of workers to try to main-

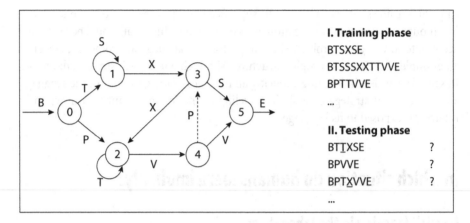

Fig. 1 - Example of a finite-state grammar (*left*), which generates letter sequences such as those shown on the right. In the first (training) phase of an artificial grammar learning (AGL) experiment, participants study some of these grammatical sequences. Then, in a subsequent testing phase, they are required to judge the grammaticality of new sequences, which can be either grammatical (e.g., BPVVE) or non-grammatical (e.g., BTTXSE, where T cannot be repeated at this position).

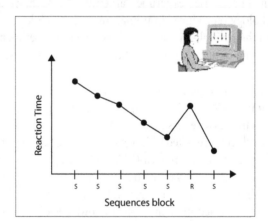

Fig. 2 - A typical learning curve in a serial reaction time (SRT) task, in which participants are required to press a button on the keyboard corresponding to the position of a target appearing on a computer screen as quickly as possible (*insert*). During the first few exposure to a given standard sequence of locations, reaction times decrease, indicating a simple practice effect. However, after a few trials, if a random sequence occurred, reaction times drastically increase, which indicates learning of the standard sequence (S = sequence, R = random).

tain the level of sugar production at a target value. The critical point is that the underlying equation linking current sugar production to the number of workers and past sugar production is unknown to the participants. The authors reported that participants trained on this task improved their ability to control the system, but not the ability to answer questions about how the system worked. Moreover, when they were asked to attempt to consciously extract the rule, learning was impaired.

Implicit learning was also observed for motoric task. Pew (51) was the first to use a pursuit visuomotor tracking task to demonstrate that complex motor learning could also occur without awareness. In this study, participants had to track with a joystick a cursor appearing on the screen of an oscilloscope. Each trial began and ended with a random trajectory of the cursor, whereas the middle trajectory was repeated among trials. This regularity was, of course, unknown to the subjects. Here again, practice effects were observed after 14 days of trial, as well as a learning effect of the specific motor sequence; importantly, participants were unable to articulate their newly acquired knowledge. Implicit learning of a wide range of such motor skills was replicated with similar tasks (37, 79). For example, in the study of Shea, Wulf, and Whitacre (68), participants stood on a stabilometer and had to move their bodies so that the plateform of the stabilometer fitted with the movements of a line presented in front of them on a computer screen. The authors showed that the participants were able to learn the regularities of the target movement.

Learning contemporary musical grammar: an example of real life implicit learning

Music is an interesting medium to investigate implicit learning processes for several reasons. It is a highly elaborated structure of our environment that is too complex to be apprehended through explicit thought and deductive reasoning. The psychological effect of musical sounds comes from the complex multilevel relationships they pertain in a given piece (34, 42). The abstract associative and architectonic relations that pertain between events that are not necessarily close in time define the relevant structures in music. These relations are difficult to articulate in an explicit way. Despite a considerable tradition in music history, as well as in contemporary music theory, to formalize the relevant structure of Western music (see 33, 34, 43), none of these frameworks provides a complete and satisfactory account of the Western tonal musical grammar. A further interesting feature of music for research on implicit learning is that musical structures are not conceived for explicit processing. It is even important for composers that listeners are sensitive to the structures that underlie a musical piece while still being unaware of them. In fact, the most common feeling among a general audience is of being unable to describe verbally what they perceive. In some instances, people are even convinced that they do not perceive any underlying structure. The fact that musical events do not refer to any specific object in the external world probably contributes to the difficulty of apprehending musical structures in an explicit way.

A final interesting feature is that musical systems constantly evolve toward new musical grammars. Being faced with masterpieces that derive from an entirely new musical system is not an artificial situation for contemporary listeners, and this raises a challenging issue for implicit learning theories. The considerable and persistent confusion reported by listeners to contemporary music suggests that some musical grammars may be too artificial to be internalized through passive exposure (38). To the best of our knowledge, very few researches have directly addressed implicit learning with musical material (6, 16, 30, 31). Much research in music cognition, however, indirectly deals with implicit learning processes by showing that explicit learning is not necessary for the development of sensitivity to the underlying rules of Western music[2] (for a review, see 7). This implicit learning is mostly influenced by the statistical regularities found in the temporal organization of musical events. A self-organizing connectionist model simulates this learning through the progressive adaptation of the weights of connections between the three key elements of the Western musical grammar: notes, chords, and keys (24). To a certain extent, these studies of musical cognition, undertaken in a natural environment with Western tonal music, confirm the current conclusions of studies of implicit learning using artificial material in the laboratory.

Only a few studies have addressed the implicit learning of new musical systems. Most of them have focused on the learning of serial music, a system that has evolved in the West at the beginning of the twentieth century. During this period, the tonal musical system gradually waned and was overtaken by serial systems of composition developed by the so-called Second School of Vienna, and in particular by Arnold Schoenberg (22). Serial works of music obey compositional rules that differ considerably from those that govern tonal music. A serial musical piece is based on a specific temporal ordering of the 12 tones of the chromatic scale (i.e., the tones c, c#, d, d#, e, f, f#, g, g#, a, a#, and b), irrespective of their octave placement.[3] The specific ordering of these tones defines the tone row of the piece. Each tone of the row must be played before a given tone occurs for the second time. For example, if the piece is based on the following tone row g-b-b*b*-c#-a-c-d#-d-f#-f-g#-e, the g# note must not be repeated before all the other notes have been sounded, irrespective of the octave placement. The serial musical system defines several types of transformations that can be applied to the tone row. First, the tone row can be transposed to each of the 12 tones it contains. For example, the following set of tones b-d#-d-f-c#-e-g-f#-b*b*-a-c-g# is a simple transposition of the previous set row, starting on b. The second transformation in serial music consists in playing the row in retrograde. For example, the set of tones e-g#-f-f#-d-d#-c-a-c#-b*b*-b-g is a retrograde form of our example row. Third, a tone row can be transformed by inversion. That is, a given interval[4] in the row (say an ascending major third g-b) can be transformed into a descending major third (g-e*b*). The inverse transformation of the example tone row is g-e*b*-e-c#-f-d-b-c-g#-a-f#-b*b*. Fourth, a tone row can be inversed

---

2. The tonal system designates the most usual style of music in the West, including baroque (e.g., Bach), classic (e.g., Mozart), and romantic (e.g., Chopin) styles, as well as folk music such as pop music, jazz, and Latin music.

3. The 12 tones of the chromatic scale are repeated at different pitch heights, spaced by the interval called an octave. A lower C and a higher C both belong to the same pitch class C. Listeners perceive tones of the same pitch class as perceptually equivalent.

and played in retrograde, resulting in a retrograde inversion of the original row. In this case, the retrograde inversion of our example is Bb-f#-a-g#-c-b-d-f-c#-e-eb-g.

Each serial composition results from a complex combination of all of these transformations that are applied to a specific tone row. Schoenberg argued that these manipulations would produce an interesting balance between perceptual variety and unity. Several experimental studies have addressed the psychological reality of the organization resulting from the serial musical grammar with explicit tasks. Most of the researchers suggest that the serial rules are *not* perceptible and not even learnable by musical experts (16, 19). Using an implicit task derived from Reber's study led to a quite opposite finding. In our study, participants were first required to listen to musical pieces derived from a 12-tone row. In this familiarization phase, they were asked to detect pieces that occurred twice. Their performance resulted in a memory score. In a testing phase, participants were then presented with pairs of new musical pieces. In each pair, one piece obeyed the previously learned row while the other piece (the foil) obeyed another row. In each pair, the two pieces were matched according to all surface features such as rhythm, pitch range, and melodic contour (**Fig. 1**, *bottom*). Accordingly, the two pieces of each pair sounded very similar. Participants were asked to identify which piece followed the same compositional rules as the pieces previously heard in the learning phase. Their responses resulted in a grammatical score. The musical stimuli were written by a composer who was encouraged to define musical pieces of aesthetic quality and interest, and that exhibited the complex rhythm and broken melodic contours, which are typical of serial music. Three experiments demonstrated that participants actually acquired some knowledge during the hearing of serial pieces. This knowledge enabled them to differentiate at a level above chance those that violate the basic rules of the learned tone row. The present finding also sheds light on the implicit versus explicit nature of the acquired knowledge, and the content of the information internalized through hearing the pieces. The outcome has several implications for research on implicit learning as well as for music cognition and composition. This finding is consistent with other researches involving the implicit learning of new musical grammars (6) and with research done on the implicit learning of Western tonal music.

What is the nature of the knowledge acquired through implicit learning?

Three main models have been distinguished (40) that can account for the performance of participants in AGL tasks. The **abstractionist** view defended by Reber (55, 57, 58)

---

4. A pitch interval designates the separation in frequency between two tones. In Western music theory, these frequency separations are represented by the number of semitones that separate the tones. A minor second represents one semitone; a major second, two semitones; a minor third, three semitones; a major third, four semitones; and so on.

proposes that implicit learning rests on unconscious mechanisms of rules abstraction, triggered when we are exposed to complex stimulations (such as the sequences produced from an artificial grammar), the complexity of which avoids the discovery and the use of simple explicit rules. Evidence in favor of Reber's abstractionist position mostly comes from transfer experiments (20, 21, 56). It has been observed that, in an AGL paradigm, the structure learned for a given alphabet can be transferred to another alphabet that was not previously presented to participants (56). This transfer of knowledge can also occur between different sensory modalities (2). Overall, this highlights the abstract nature of the internalized knowledge. However, the very content of this abstract knowledge is contentious. A strict abstractionist view posits that the rules of the finite state grammar are mentally represented, but this position has been challenged by simpler accounts (11, 28, 50, 60).

A radically different account of Reber's claims for the implicit abstraction of structure in AGL tasks was first provided by Brooks (10), who offered an early memory-for-instances model of learning. In its weaker form (11), this **exemplar** approach posits that participants do not infer abstract representations from the stimuli, but they memorise specific exemplars in episodic memory during the learning phase. In the subsequent test phase, participants would then judge the *similarity* of new items with the stored ones, instead of judging the abstract grammaticality of the sequences. Numerous studies manipulated conjointly the grammaticality and the similarity of test items with the learned sequences, and showed that participants' responses were influenced by both factors, supporting both abstract and exemplar hypotheses (39, 41, 78). Knowlton and Squire (28) suggested that similarity and grammaticality compete with each another such that the similarity strategy tends to override the use of grammaticality when both cues are present in the test items.

Originally concerned with methodological issues observed in AGL tasks by Perruchet (48), the **fragmentarist** model posits that participants learn some local structures that are salient in the stimuli, instead of whole sequences. For example, test sequences that contain bigrams and trigrams (two- and three-letter chunks) that appeared frequently in the training exemplars are more likely to be endorsed as grammatical as test items that do not contain frequently chunks, as shown by Perruchet and Pacteau (49). Thus, sensitivity to the frequency of occurence of these local structures could allow participants to discriminate between grammatical and nongrammatical items in the absence of abstract knowledge of the rules. It is worth noting that this approach cannot account for the transfer effects observed in AGL tasks.

In sum, none of these three models is exclusive. Different mechanisms could be involved in different experimental situations, and it is likely that all may contribute to learning in real life (11, 28, 39).

Conclusion

In the present chapter, implicit leaning processes were illustrated in a large variety of situations for a large variety of participants. Humans manage to internalize the statistical regularities that govern their environment through exposure to complex stimuli. This implicit knowledge is transferable to other types of stimulations, a fact which opens several possibilities for reeducation strategies, as developed in Chapters 7 and 10. *Response p. 99: column 2.*

References

1. Abrams M, Reber AS (1988) Implicit learning: robustness in the face of psychiatric disorders. J Psycholinguist Res 17:425-439
2. Altmann G, Dienes Z, Goode A (1995) On the modality independence of implicitly learned grammatical knowledge. J Exp Psychol Learn Mem Cogn 21:899-912
3. Aslin RN, Saffran JR, Newport EL (1998) Computation of conditional probability statistics by human infants. Psychol Sci 9:321-324
4. Baars BJ (1998) Metaphors of consciousness and attention in the brain. Trends Neurosci 21(2):58-62
5. Berry DC, Broadbent DE (1984) On the relationship between task performance and associated verbalisable knowledge. Q J Exp Psychol 36:209-231
6. Bigand E, Perruchet P, Boyer M (1998) Implicit learning of artificial grammar of musical timbres. Curr Psychol Cogn 17:577-600
7. Bigand E, Poulin-Charronnat B (2006) Are we "experienced listeners"? A review of the musical capacities that do not depend on formal musical training. Cognition 100(1):100-130
8. Bigand E, Poulin-Charronnat B, Tillmann B, et al. (2003) Sensory versus cognitive components in harmonic priming. J Exp Psychol Hum Percept Perform 29:159-171
9. Bigand E, Tillmann B, Poulin-Charronnat B, et al. (2001) The effect of harmonic context on phoneme monitoring in vocal music. Cognition 81(1):11-20
10. Brooks LR (1978) Non-analytic concept formation and memory for instances. In: Rosch E, Lloyd B (eds) Cognition and concepts, pp. 169-211. Erlbaum, Hillsdale, NJ
11. Brooks LR, Vokey JR (1991) Abstract analogies and abstracted grammars: a comment on Reber, and Mathews et al. J Exp Psychol Gen 120:316-323
12. Clarapède E (1911) Récognition et moiité. Archives de Psychologie 11:79-90
13. Cleeremans A, Jiménez L (2002) Implicit learning and consciousness: a graded, dynamic perspective. In: French RM, Cleeremans A (eds) Implicit learning and consciousness: An empirical, computational and philosophical consensus in the making. Psychology Press, Hove, UK
14. Cohen NJ, Squire LR (1980) Preserved learning and retention of pattern-analyzing skill in amnesia: dissociation of knowing how and knowing that. Science 210:207-210
15. Dalla Bella S, Peretz I, Rousseau L, Gosselin N (2001) A developmental study of the affective value of tempo and mode in music. Cognition 80(3):B1-B10

16. Dienes Z, Longuet-Higgins HC (2004) Can musical transformations be implicitly learned? Cogn Sci 28:531-558

17. Ey H (1975) Des idées de Jackson à un modèle organo-dynamique en psychiatrie. Privat, Toulouse

18. Fodor J (1983) The modularity of mind: an essay on faculty psychology. MIT Press, Cambridge, MA

19. Francès R (1958) La perception de la musique. Vrin, Paris

20. Gomez RL, Gerken L (1999) Artificial grammar learning by 1-year-olds leads to specific and abstract knowledge. Cognition 70:109-135

21. Gomez RL, Gerken L, Schvaneveldt R (2000) The basis of transfer in artificial grammar learning. Mem Cognit 28:253-263

22. Griffiths P (1978) Histoire concise de la musique moderne. Fayard, Paris

23. Hauser MD, Newport EL, Aslin RN (2001) Segmentation of the speech stream in a non-human primate: statistical learning in cotton-top tamarins. Cognition 78:B41-B52

24. Helmholtz H (1867) Handbuch der physiologischen Optik. Leopold Voss, Leipzig

25. Hull CL (1920) Quantitative aspects of the evolution of concepts. Psychol Monogr 28(1)-85 pp

26. Kahneman D, Tversky A (1982) On the study of statistical intuitions. Cognition 11(2):123-141

27. Kirkham NZ, Slemmer JA, Johnson SP (2002) Visual statistical learning in infancy: evidence for a domain general learning mechanism. Cognition 83(2):35-42

28. Knowlton BJ, Squire LR (1996) Artificial grammar depends on implicit acquisition of both abstract and exemplar-specific information. J Exp Psychol Learn Mem Cogn 22:169-181

29. Korsakoff S (1889) Etude médico-psychologique sur une forme des maladies de la mémoire. Revue Philosophique de la France et de l'Etranger 28:501-530

30. Kuhn G, Dienes Z (2005) Implicit learning of nonlocal musical rules: implicitly learning more than chunks. J Exp Psychol Learn Mem Cogn 31(6):1417-1432

31. Kuhn G, Dienes Z (2008) Learning non-local dependencies. Cognition 106:184-206

32. Leiguarda RC, Marsden CD (2000) Limb apraxias: higher-order disorders of sensorimotor integration. Brain 123:860-879

33. Lerdahl F (2001) Tonal Pitch Space. Oxford University Press, Oxford

34. Lerdahl F, Jackendoff R (1983) A generative theory of tonal music. MIT Press, Cambridge, MA

35. Lewicki P, Hill T (1987) Unconscious processes as explanations of behavior in cognitive, personality, and social psychology. Pers Soc Psychol Bull 13:355-362

36. Lewicki P, Hill T, Bizot E (1988) Acquisition of procedural knowledge about a pattern of stimuli that cannot be articulated. Cogn Psychol 20:24-37

37. Magill RA, Hall KG (1989) Implicit learning in a complex tracking skill. Paper presented at the 30th Annual Meeting of the Psychonomic Society, Atlanta

38. McAdams S (1989) Contraintes psychologiques sur les dimensions porteuses de forme en musique. In: McAdams S, Deliège I (eds) La musique et les sciences cognitives, pp. 257-284. Mardaga, Bruxelles

39. McAndrews MP, Moscovitch M (1985) Rule-based and exemplar-based classification in artificial grammar learning. Mem Cognit 13(5):469-475

40. Meulemans T (1998) L'apprentissage implicite: Une approche cognitive, neuropsychologique et développementale. Solal, Marseille
41. Meulemans T, Van der Linden M (1997) Associative Chunk Strength in Artificial Grammar Learning. J Exp Psychol Learn Mem Cogn 23(4):1007-1028
42. Meyer LB (1956) Emotion and Meaning in Music. Chicago University Press, Chicago
43. Narmour E (1990) The analysis and cognition of basic melodic structures: the implication-realization model. University of Chicago Press, Chicago
44. Nisbett R, Wilson T (1977) Telling more than we can know: verbal reports on mental processes. Psychol Rev 84:231-259
45. Nissen MJ, Bullemer P (1987) Attentional requirements of learning: evidence from performance measures. Cogn Psychol 19:1-32
46. Peretz I, Belleville S, Fontaine F (1997) Dissociation entre musique et langage après atteinte cérébrale: un nouveau cas d'amusie sans aphasie. Revue Canadienne de Psychologie Expérimentale 51:354-367
47. Peretz I, Gagnon L, Bouchard B (1998) Music and emotion: perceptual determinants, immediacy, and isolation after brain damage. Cognition 68:111-141
48. Perruchet P (1994) Defining the knowledge units of a synthetic language: comment on Vokey and Brooks (1992) J Exp Psychol Learn Mem Cogn 20:223-228
49. Perruchet P, Pacteau C (1990) Synthetic grammar learning: implicit rule abstraction or explicit fragmentary knowledge? J Exp Psychol Gen 119:264-275
50. Perruchet P, Vinter A (2002) The self-organizing consciousness. Behav Brain Sci 25(3):297-330
51. Pew RW (1974) Levels of analysis in motor control. Brain Res 71:393-400
52. Pinker S (1997) How the Mind Works. Norton, New York
53. Posner MI, Keele SW (1970) Retention of abstract ideas. J Exp Psychol Gen 83:304-308
54. Poulin-Charronnat B, Bigand E, Madurell F, Peereman R (2005) Musical structure modulates semantic priming in vocal music. Cognition 94:67-78
55. Reber AS (1967) Implicit learning of artificial grammars. J Verb Learn Verb Behav 6:855-863
56. Reber AS (1969) Transfer of syntactic structure in synthetic languages. J Exp Psychol Gen 81:115-119
57. Reber AS (1989) Implicit learning and tacit knowledge. J Exp Psychol Gen 118:219-235
58. Reber AS (1992) The cognitive unconscious: an evolutionary perspective. Conscious Cogn 1:93-133
59. Reber AS, Walkenfeld FF, Hernstadt R (1991) Implicit and explicit learning: individual differences and IQ. J Exp Psychol Learn Mem Cogn 17:888-896
60. Redington M, Chater N (1996) Transfer in artificial grammar learning: a reevaluation. J Exp Psychol Gen 125:123-138
61. Revonsuo A (1995) Words interact with colors in a globally aphasic patient: evidence from a Stroop-like task. Cortex 31(2):377-386
62. Rozin P (1976) The selection of food by rats, humans and other animals. In: Hinde RA, Beer C, Shaw E (eds) Advances in the Study of Animal Behavior, vol. 6, pp. 22-76. Academic Press, New York
63. Saffran JR (2003) Statistical language learning: mechanisms and constraints. Curr Dir Psychol Sci 12:110-114

64. Saffran JR, Johnson EK, Aslin RN, Newport EL (1999) Statistical learning of tone sequences by human infants and adults. Cognition 70:27-52
65. Saffran JR, Newport EL, Aslin RN (1996) Word segmentation: the role of distributional cues. J Mem Lang 35:606-621
66. Saffran JR, Newport EL, Aslin RN, et al. (1997) Incidental language learning: listening (and learning) out of the corner of your ear. Psychol Sci 8:101-105
67. Schacter DL (1987) Implicit memory: history and current status. J Exp Psychol Learn Mem Cogn 13:501-518
68. Shea CH, Wulf G, Whitacre CA (2001) Surfing the implicit wave. Q J Exp Psychol 54(3):841-862
69. Skinner BF (1938) The behavior of organisms. Appleton-Century-Crofts, New York
70. Smith JG, Siegert RJ, McDowall J (2001) Preserved implicit learning on both the serial reaction time task and artificial grammar in patients with Parkinson's disease. Brain Cogn 45:378-391
71. Squire LR, Frambach M (1990) Cognitive skill learning in amnesia. Psychobiology 18:109-117
72. Tillmann B, Bharucha JJ, Bigand E (2000) Implicit learning of tonality: a self-organizing approach. Psychol Rev 107:885-913

73. Tillmann B, Peretz I, Bigand E, Gosselin N (2007) Harmonic priming in an amusic patient: the power of implicit tasks. Cogn Neuropsychol 24(6):603-622
74. Tolman EC (1948) Cognitive maps in rats and men. Psychol Rev 55:189-208
75. Tooby J, Cosmides L (2005) Evolutionary psychology: conceptual foundations. In: Buss DM (ed) Evolutionary Psychology Handbook. Wiley, New York
76. Ulman JS, Bargh JA (1989) Unintended Thought. The Guildford Press, New York
77. Vicari S, Marotta L, Menghini D, et al. (2003) Implicit learning deficit in children with developmental dyslexia. Neuropsychologia 41(1):108-114
78. Vokey JR, Brooks LR (1992) Salience of item knowledge in learning artificial grammars. J Exp Psychol Learn Mem Cogn 18:328-344
79. Wulf G, Schmidt RA (1997) Variability of practice and implicit motor learning. J Exp Psychol Learn Mem Cogn 23:987-1006

Implicit learning, development, and education

A. Vinter, S. Pacton, A. Witt and P. Perruchet

Introduction

The present chapter focuses on implicit learning processes, and aims at showing that these processes could be used to design new methods of education or reeducation. After a brief definition of what we intend by implicit learning, we will show that these processes operate efficiently in development, from infancy to aging. Then, we will discuss the question of their resistance to neurological or psychiatric diseases. Finally, in a last section, we will comment on their potential use within an applied perspective.

The fundamental role of learning, once neglected by cognitive psychologists a few decades ago, is now acknowledged in most areas of research, including language, categorization and object perception (2). Of course, nobody has ever claimed that language development is independent of infants' experience. However, the dominant Chomskian tradition has confined learning to subsidiary functions, such as setting the values of parameters in a hardwired system. Recent work shows that fundamental components of language such as word segmentation (69) can be learned in an incidental way similar to that involved in the acquisition of other human abilities. Likewise, it has never been denied that learning plays a role in categorization and object perception, but acquisition processes were thought to be limited to new combinations of preestablished features (7). However, Schyns and Rodet (77) have shown that elementary features can themselves be created with experience (for a review, see 74, 75).

The type of learning process that receives the most attention in the current literature relates to implicit learning. Different definitions of implicit learning have been proposed (63, 4), most of which involving the idea that implicit learning contributes to the formation of an implicit knowledge base, dissociated from explicit knowledge (see 76, for a review subscribing to this view). We propose a definition that is neutral with regard to the issue of the nature of the resulting knowledge. In our view, implicit learning covers all forms of unintentional learning in which, as a consequence of repeated experience, an individual's behavior becomes sensitive to the structural features of an experienced situation, without, at any time, being told to learn anything about this situation and without the adaptation being due to an intentional exploitation of some pieces of explicit knowledge about these features (58). Although there is little consensus within the literature, these two components – the behavioral sensitivity to the structure of the situation and the lack of intentional causes for this sensitivity – have been included in virtually all definitions of implicit learning (11, 65).

Many contributors to this area have added additional criteria. For instance, several researchers emphasize the point that explicit knowledge about the training situation is lacking or at least limited. Including this property in the implicit learning concept is obviously possible, insofar as terminology issues are arbitrary, but, as a matter of fact, doing so may well make the very existence of the phenomenon controversial (73). The exclusive reliance on a lack of intentional exploitation of explicit knowledge, on the other hand, makes the existence of the phenomenon "real" at the phenomenological, introspective level, and it is confirmed by a large number of experimental investigations. In our view, this type of learning is based on the action of unconscious processes, basically associative learning processes that progressively transform the individual's behavior, without noticing this transformation (59, 60).

Most of the studies in implicit learning area of research are laboratory studies run with adults. A prototypical paradigm in implicit learning is the artificial grammar paradigm (62). In this paradigm, participants are usually exposed to a subset of grammatical strings generated by a finite-state grammar, where the strings can be composed of printed consonants for instance. The grammar defines the transition rules between events. Participants are then tested to see whether they can discriminate between new grammatical and non-grammatical strings. The results show that participants recognize grammatical strings at a significantly above-chance level, as if they had discovered the rules of the grammar. We suggest that, through the action of unconscious processes, the participants develop, in the course of the training phase, a behavioral sensitivity to the structure of the situation so that they become "familiar" to the "look" of the grammatical strings, whether these strings have been specifically seen during training or not (new grammatical strings). This feeling of familiarity does not require possessing any knowledge about the genuine structure of the strings. Implicit learning shapes the perceptions a participant develops of a situation through the direct and continuous tuning of the processes devoted to the treatment of incoming information. These processes provoke changes in the way information is encoded, and these changes directly affect the participant's phenomenal experience (61, 59). We will turn to this interpretation later in the chapter.

Implicit learning processes in development

Examining the characteristics of the experimental situation usually involved in this field of research helps to understand why implicit learning is, a priori, relevant for development. First, implicit learning is generally observed while participants are not asked to discover the structure of the situation they are confronted to. Instead, participants are generally instructed to engage in any activity ensuring attentional processing of the training display but diverting them from tacking an analytical approach. Second, only well-structured patterns are displayed. For instance, in the artificial grammar paradigm, only positive instances of the material to be learned (i.e., only grammatical strings) are shown to the participants during training. As we will discuss later, this characteristic is a prerequisite for incidental conditions of learning because showing errors or negative instances of a rule, for instance, may well cause a shift within the learner toward adopting a problem-solving attitudinal set and/or may cause interferences that are detrimental to learning. The third characteristic of implicit learning situations is their relative complexity. It has been shown that participants are able to learn implicitly highly complex material that they would not be able to easily learn explicitly. Thus, on the whole, the implicit learning conditions are close to most real-life situations encountered by children or adults during their life. Implicit learning processes are indeed thought to be fundamental throughout life, supporting continuous behavioral adaptation to changing environmental conditions (65, 34).

Clearly, a large proportion of the motor, perceptive, and cognitive acquisitions made by children in the course of development result from learning, and more specifically from implicit learning processes. Implicit learning has been seen as responsible for at least some aspects of first-language (9) and second-language learning (8), category elaboration, reading and writing acquisition (56), adaptation to the physical constraints of the world (41), and acquisition of social skills (65). Most of this learning takes place during infancy and childhood, and constitutes the essential core of what a newborn must acquire to become an adult. This is why the idea of the primacy of implicit learning processes, initially claimed by Reber (65), has been by and large tacitly adopted by most authors working in the implicit learning domain. However, clearly, implicit learning processes do not operate only during infancy or childhood but are responsible for the continuous behavioral adaptation of humans during their entire life, as we will show it.

Developmental psychologists also consider that implicit learning processes play an important role in development. Karmiloff-Smith's model (38) postulates that the first phase achieved in each domain of competence corresponds to a level of behavioral mastery involving implicit knowledge, formed by data-driven processes. Explicit knowledge would be developed during a second phase through the action of an endogenous process of representational redescription. The distinction between implicit and explicit knowledge is present in several other developmental models (for a review, see 45) and appears to be basic to developmental studies of memory (36). Moreover, highlighting the fundamental role of bottom-up processes, as can be observed in the dynamical theories (82) or in connectionist modeling (16, 51), also attests to the major interest that developmental psychologists attribute to implicit learning processes in the formation of new adaptive behavior.

However, despite this role given to implicit learning processes, the developmental literature on this domain remains sparse. Moreover, nothing clear is known about the possible age-related specificity of implicit learning processes. Reber (65) has made the assumption that these processes are age independent, but the results of the current studies appear contradictory in this respect.

Implicit learning processes in infancy, childhood, and aging

Gomez and Gerken (24) used the classical paradigm in implicit learning of the artificial grammar paradigm (62), with infants aged approximately 12 months. To adapt this approach (see above) for use with infants, Gomez and Gerken's study used auditory syllables instead of printed letters. These syllables were combined according to the rules of an artificial grammar to form legal sequences that were repeated several times during training. Infants were tested with familiar or new legal sequences, and illegal sequences. The results showed that the infants displayed longer orientation times toward familiar or new legal strings than toward nongrammatical strings, suggesting that they became sensitive to at least some aspects of the structure of the training set. Note that this study not only demonstrates that the implicit learning of an artificial grammar is efficient at a very early age but also suggests that these learning processes are probably involved in language acquisition. A similar conclusion can be achieved from a study of incidental learning of word segmentation conducted by Saffran *et al.* (69). Saffran, Johnson, Aslin, and Newport (68) have shown that eight-month-old infants are able to use the same learning mechanisms to segment sequences of nonlinguistic stimuli. The efficiency of implicit learning processes early in development (four to five years) has also been revealed in two other studies, one performed by Lewicki (43) and one by Czyzewska *et al.* (1991), quoted in Lewicki, Hill, and Czyzewska (44). More recently, two-year-old children have been shown to be successful in learning implicitly a sequence of spatial locations (5).

With regard to older children, Meulemans, Van der Linden, and Perruchet (50) compared the performance of children aged 6 to 7 years and 10 to 11 years and adults in an implicit learning task. They used the classical serial reaction time task (53), where participants had to respond as quickly as possible to the appearance of a target at one of four locations on a screen by pressing one of four keys corresponding to the position of the target. Without them knowing it, participants were shown a repeating sequence of target appearances, with some intermixed random trials. Regardless of age, reaction times improved on the repeated sequence when compared to the random parts, thus demonstrating that six-year-old children learned the sequence as well as adults did. Moreover, children and adults improved their performance on the same parts of the sequence, a finding that gives additional support to the claim that implicit learning is age insensitive. A study performed by Roter (1985), quoted in Reber (65), also confirms this view. No age-related differences in an artificial grammar task were obtained in connection with implicit performance in children aged 6 to 7 years, 9 to 11 years, and 12 to 15 years.

However, contradictory results are provided by Maybery, Taylor, and O'Brien-Malone's study (47), which was directly inspired by Reber's assumptions (65) of age independence. These authors compared two groups of children, one aged 5 to 7 years and the other one aged 10 to 12 years. An incidental covariation task adapted from Lewicki (43) was used, where children had to learn a covariation between the location of a picture in a 4 ∞ 4 matrix and two other features, the side from which the experimenter approached them and the color of the matrix board and cover. After training, 10- to 12-year-old children were better at guessing the location of the pictures in a subsequent test phase than were 5- to 7-year-olds. Moreover, the performance displayed by the younger children was not above chance, indicating that these children did not implicitly learn the covariations. A few age-related differences are also reported in a serial time reaction task in children and adolescents under incidental learning condition, although these differences were much higher and systematic under explicit learning condition (37).

To sum up, the literature reports contradictory results with regard to the age independence of implicit learning processes. Mayberry and O'Brien-Malone (46) consider that empirical evidence for this assumption is up to now limited. One possible explanation is that the age effect observed in the Mayberry, Taylor, and O'Brien-Malone's study was due to a contamination effect of explicit knowledge on performance in the implicit task. The intentional exploitation of explicit knowledge can never be totally ruled out in classical implicit learning paradigms (73). Also, of course, if such explicit factors intervene during implicit learning, a global age effect can be expected in performance improvement. It thus appears crucial to use a method avoiding any contamination effect. To this end, Vinter and Perruchet (84) developed the "neutral parameter procedure," which had been devised to minimize the intervention of explicit influences on performance. This procedure is based on two criteria. The task demands criterion requires that instructions lead participants to focus on behavioral components other than those on which the unconscious influences are assessed, and the neutral effect criterion stipulates that unconscious effects must be assessed on the basis of a behavioral parameter that is neutral with regard to task achievement. Applying this procedure, Vinter and Perruchet (85) have shown that children between the ages of 4 and 10 years are able to modify implicitly their usual drawing behavior, without them aiming at this change. More important with respect to the topic discussed here, no age-related differences appeared in these experiments run with the "neutral parameter procedure." For the authors, it means that implicit learning processes are age independent, as claimed by Reber (65), but age effects are likely to appear as soon as explicit influences can intervene on the participant's performance. Other factors may cause the emergence of age-related differences, as clear from the literature on implicit learning in aging.

Indeed, the postulate of age independency appears to be more controversial with respect to aging. On the one hand, equal amounts of implicit learning were found when young and old people were compared in several studies (21, 28, 29, 72). No age-related decline in performance was reported in a recent study where old participants were asked to learn letter strings with a given letter always appearing at the same position (31). Young and old adults learned implicitly this regularity equally well. The authors demonstrated that learning occurred during the encoding phase. This study, and others, testifies for the preserved capacity of older people to adapt efficiently to environmental regularities.

On the other hand, a decline in implicit performance was revealed in other studies when complex learning material was used or when low-ability elderly people were tested (10, 12, 32, 30). French and Miner (21) demonstrated that age differences between young and old participants emerged in implicit learning when a dual-task condition was used but not under a single-task condition. The same conclusion was achieved in a more recent study by Nejati *et al.* (53), who showed that implicit learning in elderly adults was affected by an increased attentional load introduced by a condition of dual-task interference. Age-related deficits were also observed within a restricted age range, when elderly individuals of different ages were compared in a complex task (32). This study, which contrasted young-old (65- to 73-year-old) and old-old (76- to 80-year-old) people, revealed a decline in implicit learning performance within aging itself. However, older adults seemed to remain sensitive to highly complex sequential regularities, although they learned those less than younger adults (3).

Howard and Howard (32) suggested that processing material with high-level structure places high demand on working memory, which is known to decline with aging (71). Indeed, they reported a significant positive correlation between working memory span and both speed and accuracy of implicit learning. These authors appealed to the concept of the simultaneity mechanism of cognitive aging developed by Salthouse (70) to account for this result. The more complex the material to process is, the more events people have to keep activated simultaneously in their working memory in order to learn how they relate to one another. A decline in working memory capacity should therefore provoke deficits in implicit learning tasks when they are structured at a complex level. It is this decline that might account for the age-related differences observed in implicit learning between young and old people as well as between young-old and old-old people.

It could be argued, however, that these age effects are at least partly due to the difference of timing in overt performance between young and old people, old people showing a global slowdown in their responses to stimuli, whatsoever. Howard, Howard, Denis, and Yankovich (33) have thus built an implicit learning situation where event timing mimicked that experienced by older adults in this situation and have confronted young adults to such slowdown implicit learning condition. Their results indicated that these artificially "aged" young adults still learned implicitly in a complex situation, but both performed lower than young control adults and better than old control adults. The pattern of performance deficits displayed by old adults still appeared different from that observed in the "aged" young adults. These results rule out the idea that event timing alone may be responsible for the age effects shown in old people, when they learned implicitly from complex situations.

To sum up, implicit learning processes operate efficiently all along life, ensuring the progressive and continuous adaptation of human behavior to the environment. These processes are globally not sensitive to age effects, although clear limits in this age independency postulate seem to appear. The more demanding in attentional cognitive resources a learning task is, the more complex the information to be learned is, and the more permeable to explicit influences the learning procedure is, the more likely age-related differences are to emerge.

Implicit learning processes and pathology

Considering that, from the phylogenetic viewpoint, the implicit mode of learning precedes the explicit mode, Reber (64, 65) claimed that implicit learning should be independent of IQ and should be able to withstand neurological or psychological damage.

The question of IQ independency

The literature supports globally the IQ-independence postulate. Reber, Walkenfeld, and Hernstadt (66) found a nonsignificant correlation between IQ and implicit performance in an artificial grammar task in young adults, while significance was reached when IQ was correlated with an explicit learning performance score. The same conclusion was proposed by Myers and Conner (52) in a computer-control task and by McGeorge, Crawford, and Kelly (48) in an artificial grammar task. The independence of implicit learning with psychometric intelligence has been proved in an impressive study carried out by Gebauer and Makintosh (23) on a very large sample of participants. These authors failed to report any significant correlations between various measures of intelligence and different measures of implicit learning performance. However, this study was not concerned with persons with low IQs.

Using a covariation task, Maybery, Taylor, and O'Brien-Malone (47) did not find any relationship between IQ and implicit performances in children with an average age of 6 to 11 years and divided into low IQ (78 to 97), medium IQ (100 to 110) and high IQ (110 to 125) groups. They reported that implicit learning improved with age and that explicit learning, assessed through a task presenting a logical structure similar to the implicit task, improved with age and with intelligence. Atwell, Conners, and Merrill (1) also compared the impact of implicit and explicit learning in individuals with intellectual disability, with IQs varying only from 50 to 75, using an artificial grammar learning paradigm. Their conclusion agreed with Reber's postulate that implicit learning is largely preserved in intellectually disabled persons.

However, this conclusion has been challenged by Fletcher, Maybery, and Bennett (20), who compared a group of gifted children aged 9 to 10 years (IQ of around 120) with a group of mentally retarded children (IQ of around 60) using a task where participants had to learn implicitly a covariation. Implicit performance was below chance in intellectually disabled children and above chance in the gifted children. These results suggest that implicit learning processes might be inoperative in children with mental retardation. But this negative result may again be due to the fact that explicit influences have contaminated the children's performance in the learning task. Indeed, adopting the neutral parameter procedure suggested by Vinter and Perruchet (84) in a task where participants are incidentally led to modify their graphic behavior, Vinter and Detable (86) have shown that the impact of implicit learning was not a function of IQ in adolescents with IQs varying from 30 to 70.

The question of resistance to neurological or psychological damages

The robustness of implicit learning processes has been assessed in regard to various kinds of neurological and psychological or psychiatric diseases. It is out of the scope of this chapter to review this literature; we will just give a brief overview of the main results.

It was of course very tempting to investigate whether amnesic patients are still able to learn implicitly because learning can hardly be dissociable from memory, and contamination of performance by explicit influences can hardly be suspected in these patients. A large body of research conducted with amnesic patients concerns implicit sequence learning. Globally, their capabilities to learn implicitly sequences are shown to be preserved, whether Korsakoff's or Alzheimer's patients are considered (54, 55, 17, 39). This result demonstrates that implicit sequence learning does not require the brain areas that are necessarily involved in explicit memory. However, implicit performance was sometimes superior in controls than in amnesic patients (54) but not systematically at a significant level (67). It has been suggested that amnesic patients may encounter more difficulties than controls when higher order of information has to be learned (13), although again they did learn such complex information (12). However, this issue remains controversial. In a sequence learning paradigm, Vandenberghe, Schmidt, Fery, and Cleeremans (83) recently showed that amnesic patients learned a sequence that followed deterministic rules but not probabilistic ones, while control participants succeeded in both sequence structures.

The investigation of implicit learning processes in patients with Huntington's disease or with Parkinson's disease (PD) reveals that implicit sequence learning may be partly damaged in these patients (17, 35). These results are not clear cut; however, only a third of the patients with Huntington's disease tested by Knopman and Nissen (39) did show impaired performance. Siegert, Taylor, Weatherall, and Abernethy (79) carried out a meta-analysis of a series of studies run with PD patients, and that have investigated implicit sequential learning. Their conclusion was that implicit sequence learning appears to be impaired in these patients. What aspects of performance are more precisely impaired? Seidler, Tuite, and Ashe (77) revealed that PD patients did not fail to learn implicitly sequential information, but that they were impaired in managing to translate sequence knowledge into rapid motor performance. This conclusion may suggest that at least part of the deficits shown in PD patients may come from the use of overt motor responses in these implicit learning tasks. Indeed, Smith, Siegert, and McDowall (81) did not report any differences between PD patients and controls when tasks involving verbal responses were used, such as an artificial grammar task or a verbal version of the serial reaction time task. Other studies converge in reporting rather intact implicit learning capacities in PD patients in an artificial grammar task (49, 87). However, when the learning procedure included a trial-by-trial feedback, the PD patients exhibited deficits in category learning task (80), as well as when a complex relationship between stimulus dimensions was used to define category membership in an implicit category learning task (19). In summary, this literature tends to confirm that the implicit learning processes are globally preserved in patients with Huntington's disease or with PD, as long as the task does not rely too strongly on overt motor responses and on integrative processes, and possibly does not require processing too complex information.

A growing body of research is devoted to the study of implicit learning processes in psychiatric diseases, in particular in schizophrenic patients. The conclusions that can be drawn from this literature are very similar to those mentioned in the previous areas of research. On the one hand, implicit learning processes appear to be intact in patients with schizophrenia at least when assessed with an artificial grammar learning task (14,

27). On the other hand, a moderate impairment of their performance in serial reaction time tasks has been recently confirmed by Siegert, Weaterall, and Bell (78), who performed a meta-analysis of results collected in more than 200 patients. These tasks are usually based on visuospatial cues. When nonspatial sequences are introduced, a smaller learning effect is still observed in patients with schizophrenia in comparison to healthy controls, although both groups do display learning. Thus, the moderate deficit shown in these patients in regard to sequential learning could be due to a minor sensitivity to regularly occurring sequences of events in the environment.

In sum, the current literature provides a global support to the postulate expressed by Reber (65), stipulating that implicit learning processes are resistant to both neurological and psychiatric diseases. Differences with control participants may, however, emerge, depending on the type of tasks used, on the type of responses measured and possibly on the complexity of the material to be learned.

Implicit learning processes and education or reeducation

This last section will examine whether the demonstration that implicit learning processes are relatively robust to age and pathology may open new ways to approaching educational or reeducational methods. It is, however, important to point out that such a section can only be speculative because of a global lack of systematic researches carried out within such an applied perspective. We will also limit our speculative considerations to the educational (scholastic) domain, with the hope that some reflections are general enough to be extended to broader preoccupations related to remediation in diverse pathological contexts.

Implicit learning processes outside of laboratory

To provide support to the view that implicit learning can constitute an interesting way to approaching education or reeducation, it is pertinent to show that this mode of learning contributes naturally to human development, that is, out of laboratory, although the body of research devoted to this question is not large. The only domain in which a sizeable amount of literature has emerged concerns the relationships between implicit learning and oral or written language acquisition (25). The practical applications of implicit learning appear to be still sparser. Some methods have evolved that exploit principles that can be a posteriori related to implicit learning principles, such as using conditions as similar as possible to natural learning to reach second language or reading (26, 40). An extensive literature also concerns the use of errorless learning for reeducative purposes in a neuropsychological perspective (see 18). The explanations for this relative paucity are certainly manifold. One of the most important may be that learning in real-world situations most often involve some mixture of implicit (or incidental) and explicit (or intentional) learning. Similarly, for reeducative purposes, a mixture of incidental and explicit learning is possibly preferable because behavioral acquisitions obtained through implicit learning processes do not contribute to knowledge formation as explicit learning processes do. This point warrants to be made clearer.

Our own understanding of how implicit learning processes operate has been developed in details elsewhere (59, 60). A few points are nevertheless worth mentioning in order to facilitate the understanding of how we conceive of the potential interest of implicit learning for (re)educational procedures. Implicit learning occurs whenever we can suspect that unconscious processes have led to participant's behavioral modifications, such that these changes reflect the structural characteristics of the situation with which the participant repeatedly interacts, without intentionally looking for such an adaptation. It is from the direct interactions between some properties of the subject's attentional and memory systems (more precisely, a limited attentional focus size, a tendency to associate automatically elements that enter together in a same attentional focus, and a tendency for memory traces to be subject to reinforcement, forgetting, and interference) and some structural properties of the material to be learned (for instance, their statistical distribution) that the progressive behavioral adaptation emerges. In other words, implicit learning does not lead, in our view, to the acquisition of unconscious knowledge about the structural characteristics of the learning situation. Instead of developing (unconscious) knowledge about the learning situation, implicit learning processes directly shape the participant's behavior and concomitant phenomenological apprehension of the situation, thanks to the formation of cognitive units that progressively become isomorphic to the structure of the situation. In an artificial grammar learning task, for instance, the participants would not unconsciously abstract the unknown grammatical rules that structure the material they are confronted with, but would become progressively sensitive to the structural features of this material, such as its statistical properties and its salient features. The more salient a feature is, the more likely it can draw attention and consequently create a memory trace that shapes the individual's phenomenological experience. Furthermore, the more frequent this feature is, the stronger its memory trace is consolidated. In our view, these basic functional laws of attention and memory, in interaction with the specific properties of the material to be learned, account for the progressive adaptation of the participant's behavior to the rules of the grammar (or to the products of the rules), without any need of abstracting the rules themselves.

Thus, if the educator or reeducator aims at helping subjects to acquire rule-based knowledge about a precise situation, methods based upon implicit learning processes would not be appropriate. But if the objective is to help subjects to develop adapted behaviors to their environment, these methods are of interest, according to us.

We propose to examine now how to build a learning situation based on implicit processes.

A rationale for building implicit learning situations

Considering our understanding of how implicit learning processes operate both inside and outside laboratory, we can try to delineate what are the main characteristics that learning situations have to present in order to elicit at best these processes. In some way, this turns out to build a rationale for designing any learning situation that aims at eliciting implicit processes.

During the learning phase, the participant must be confronted only to positive instances of the rule or of the regularity (or of the behavior) that have to be learned. Including errors (or counterexamples of the regularity) in the material manipulated during learning must be avoided. This condition contrasts with more classical learning situations such as those used by teachers at school, where the students are, for instance, required to identify grammatical errors in a text or to select the good response among three false ones. These types of exercises aim at testing whether the student is able to correctly apply and generalize a rule that has previously been explicated. In an implicit learning approach to the question of orthographic acquisition, the participant would be directly confronted with a series of positive instances of the rule (the difficulty in this case would be to imagine a task that obliges the participant to process attentively all the orthographically well formed sentences several times). The repeated exposition to such a structured material will elicit associative processes so that the elements that enter together into an attentional focus will be associated. However, these associative processes are rather blind, and they function whether the material contains errors or not. It is for this reason that introducing errors into the material may have detrimental effects on learning: The learners may become familiarized as much with false as with correct associations. This point can be illustrated indirectly by an anecdotal observation. An interesting spelling error can be observed in French researchers who are familiar with the English language, when they write the French word *adresse*. This word is often spelled *addresse* because of the repeated confrontation with the English spelling of the same word. Similar negative effects of the exposition to errors in relation to spelling or other abilities have been shown in the literature (6, 15, 22, 57). The success of the use of errorless learning methods for reeducative purposes also testifies for the value of an approach founded on the withdrawal of the confrontation to errors (18).

A second important feature of implicit learning tasks is the fact that the regularity or the rule that is of interest must be "isolated" at best. We have pointed out the important role played by attention in the formation of the associations between the material's elements, these associations constituting the substance of the learning processes. However, the child's or adult's attentional focus is limited and cannot capture a large number of elements together. Moreover, this focus is constrained in time and in space, and the elements to be associated cannot be too distant or separate, whether time or space is considered. Indeed, the possibility to establish an association decreases rapidly when the distance between elements increases (11). For these reasons, it is better to isolate the regularities of interest in the learning situation. We can again give an indirect illustration to this point, showing that when regularities occur within a limited space and time, they provoke the formation of automatisms that express themselves even if they do not correspond to an adapted behavior. An illustration can be found in some aspects of orthographic acquisition, such as how to mark the plural of nouns. Consider the following few examples of French expressions that a child may read in a text: *il cher-*

che ses clés (he's looking for his keys), *tu prends tes jouets* (you take your toys), and *elle coupe des fleurs* (she's cutting flowers). The association between the "s" at the end of the article and the "s" at the end of the noun is regular and frequent, and it occurs within a reduced space and time, rendering their association into a same attentional focus very likely. This association is consolidated through experience and can form the basis of an automatism. This is suggested by the work of Largy *et al.* (42). They asked French university students to recall sentences by writing them down. These sentences included homophonous words such as *asperge*, which means "to sprinkle" as a verb and "asparagus" as a noun. To increase task demands, participants were also asked to memorize nouns and to write them down when they had finished writing the sentence (on another page so that they could not correct possible misspellings). The target sentences were sentences such as *L'éléphant voit les clowns et il les asperge* ("The elephant sees the clowns and sprinkles them"). French children and adults tended to add –s more or less systematically at the end of *asperge*, as if it were a noun. Erroneous addition of –s increased even further when the personal pronoun *il* in the sentences stood for a noun that lexically primed the nominal form of a noun-verb homophonous pair. For example, *il* in the sentence *Le jardinier sort les legumes et il les asperge* ("The gardener takes the vegetables out and sprinkles them") refers to the "gardener" who is related to the homophonous noun form "asparagus," but *il* refers to a word that primes the verbal form of *asperge* in the sentence *L'éléphant voit les clowns et il les asperge* ("The elephant sees the clowns and sprinkles them"). These errors can be seen as a product of the action of unconscious associative processes that have easily captured the association between the article (plural) and the noun (plural), thanks to their close occurrence in time and space, the unit *les asperges* (the asparagus) being furthermore much more frequently encountered than the unit *les asperge* (sprinkles them).

Thus, in order to facilitate the attentional capture of the relevant elements that must be associated, it is better to withdraw from the learning situation all elements that may make less salient the to-be learned association and could attract the participant's attention.

A third important characteristic of a learning condition based on implicit processes is the fact that the material to be learned must be repeatedly presented to the learners. Associations take time to emerge, and this is why the repetition of the presentation of the learning condition is crucial. The number of repetitions, the number of learning sessions, and their mode of presentation (distributed or not for instance) depend on several factors and cannot probably be determined with security in advance. This uncertainty, as well as the fundamental role of time, may contribute to increase the difficulty of relying on implicit learning processes in an applied perspective. Reeducating through implicit learning processes requires time, probably more time than explicit methods would need.

Finally, the last feature that we would like to point out is related to an important aspect of the very definition of implicit learning. The learning condition must be designed so that the learner is brought to process attentively the relevant information without making explicit at all what he or she is supposed to learn. For instance, if one aims at developing in children a behavioral sensibility to some orthographical rules, the person can imagine to ask them to spell out words, without never mentioning the rule that is of interest. Spelling out words requires an attentional processing of the words, which is a prerequisite for capturing any regularity occurring in these words (and of course, a rule provokes inevitably regularities at the material's surface).

Conclusion

In conclusion to this chapter, it is probably important to point out that our proposals concerning the use of implicit processes for educative or reeducative purposes should be taken with caution. Clearly, the gap may be large between, on the one hand, general learning principles that globally apply to human behavior and, on the other hand, specific reeducational methods that should be dedicated to specific human behavioral disorders. Furthermore, implicit learning processes shape the individual's behavior in resonance with the structure of a learning situation but do not lead to any explicit knowledge of this very structure. For instance, if one aims at teaching orthographical rules, implicit learning processes would not be appropriate to this scope because they can only develop in individuals a behavioral tendency to adapt to the frequent and salient regularities that reflect the rules. Consequently, the performance cannot attain perfection (as would be the case if one would apply the rules), and it is permeable to errors each time a frequent association enters in conflict with a much less frequent association displaying another rule, as we have seen it before with our example of article-noun plural rule. However, we do believe that testing whether implicit learning processes may provide even partial solutions for remediation is worth trying.

References

1. Atwell JA, Conners FA, Merrill EC (2003) Implicit and explicit learning in young adults with mental retardation. Am J Ment Retard 1:5668
2. Bates E, Elman J (1996) Learning rediscovered. Science 274:1849
3. Bennett IJ, Howard JH Jr., Howard DV (2007) Age-related differences in implicit learning of subtle third-order sequential structure. J Gerontol 62B:98-103
4. Berr y DC, Dienes Z (1993) Implicit learning: theoretical and empirical issues. Lawrence Erlbaum Associates, Hove
5. Bremner AJ, Mareschal D, Destrebecqz A, Cleermans A (2007) Cognitive control of sequential knowledge at 2 years of age: Evidence from an incidental sequence learning and generation task. Psychol Sci 18:261-266
6. Brown AS (1988) Encountering misspellings and spelling performance: why wrong isn't right. J Educ Psychol 80:488-494
7. Bruner JS, Goodnow JJ, Austin GA (1956) A study of thinking. Wiley, New York

8. Carr TH, Curran T (1994) Cognitive factors in learning about structured sequences. Stud Second Lang Acquis 16:205-230

9. Chandler S (1993) Are rules and modules really necessary for explaining language? J Psycholinguist Res 22:593-606

10. Cherry KE, Stadler, MA (1995) Implicit learning of a nonverbal sequence in younger and older adults. Psychol Aging 10:379-394

11. Cleeremans A (1993) Mechanisms of implicit learning: a connectionist model of sequence processing. MIT Press: Bradford Books, Cambridge, MA

12. Curran T (1997) Effects of aging on implicit sequence learning: accounting for sequence structure and explicit knowledge. Psychol Res 60:24-41

13. Curran T, Schacter DL (1997) Implicit memory: what must theories of amnesia explain? Memory 5:37-47

14. Danion JM, Meulemans T, Kauffmann-Muller F, Vermaat H (2001) Intact implicit learning in schizophrenia. Am J Psychiatry 158:944-948

15. Dixon, M, Kaminska, Z (1997) Is it misspelled or is it mispelled? The influence of fresh orthographic information on spelling. Read Writ 9:483-498

16. Elman JL, Bates EA, Johnson MH, et al. (1996, eds) Rethinking innateness. MIT Press, Cambridge, MA

17. Ferraro FR, Balota DA, Connor LT (1993) Implicit memory and the formation of new associations in nondemented Parkinson's disease individuals and individuals with senile dementia of the Alzheimer type: a serial reaction time investigation. Brain Cogn 21:163-180

18. Fillingham JK, Hodgson C, Sage K, Lambon Ralph MA (2003) The application of errorless learning to aphasic disorders: A review of theory and practice. Neuropsychol Rehabil 13:337-363

19. Filoteo JV, Maddox WT, Salmon DP, Song DD (2007) Implicit category learning performance predicts rate of cognitive decline in nondemented patients with Parkinson's disease. Neuropsychology 21:183-192

20. Fletcher J, Maybery MT, Bennett S (2000) Implicit learning differences: a question of developmental level? J Exp Psychol Learn Mem Cogn 26:246-252

21. French PA, Miner CS (1994) Effects of presentation rate and individual differences in short-term memory capacity on an indirect measure of serial learning. Mem Cognit 22:95-110

22. Gathercole SE, Baddeley AD (1993) Working memory and language. Lawrence Erlbaum, Hove

23. Gebauer GF, Mackintosh NJ (2007) Psychometric intelligence dissociates implicit and explicit learning. J Exp Psychol Learn Mem Cogn 33(1):34-54

24. Gomez RL, Gerken L (1999) Artificial grammar learning by 1-year-olds leads to specific and abstract knowledge. Cognition 70:109-135

25. Gomez RL, Gerken, L (2000) Infant artificial language learning and language acquisition. Trends Cogn Sci 1:178-186

26. Graham S (2000) Should the natural learning approach replace spelling instruction? J Educ Psychol 92:235-247

27. Horan WP, Green MF, Knowlton BJ, et al. (2008) Impaired implicit learning in schizophrenia. Neuropsychology 22:606-617

28. Howard DV, Howard JH Jr. (1989) Age differences in learning serial patterns: direct versus indirect measures. Psychol Aging 4:357-364

29. Howard DV, Howard JH Jr. (1992) Adult age differences in the rate of learning serial patterns: evidence from direct and indirect tests. Psychol Aging 7:232-241

30. Howard DV, Howard JH Jr. (2001) When it does hurt to try: adult age differences in the effects of instructions on implicit pattern learning. Psychon Bull Rev 8:798-805

31. Howard DV, Howard JH Jr., Dennis NA, et al. (2008) Aging and implicit learning of an invariant association. J Gerontol 63B:100-105

32. Howard JH Jr., Howard DV (1997) Age differences in implicit learning of higher order dependencies in serial patterns. Psychol Aging 12:634-656

33. Howard JH Jr., Howard DV, Dennis NA, Yankovith H (2007) Event timing and age deficits in higher-order sequence learning. Aging Neuropsychol Cogn 14:647-668

34. Hoyer WJ, Lincourt AE (1998) Aging and the development of learning. In: Stadler M, Frensch P (eds) Handbook of implicit learning, pp. 445-470. Sage Publications, Thousand Oaks

35. Jackson SR, Morris DL, Harrison J, et al. (1995) Parkinson's disease and the internal control of action: a single-case study. Neurocase 1:267-283

36. Kail RV (1990) The development of memory in children. Freeman, New York

37. Karatekin C, Marcus DJ, White TJ (2007) Oculomotor and manual indices of incidental and intentional spatial sequence learning in middle childhood and adolescence. J Exp Child Psychol 96:107-130

38. Karmiloff-Smith A (1992) Beyond modularity: a developmental perspective on cognitive science. MIT Press, Cambridge, MA

39. Knopman D, Nissen MJ (1991) Procedural learning is impaired in Huntington's disease: Evidence from the serial reaction time task. Neuropsychologia 29:245-254

40. Krashen S (1981) Second language acquisition and second language learning. Prentice Hall International, New York

41. Krist H, Fieberg EL, Wilkening F (1993) Intuitive physics in action and judgment: The development of knowledge about projective motion. J Exp Psychol Learn Mem Cogn 19:952-966

42. Largy P, Fayol M, Lemaire P (1996) On confounding verb/noun inflections. A study of subject-verb agreement errors in French. Lang Cogn Process 11:217-255

43. Lewicki P (1986) Nonconscious social information processing. Academic Press, Orlando

44. Lewicki P, Hill T, Czyzewska M (1992) Nonconscious acquisition of information. Am Psychol 47:796-801

45. Mandler JM (1998) Representation. In: Kuhn D, Siegler R (eds) Cognition, perception and language, vol. 2., of Damon W (ed) Handbook of child psychology, Lavoisier, Paris

46. Maybery M, O'Brien-Malone A (1998) Implicit and automatic processes in cognitive development. In: Kirsner K, Speelman C, Maybery M, et al. (eds) Implicit and explicit mental processes. Lawrence Erlbaum, Mahway, NJ

47. Maybery M, Taylor M, O'Brien-Malone A (1995) Implicit learning: sensitive to age but not IQ. Aust J Psychol 47:8-17

48. McGeorge P, Crawford JR, Kelly SW (1997) The relationships between psychometric intelligence and learning in an explicit and an implicit task. J Exp Psychol Learn Mem Cogn 23:239-245

49. Meulemans T, Peigneux P, Van der Linden M (1998) Brain Cogn 37:109-112
50. Meulemans T, Van der Linden M, Perruchet P (1998) Implicit sequence learning in children. J Exp Child Psychol 69:199-221
51. Munakata Y, McClelland JL, Johnson MH, Siegler, RS (1997) Rethinking infant knowledge: Toward an adaptive process account of successes and failures in object permanence tasks. Psychol Rev 104:686-713
52. Myers C, Conner M (1992) Age differences in skill acquisition and transfer in an implicit learning paradigm. Appl Cogn Psychol 6:429-442
53. Nejati V, Farshi MT, Ashayeri H, Aghdasi MT (2008) Dual task interference in implicit sequence learning by young and old adults. Int J Geriatr Psychiatry 23:801-804
54. Nissen MJ, Bullemer P (1987) Attentional requirements of learning: evidence from performance measures. Cogn Psychol 19:1-32
55. Nissen MJ, Willingham D, Hartman M (1989) Explicit and implicit remembering: When is learning preserved in amnesia? Neuropsychologia 27:341-352
56. Pacton S, Perruchet P, Fayol M, Cleeremans A (2001) Implicit learning out of the lab: the case of orthographical regularities. J Exp Psychol Gen 130:401-426
57. Perruchet P, Rey A, Hiver E, Pacton S (2006) Do distractors interfere with memory for study pairs in associative recognition? Mem Cognit 34:1046-1054
58. Perruchet P, Vinter A (1998) Learning and development. The implicit knowledge assumption reconsidered. In: Stadler M, Frensch P (eds) Handbook of implicit learning, pp. 495-532. Sage Publications, Thousand Oaks
59. Perruchet P, Vinter A (2002) The self-organizing consciousness. Behav Brain Sci 25:297-388
60. Perruchet P, Vinter A (2008) La conscience auto-organisatrice. L'Année Psychologique 108:79-106
61. Perruchet P, Vinter A, Gallego J (1997) Implicit learning shapes new conscious percepts and representations. Psychon Bull Rev 4:43-48
62. Reber AS (1967) Implicit learning of artificial grammars. J Verbal Learn Verbal Behav 6:855-863
63. Reber AS (1989) Implicit learning and tacit knowledge. J Exp Psychol Gen 118:219-235
64. Reber AS (1992) The cognitive unconscious: an evolutionary perspective. Conscious Cogn 1:93-113
65. Reber AS (1993) Implicit learning and tacit knowledge. Oxford University Press, Oxford, UK
66. Reber AS, Walkenfeld FF, Hernstadt R (1991) Implicit and explicit learning: individual differences and IQ. J Exp Psychol Learn Mem Cogn 17:888-896
67. Reber PJ, Squire LR (1994) Parallel brain systems for learning with and without awareness. Learn Mem 1:217-229
68. Saffran JR, Johnson EK, Aslin RN, Newport EL (1999) Statistical learning of tone sequences by human infants and adults. Cognition 70:27-52
69. Saffran JR, Newport EL, Aslin RN, et al. (1997) Incidental language learning. Psychol Sci 8:101-105
70. Salthouse TA (1996) The processing-speed theory of adult age differences in cognition. Psychol Rev 103:403-428
71. Salthouse TA, Babcock RL (1991) Decomposing adult age differences in working memory. Dev Psychol 27:763-776

72. Salthouse TA, McGuthry KE, Haambrick DZ (1999) A framework for analyzing and interpreting differential aging patterns: application to three measures of implicit learning. Aging Neuropsychol Cogn 6:1-18

73. Shanks DR, St. John M (1994) Characteristics of dissociable human learning systems. Behav Brain Sci 17:367-447

74. Schyns PG, Rodet L (1997) Categorization creates functional features. J Exp Psychol Learn Mem Cogn 23:681-696

75. Schyns PG, Goldstone RL, Thibaut JP (1998) The development of features in object concepts. Behav Brain Sci 21(1):1-17; discussion 17-54

76. Seger CA (1994) Implicit learning. Psychol Bull 115:163-196

77. Seidler RD, Tuite P, Ashe J (2007) Selective impairments in implicit learning in Parkinson's disease. Brain Res 1137:104-110

78. Siegert RJ, Weatherall M, Bell EM (2008) Is implicit sequence learning impaired in schizophrenia? A meta-analysis. Brain Cogn 67:351-359

79. Siegert RJ, Taylor KD, Weatherall M, Abernethy DA (2006) Is implicit sequence learning impaired in Parkinson's disease? A meta-analysis. Neuropsychology 20:490-495

80. Smith J, McDowall J (2006) When artificial grammar acquisition in Parkinson's disease is impaired: the case of learning via trial-by-trial feedback. Brain Res 1067:216-228

81. Smith J, Siegert RJ, McDowall J (2001) Preserved implicit learning on both the serial reaction time task and artificial grammar in patients with Parkinson's disease. Brain Cogn 45:378-391

82. Thelen E, Smith LB (1994, eds) A dynamic systems approach to the development of cognition and action. MIT Press, Cambridge, MA

83. Vandenberghe M, Schmidt N, Fery P, Cleeremans A (2006) Can amnesic patients learn without awareness? New evidence comparing deterministic and probabilistic sequence learning. Neuropsychologia 44:1629-1641

84. Vinter A, Perruchet P (1999) Isolating unconscious influences: the neutral parameter procedure. Q J Exp Psychol A 52:857-875

85. Vinter A, Perruchet P (2000) Implicit learning in children is not related to age: evidence from drawing behavior. Child Dev 71:1223-1240

86. Vinter A, Detable C (2003) Implicit learning in children and adolescents with mental retardation. Am J Ment Retard 108:94-107

87. Witt K, Nuhsman A, Deuschl G (2002) Intact artificial grammar learning in patients with cerebellar degeneration and advanced Parkinson's disease. Neuropsychologia 40:1534-1540

Implicit learning and implicit memory in moderate to severe memory disorders

A. Moussard and E. Bigand

Introduction

Numerous experimental psychology studies have established firmly that important parts of the human cognitive process operate automatically without the conscious or explicit control of the subjects (9). Such processes can concern memorization of episodes from life in a way that will subsequently have an implicit influence on our behavior (such as decision-making or reaction time). They can equally assist acquisition of more complex knowledge from our surroundings, by the automatic capture of the statistical regularities found in them (see Chapter "Introducing implicit learning: from the laboratory to the real life", E. Bigand and C. Delbé). This is the way, for example, that a baby learns to speak its mother tongue. Without intent, and not consciously, it extracts, progressively, different words from the flow of an adult's speech; then it learns the rules of grammar, from which it is able to use the words in a sentence. This type of learning can be considered as a method by which the individual adapts to his or her environment (42) and, according to Reber (45), must derive, in evolutionary terms, from a very old mechanism appearing before the emergence of consciousness. This evolutionary hypothesis relies on several different properties of implicit processes.

First, the mechanisms that are the oldest in the evolution of a species show only slight differences from one individual to another within the population, and such is the case with those implicit processes that have been tested in the laboratory. For example, Reber and his collaborators (46) showed that performance in learning an artificial grammar is not correlated with IQ. Other studies have provided evidence that implicit learning capabilities are independent of a person's age. Indeed, eight-month-old babies are capable of extracting pseudo-words repeated in artificial speech of no meaning (51, 52). Similarly, both young and mature adults show the same results in learning a series of complex events (21).

Second, the hypothesis of the great evolutionary age of implicit cognitive mechanisms depends on the lack of association between these implicit processes and those that are implicated in explicit learning or declarative memory. Thus, if implicit learning is a result of a form of knowledge acquisition anterior to the appearance of conscious cognition, it cannot call on the same mechanisms. Several studies indeed show that, for an identical task, parameters of implicit and explicit functions are not correlated (32). Put another way, a subject's score in one parameter does not provide a forecast of the score in the other. These results suggest that implicit and explicit cognitive processes arise from distinct and independent systems.

Third, the precedence of implicit learning capacity must mean it is pathologically more robust: capabilities that arose later and are more sophisticated, such as the linguistic, are the more vulnerable, while the anterior and more automatic are those that decay last. Neuropsychological experiments confirm both the nonassociation of implicit and explicit processes and the greater pathological robustness of the implicit. They have shown intact implicit learning capacities in a variety of cognitive disorders: amnesia, Alzheimer's disease (AD), parkinsonism, Huntington's chorea, developmental dyslexia, Williams-Beuren syndrome, multiple sclerosis, schizophrenia, and so on. We shall tackle in the first part of this chapter the survival of implicit learning and implicit memory in those diseases that affect declarative memory and new learning. Two illustrations of the problem will be given from those cases most often appearing in the scientific literature: amnesia and AD. The consequences for clinical rehabilitation are important. Those methods that support preserved mechanisms, and new perspectives on rehabilitation, will be discussed in the second part of this chapter.

Implicit learning and implicit memory in pathological conditions

Amnesia

Amnesia is defined as severe and permanent memory loss, stable over time, and characterized by the sufferer's inability either to acquire new memories (anterograde amnesia) or to recall memories acquired before the onset of cerebral damage (retrograde amnesia) (34). There is a variety of causes, but memory malfunction can arise without other symptoms appearing: intellectual habits and working memory are preserved in most instances. The study of amnesiacs has contributed greatly to our understanding of human memory, most notably in distinguishing several independent memory functions, some of which can be altered while, as we shall see, the rest remain functional.

Toward the end of the nineteenth century, several different levels of consciousness became recognized, through studies of memory processes. Claparède (1873-1940), a Swiss doctor and psychologist, reported an anecdote that would become the basis of studies of implicit memory. One day, he hid a pin in the hand he used to greet and shake the hand of an amnesic female patient. Later, when the patient had no memory of the pinprick, nor even remembered meeting the doctor that day, she withdrew her hand, as a reflex, when he extended his to shake it, and was unable to explain why she did so. For Claparède, "implicit recognition" was "that which determines a subject's behavior in a way implying that the subject recognizes objects previously encountered, without feeling that he or she knows them. It is, if you like, an unconscious recognition." He contrasted this with "explicit recognition," "characterized by the full awareness of what is already experienced" (Claparède, cited in 12). This distinction between implicit and explicit memory processes, proposed also by several famous researchers on memory such as Ribot, Ebbinghaus, or Korsakoff (see 39), was supported in the 1960s with the birth of neuropsychology and the publication of case HM (36).

When aged 27, HM had a bilateral section of the median temporal lobe, in consequence of an epilepsy that had proved difficult to treat pharmacologically, and particularly handicapping. After the operation, he presented severe and isolated problems of anterograde episodic memory, and to a lesser degree also retrograde. Incapable of explicit new learning, HM nevertheless went on to show capability of acquiring new memories by implicit methods, notably by procedural memory. In a mirror-image drawing task, the subject draws a single-line six-pointed star, looking at his hand, and the star only in a mirror. At first, at each change of direction of the pencil, the subject tries to draw in the opposite direction, and thereby makes a number of errors that can eventually be stamped out by practice. After 30 attempts in 3 days, HM showed himself capable of correctly executing the drawing using the mirror and started each new attempt at the skill level he had achieved by the end of the previous attempt. However, he never had any recollection of previously attempting this exercise: his learning the exercise had occurred without his having any familiarity with it (37). A further study, carried out almost 30 years later, was even more surprising in showing that HM retained his capability for this task over the long term: one week, two weeks, and even a year after learning it (15). Moreover, the study, testing two further amnesic patients, showed that all three were capable of transferring their new skill to drawing via the mirror another geometric shape – a double hexagon composing the same number of sides and angles as the six-branched star.

Several years later, preservation of another implicit memory system – called perceptual learning by Milner (37) – was demonstrated in HM's results in a priming task. In this test, the subject is asked to identify images or words of which the contours have been rubbed out and are gradually filled in, until the subject can recognize them. An hour later, in a second presentation of the fragmented images, it is observed that the subject needs less contour information to successfully identify the images, compared to the first time the test was tried. The same result was found for HM, even though he retained no memory of having seen the images previously. Furthermore, HM showed residues of this learning up to four months after the first session (37).

The same perceptive priming effect was evidenced a little later in a second amnesic patient, KC (see 50, for a review of studies bearing on the case). KC developed an amnesic syndrome strongly comparable to that of HM, in consequence of a motorcycle accident when he was 30. His set of cognitive functions was evaluated normal, with the exception of a slight problem in the recognition of colors, and more severe problems in anterograde memory (in both verbal and nonverbal material) and retrograde memory (with the incapacity to order correctly in space and time the things he had experienced). Like HM, KC showed a perceptive priming effect comparable to those of other subjects, measured by a word completion test. In this test, pairs of nonrelated words (e.g., window, reason; jail, strange) are presented to the subject. Then, pairs in which the second word is incomplete are presented, and the subject is asked to write the first word to come to him in the spirit of completing the pair. These incomplete pairs are sometimes the same as were first presented (such as window, rea....), sometimes different (such as jail, rea....). The results show that participants, including KC, tend more often, if the pair is the same, to provide the word to which they had formerly been exposed, than if the pair is different. In the same way, in a lexical decision task, wherein the subject should say as quickly as possible whether pairs of sets of letters presented constitute words or not, KC, in common with other participants, took less time to decide in the case of words previously studied than of pairs not studied or pairs of nonwords. In all these situations, KC failed a direct recognition test of the words, simply ignorant of having studied the pairs of words 30 minutes before.

There is therefore no doubt in the fact that there exists a system of memory permitting the recording of certain events, of acquiring procedural skills, or of making simple associations between two elements, independently of explicit memory capacity, of the intention to learn, or even of the awareness of having learned something.

What happens with these patients in more complex implicit learning tasks? We can study this question through several exemplars of statistical implicit learning. Three will be tackled here: artificial grammar learning, categorization of objects, and serial reaction time (SRT; for an introduction to the exemplars, and to theories of implicit learning, see Chapter "Introducing implicit learning: from the laboratory to the real life", E. Bigand and C. Delbé).

The paradigm of artificial grammar learning (see , for a review) allows small-scale laboratory reproduction of the conditions pertaining to the acquisition of certain linguistic regularities. Complex rules, defined by an invented grammar, generate a series of letters without meaning – for example, MTVXXT. A large number of these "grammatical items" are shown to the subject. He is not told that there is in fact an underlying structure to the items, but is asked simply to reproduce them. Then, he is informed that the stringing together of the letters is subject to rules, and he is shown further grammatical items, different from those first seen but built from the same rules. Mixed in with these items are some nongrammatical ones – items whose construction is in breach of the rules. The subject's task is to decide which items are grammatically correct. Knowlton, Ramus, and Squire (26) compared the performances in this task of a group of 13 amnesic patients and a group of 8 normal subjects, equivalent in age and scholarly achievement to the patients. The patients achieved classification scores equivalent to those of the normal group, even though they could not describe the grammatical rules, and their performance was worse when asked to specify whether or not they had seen the items during the exposition phase of the experiment (an explicit memory task). In another experiment in this series, the patients performed less well than the normal subjects in a classification task that asked them to base their judgment of grammatical correctness on a comparison of the new items with those of the exposition phase, therefore representing a more explicit requirement. Finally, there was no correlation between classification scores and intelligence test scores.

Meulemans and Van der Linden (35) replicated these results on nine amnesic patients, showing that patients' performance was weaker in an explicit task of item generation, wherein participants had to create for themselves letter sets that followed the grammatical rules. And again, implicit classification scores did not correlate with the explicit scores from item generation. Further, in this study, the frequency of appearance of bigrams and trigrams (items of two and three letters only) was the same for the grammatical and nongrammatical items, indicating that the classification task could not have been done on the basis simply of knowledge of the letter groupings. Thus, the patients, like the normal group, seem to have extracted abstract rules for the construction of items, without being able to say they had done so – their answers tended to be along the lines of a feeling of familiarity, with an impression of "replying at random." Another proof that the participants, both patients and the normal group, had extracted the rules and not simply remembered the superficial characteristics of the items studied is that they were capable of transferring their knowledge to different sets of letters – for example, BDCFFD, not given in the exposition phase, but grammatically correct, replacing MTVXXT (28, study of nine amnesic patients).

We note, although it is not the purpose of this chapter, how much the study of amnesic patients has contributed to the development of our knowledge of the functioning of normal learning. The work has, for example, supported the conclusion that classification tasks, at the functional level, depend on processes other than those of explicit memory and explicit recognition and, at the atomic level, on structures other than those damaged in the amnesic syndrome (such as the hippocampus and diencephalon).

The second paradigm of implicit processes is that of categorization, fundamental to our understanding of the world around us. It allows us to organize the different elements we encounter as a function of their nearness and their resemblance to a prototype. For example, categorization is that which allows us to recognize an animal as belonging to the set of dogs, or a piece of furniture as being a table, even though we might never have seen before *this* dog or *that* table. And this is on the basis of the information we possess of the different categories – for the table, perhaps, a board supported by four legs. The process of category formation works directly, and we encounter a set of elements grouped by characteristics common to all of them, from which we can gain a global knowledge of these elements. Much studied in experimental psychology, this type of learning has been replicated in normal and brain-damaged subjects by various experimental procedures. Squire and his collaborators (27, 49, 56) have contributed much to the field through the study of amnesiac patients.

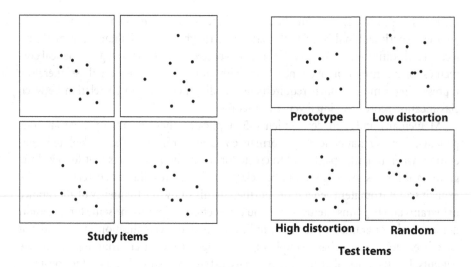

Fig. 1 - Examples of geometric point patterns used in the exposition phase and the test, by Knowlton and Squire (27). The exposition patterns were heavily distorted forms of the prototype; test patterns were heavily or lightly distorted forms or random patterns.

In the 1993 study by Knowlton and Squire (27), 10 amnesic patients and 12 normal subjects were shown several patterns of dots, in different arrangements, varied by their degree of similarity one to another as shown in **Fig. 1**. Following this exposition phase, new patterns were created, more or less different from the prototype from which they were generated, and mixed with patterns of dots in random formation. The subjects were asked to classify the new patterns as belonging, or not, to the set of patterns that they had initially been shown.

The results indicated that the amnesic patients achieved a classification score equivalent to that of the normal participants, even though their performance in explicitly recognizing the items already presented to them was weaker. It seems that they had acquired implicitly knowledge of the structures of the patterns that they had been shown. However, one debating point remains unaddressed: it might be that recognition performance is inferior to classification performance because of the greater difficulty of the task of recognition, which required a great number of examples to be remembered, while it required only one example (the most typical) to be remembered effectively to carry out the classification task. Despite their amnesia, the patients might have benefited from sufficient residual memory to enable them to carry out the classification, less demanding of memory. One patient presented with particularly severe amnesia – EP, 73 years old, a victim of herpes encephalitis 3 years before the study – and facilitated testing of this point. Squire and Knowlton (56) devised a recognition test to see if recognition could be effected on the basis of a single example: the same pattern of dots was presented to EP 40 times in succession. Then, EP was asked to recognize this pattern among a selection of patterns. Despite the extreme ease of the task, EP showed poor performance about the level of purely chance results. However, his score in a classification test of new items was normal. Thus the study confirmed that the categorization process (1) is independent of declarative memory and operates independently of memorization of one or more particular examples, rather coming through global knowledge of rules defining a particular category; (2) is independent of structures within the brain that underlie declarative memory, and that were damaged in these patients – notably the limbic system and the diencephalon; and (3) is preserved even in particularly severe pathological conditions of episodic memory – as EP's case testifies.

Another criticism that might be addressed at these studies is the not-very-common nature of the materials used. Patterns of dots are difficult to describe verbally and not decomposable into smaller elements (49). Their handling is thus not aided by a description, even purely mental, of their characteristics, in the way we can normally do with most of the objects we meet in daily life (e.g., a cat with pointed ears, four paws, and so on). Reed and his collaborators (49) proposed that, if the objects encountered are "verbalizable," their handling could with advantage call on declarative memory, while implicit learning would be the route only for those objects either more complex or of difficult explanation. Amnesic patients, deprived of declarative memory, could be called on again to test this hypothesis, in a task to classify objects similar to those we are familiar with – objects representing new types of animals (see **Fig. 2**). The eight patients participating in the study achieved once again a score equivalent to that of the normal group. The study allows us to conclude that the implicit process of categorization is common to the different experiences of daily life in which we are exposed to a large number of objects belonging to the same group.

This observation is more important for the patients because it implies that the capacity preserved could be exploited in rehabilitation, be applied to concrete daily life situations, and not merely be limited to abstract tasks in the laboratory.

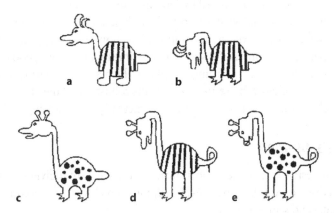

Fig. 2 - Examples of items used in the study of Reed *et al.* (49): prototype (**a**), weakly distorted (**b**), neutral (**c**), heavily distorted (**d**), and anti-prototype (**e**).

The third paradigm frequently used for testing implicit learning capacity in patients afflicted by diverse pathological conditions is the SRT task. Another type of learning parameter is measured, taking into account the sequential aspect of the events to which the patients are exposed and allowing us to gain understanding of our environment through the disposition in space and time of the elements that compose it. The SRT task (40) asks that the subject react as quickly as possible to the appearance of a marker that turns up successively in one of four possible positions on a screen. Without the participant being informed, the order of the marker's appearances is predetermined by a complex sequence, which the participant gradually learns as the test goes along: consequently, his reaction time progressively reduces. After a large number of trials, the sequence is changed (the markers appear randomly in the four possible positions), whereupon the reaction time suddenly rises, indicating that the participant had discovered certain regularities in the initial sequence, even if he or she were not conscious of it. When the initial sequence is restored, the time to react to the appearances of the marker falls rapidly anew.

A similar study on nine amnesiac patients (48) showed that the patients were capable of learning in the same way as normal participants. Their performances on explicit knowledge measures – verbalization of the characteristics of the sequence, recognition, or recreation of the learned sequence, concrete prediction of the location of the next appearance of the marker – were once again worse. However, a further interesting observation made in this study bears upon the retention, more or less long term, of the implicit knowledge gained since the patients, after the explicit tests, continued to show familiarity with the sequence learned through experience. We note that the durability of acquired implicit knowledge is essential to the question of rehabilitation, as we will discuss later.

Preservation of serial learning capacities in amnesia was, however, qualified in a study by Vandenberghe and collaborators (59). The patients were effectively confounded if the sequence was made more complex (i.e., noisy), while the normal group under the same conditions continued to demonstrate learning.

Despite this, it seems that whatever sort of paradigm is used, and whatever the cause (Korsakoff's syndrome, anoxia, cranial trauma, infection, ruptured aneurism, tumor), patients suffering from amnesia show most of the time that they have good capacity for implicit memory and implicit learning, in spite of the massive impairment of declarative memory. It is therefore interesting to study the robustness of the same capacities in another widely spread pathology of memory, particularly handicapping: AD.

Alzheimer's disease

Just as for amnesic patients, the implicit memory capacities of individuals affected by Alzheimer's disease (AD) have been explored, most notably as to procedural learning and perceptual and semantic priming.

Van Halteren-Van Tilborg and his collaborators (58) wrote a review bearing on 23 studies that tested various forms of procedural learning in AD patients. Most of the studies dealt with the acquisition of motor skills (such as tracking proficiency, mirror drawing, bimanual coordination), sometimes associated with cognitive components (such as labyrinth tests, jigsaw puzzle assembly, or SRT tasks). Independently of the test used, the studies showed, globally, that patients retained some learning capacities, whether to the same level as those of normal participants (selected for equivalence in age and academic strength) or inferior but nevertheless significant. The authors note, however, that in all these studies, those patients that failed a test were probably not included in the final analysis, a procedure that must have biased the conclusions. It is probable, however, that the failures are attributable to other difficulties connected with the disease (attention deficit, comportment and perception problems, trouble under-standing orders, and so on) and did not correspond to a general lack of procedural learning capacity (27).

Further studies were designed to test perceptual priming (14, 18, 30) and semantic priming (3). Generally, the fact of having been previously exposed to an item (for per-ceptive priming) or to an element semantically linked to it (for semantic priming) allows AD patients to handle that item subsequently more rapidly than other items. This shows that a trace of memory of the first encounter with these elements remains, even though the patients once again show no sign of conscious memory of the encoun-ter.

An interesting effect often linked to that of priming is the "mere exposure effect" (MEE), defined by the tendency of individuals generally to show a preference for, or more positive reaction to, things they know rather than new stimuli. Once again, such a reaction operates outside the consciousness of the subject and in the absence of explicit recognition or even a feeling of familiarity tied to these stimuli (62). In two studies, the MEE has been demonstrated in the visual dimension in lightly or moder-ately afflicted AD patients (61, 64). In these two studies, participants were exposed to a number of photographs of faces they did not previously know: 15 faces viewed 5 times each, and 19 viewed 3 times each. They were not asked to remember them (they had, for example, to name the color of the eyes). Then, pairs of photographs were presented, each pair containing one face already shown and one new – not seen before. The par-ticipants had to say which face they preferred. The patients, just like normal people, showed a significant tendency to prefer those faces to which they had previously been exposed. However, in a subsequent task of explicitly stating whether they recognized the faces, only the normal participants were capable of attaining more than a chance score. The effect was reproduced further in 10 AD patients in the auditory dimension, using unfamiliar melodies presented once, 5 times or 15 times (43): the AD patients demonstrated a normal MEE, even when the melodies had been presented to them in the exposition phase only once (see 19, for a study that does not highlight the exposure effect in the auditory domain in AD patients).

As to implicit statistical learning, several studies have highlighted, at least in the mild stages of AD, preservation of the capacities for learning artificial grammar (47) and for the visual categorization process (7, 23). Moussard and collaborators (38) have shown that categorization processes in the auditory dimension are equally preserved in mild to moderate stages of AD. In this study, 12 AD patients [5 in the light stage of the disease (MMSE = 21) and 7 in the moderate stage (MMSE = 20)], nonmusicians, learned implicitly to categorize musical styles. During the exposition phase, they heard 20 excerpts from the works of J. S. Bach, from the baroque period of music. In the test phase, new Bach excerpts were mixed with excerpts from two stylistically different periods: romantic (Brahms, Chopin, Schubert, and Schumann), and early twentieth century (Ravel, Debussy, Scriabin, and Prokoviev). Taking account of the difficulties certain AD patients have in verbal understanding, and of their large measure of forgetfulness (particularly with those in the moderate stage), the implicit task demanded was the simplest possible. The participants were not asked to classify the new items by function of what had been heard before but to say for each excerpt whether they had the impression they had heard the music a little earlier in the exercise. Although all the excerpts were new to them, and to them, all belonged to the general category popularly known as "classical music," both the patients and a group of control participants matched to them for age said that they had heard the Bach excerpts more often than excerpts from the other two categories.

The probabilistic classification task (29) is another type of probability learning that has been tested in AD patients (10, 11). In this task, participants must predict which of two possibilities (e.g., rain or shine) is foretold by different geometric figures displayed on cards (see **Fig. 3**).

Each figure presented on the cards (collection of circles, squares, diamonds, or triangles) is associated in a more or less robust manner with one of the two possible

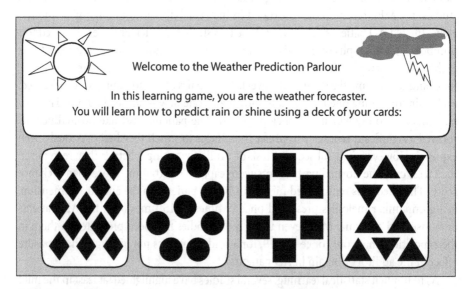

Fig. 3 - Exemple of the card sets presented to participants in the probabilistic classification task (29), after an illustration in Sage and collaborators (54).

replies, and the subject spots this association implicitly as and when in 50 attempts at the task. The predictive success increases, therefore, as the trial runs on, until the results become different from a chance response, even though the subjects are not capable of verbalizing the rules by which they respond. Eight patients with mild AD (11) and 22 in mild or moderate stages (10) showed, in the test, classification capacities equivalent to those of normal subjects. These results are often interpreted in light of the arguments they imply for the normal functioning of this type of learning, notably for the cerebral structures correspondingly implicated (and which are therefore not damaged by the AD); but they show us equally up to what point AD patients are capable of new, even complex, learning in the implicit mode.

A further statistical learning paradigm much studied in AD patients is SRT (see 26, for a review of five studies in SRT). The first of the studies was lead by Knopman and Nissen (25), who noticed that the majority of AD patients showed themselves capable of acquiring implicit sequential knowledge. Even though their reaction times were overall longer than those of control subjects, the times shrank significantly during the progress of the trials, in a way equivalent to that of normal subjects. Ferraro and his collaborators (13) compared the performances of two AD groups in this task, marked by two different states of advancement of the disease: very mild and mild (defined by scores obtained on the "Clinical Dementia Rating Scale"; 4, 22). In this study, only patients very lightly affected showed learning abilities equivalent to those of normal participants of the same age. The authors concluded that implicit learning capability deteriorated rapidly with the progression of dementia.

However, it is important to note that the SRT task is particularly demanding of both motor function and attention (40, 55). Now, AD often leads to impairment of motion (especially apraxia) and of attention capacities. Such difficulties can therefore present obstacles to a successful achievement of the task demanded, without necessarily meaning that implicit sequential learning processes have been changed. The study by Moussard and collaborators (38), for example, showed it was possible to highlight implicit learning capacities in AD patients with an MMSE score getting as low as 15/30, by adapting the task to the patient. The tasks chosen were of short duration, making simple demands and not requiring motion. Further, they were adapted to the dimension of music, in order to create a more play-like working situation, thus helping to keep the patients' attention. Also in the study, AD patients in the light or moderate stages of their illness gave results equivalent to those of a normal group, matched for age, in categorization tasks (described above) and in segmentation of flow. For the latter task (53), the participants were exposed to an artificial stream of musical tones (57). Six trigrams, each of three different tones, were repeated one after the other, without pause or repetition, for six minutes. In the test phase, the subject had to identify the original trigrams among decoys made of the same tones but ordered differently. Previous studies bearing on this paradigm, most often in the language domain and using a flow of syllables, suggest that subjects exposed to such a continuous flow learn implicitly the transition probabilities between the elements of a trigram (53; see also Chapter "Introducing implicit learning: from the laboratory to the real life", E. Bigand and C. Delbé). This process allows us to extract the units that make up the flow, even though no acoustic indicator is given to separate the trigrams that make it up.

In conclusion, implicit memory and implicit learning found in AD patients are more heterogeneous than those in amnesiac patients. The difference is perhaps to be found in that amnesics' problems with declarative memory are relatively unconnected with anything else, while memory perturbations in AD patients are associated also with other problems of cognitive, motor, or behavioral disorders, which interfere with the achievement of tasks set in the laboratory. Whatever the case, numerous studies show that AD patients demonstrate preservation of some memory capacity, even of quite complex learning. This retained skill of acquiring new information, despite severe impairment or even total loss of declarative memory (especially episodic), should be of great interest for the therapeutic management of such patients. Different applications based on theories of implicit memory have already been proposed; the therapeutic use of the capacity for statistical learning remains at the theoretical stage even today.

Implications for rehabilitation

There is some consensus nowadays to qualify the pertinence of traditional approaches to memory rehabilitation, principally those grounded in a "muscular" conception of memory (33) and especially in the case of severe confusion or advanced dementia. Until the 1980s, the dominant approach to memory reeducation consisted in trying to restore the lost function by nonspecific, repetitive exercises, as if memory were a muscle that had to be made to work to improve its efficacy. But several studies failed to show any benefit from these therapeutic strategies; at most, the progress observed was limited to the matter trained and not transferred to situations of daily life (33). The failure of traditional methods in memory rehabilitation is particularly marked in cases of severe memory damage, as for HM (50). The emergence of a multiplicity of studies showing preservation of some capacity in those patients suffering large deterioration of declarative memory has given rise to a new way of thinking about reeducation. The idea is to use those intact capacities of implicit learning and implicit memory for the acquisition of knowledge in specific domains. Various strategies derived from this principle have been elaborated in the field of associative and procedural implicit memories. Others would see the light of day in the domain of statistical learning.

Implicit memory

Various learning techniques allow the acquisition of new knowledge by implicit memory. The most documented are the following: errorless learning (6, 24, 33), vanishing cues method (24), and spaced retrieval method (60).

In errorless learning technique, the idea is that errors produced during learning interfere with correct responses. The process is all the more important to persons suffering an affliction of explicit memory because the errors are stored by way of the intact implicit memory, and the explicit processes that normally deliberately correct and strengthen correct responses are not available to these patients (2, 24). Errorless learning consists in minimizing error production by giving the correct response several times immediately after the question, instead of making the patient work it out. During the test, the subjects are also asked to give the reply so that they are certain of it (41).

The vanishing cues method consists in having the subject learn an information target (most often verbal – one word) while the characters of which it is composed are progressively shaved off (e.g., CARROT, CARRO..., and so on down to CA..., C...). Should the subject become incapable of completing the word correctly, the test is repeated from the previous step, and shaving begins anew. The technique is controversial, however: it seems that patients remain so dependent on the final character that is shown to them (so the first letter, C) that they are lost if this is also suppressed (33). In a comparative review of 27 studies, Kessels and De Haan (24) suggested that patients benefit more from the errorless learning technique than from vanishing cues, which takes more time and does not seem to improve significantly on the methods chosen as controls.

Finally, the spaced retrieval method consists in having an information target repeated (e.g., the question "Where are the keys kept?" – answer "On the hall dresser") at ever greater time intervals (e.g., 15 s, 40 s, 1 minute, 3 minutes, and 5 minutes). If the patient gets stuck, the interval is brought back to the earlier length that allowed correct recovery of the information; then it is lengthened again, as before, until the information is remembered seemingly automatically and more or less permanently.

These different techniques can be used for patients suffering from severe diseases of memory (such as amnesia and AD), for example, for acquisition of procedural knowledge. Glisky and his collaborators (16, 17) gave several amnesic patients (including KC) the opportunity to acquire, through the vanishing cues method, the necessary skills for using computer programs (handling of text – saving and printing, and so on). In another study, the spaced retrieval technique was used to teach patients in the early stage of AD to use a mobile telephone (31).

The same techniques have also been used for associative learning in implicit memory, for example, association of face and name by AD patients (5, 8, 60). The procedures were particularly helpful for the day-to-day life: they allowed, for example, the relearning of the first names of the children and grandchildren of the patient, that which the suffering tied to this loss of memory and identity concerning his or her own family. Adapting the learning situation to the needs of the patient is an essential element of these new techniques of rehabilitation. Hopper (20) gives two cases of dementia patients who underwent therapy, based on implicit memory, adapted to their own needs. Patient SB, for example, suffered confusion in communication and periods of aggression aggravated by poor hearing and his refusal to wear a hearing aid. His carers' problems lay in anticipating his aggressive behavior and in knowing whether he had understood what they said. One of the strategies put in place for SB used the spaced retrieval technique to teach him to ask his carers to repeat sentences he had not understood. In the seven training sessions, the patient held a card whereon was written "Say that again." He had to read the card each time the therapist put the question "What do you say if you don't understand me?" In association with further techniques put in place in between the patient and the carers, communication with patient SB was improved and his aggressive behavior regulated.

An important point to take into account in the study of strategies of rehabilitation is the length of time the new learning will persist. Few studies test the long-term retention of information learned by these protocols, but it seems that knowledge acquired by implicit means is relatively robust compared to knowledge acquired explicitly: a further point encouraging to the development of these strategies.

Learning statistical regularities

So far as we know, no rehabilitation technique has to date exploited a preserved capacity for statistical learning, as it has been measured by the paradigms described above (SRT, artificial grammar, categorization, or segmentation of flow). Such a therapy is rather more difficult to conceive because of the only slight connection apparent between paradigms of implicit learning and the activities of daily life of a patient suffering AD. We know, in addition, that learning in demented patients is often situation specific to the training method; knowledge gained is difficult to transfer (at least, in a spontaneous manner) to another domain or situation (33). Tasks useful for therapy must therefore be conceived to correspond as closely as possible to patients' daily lives (which is not the case with the laboratory paradigms, more abstract, described above).

To meet this condition, retained capacities for learning statistical regularities could be exploited by establishing in patients routines, automatisms, which support their functioning in their normal daily lives, especially in those AD patients who live in an institution with a regular daily rhythm (meal times, activity times, and so on). Orientation in space and time is, for example, one of the functions rapidly impaired in the early stages of dementia. Let us develop an example of a strategy that could permit patients to find markers in time. The idea is to present melodies to the patients, each melody corresponding to a specific time. The timber could give the day of the week (e.g., flute for Wednesday), and the tempo the time of day (slow for the morning, and rapid for the afternoon). In a multiple exposure to the different melodies, the patient would see, for example, a picture with a light that lit up for the half-day that corresponded to the melody heard, and should name the time of day (to be sure he or she was attentive to the task, and the picture made sense). To test afterward his implicit knowledge of the association between the indicators contained in the melodies and the 14 different times (half-days) of day, the patient should point out the square in the picture matching each melody heard. Once the association has been created, a loudspeaker will broadcast throughout the institution the melody corresponding to the half-day in course (in the manner of a carillon). The patient would then probably be capable of telling us the day of the week and the part of the day in which we found ourselves, without however having any memory of the training sessions and without even being conscious that it was the melody he heard that gave him the information. An advantage of this paradigm is that the melodic sequences could be made more complex to carry further temporal information (like the month, the season, ...).

Another idea could be to favor actions organized in fixed sequences, for those patients who give good performances in sequential learning (e.g., in the SRT task). It could be beneficial, for example, if all carers helping the task of washing the patient carried out the movements always in the same order for each patient. Washing might thus become better accepted and proceed more smoothly, the patient being capable of anticipating the sequence of movements (which would also minimize the anxiety sometimes linked to this activity).

Future research in this domain may lead to the elaboration of simple techniques, easily applied within an institution, capable of improving the quality of daily life of patients afflicted by invasive impairment of declarative memory.

Conclusion

This chapter is a nonexhaustive review of the possibilities offered by implicit learning and implicit memory in those patients afflicted by a major disorder of declarative memory. It is to be noted that we have chosen here to favor the presentation of those studies that show preservation of these implicit capacities; others qualify these effects, or do not highlight them. Whatever the case, and although there is always a debate in cognitive psychology on the nature of knowledge thus acquired (see Chapter "Introducing implicit learning: from the laboratory to the real life", E. Bigand and C. Delbé), there is no doubting the fact that, in certain situations, amnesic or AD patients show themselves capable of acquiring complex knowledge to the same degree as normal subjects (or at least in a way that is significant). Studies concerning the use of these capabilities in rehabilitation, still too few, show that the patients are capable of benefiting from those approaches based on preserved processes and the acquisition of specific knowledge. These strategies facilitate better functioning and an advantageous autonomy in their daily lives, sometimes sufficient to lead to professional reinstatement (1). They must be further studied and their practice extended progressively to a large number of institutions taking into care this type of patient. Let us note finally that the accent should always be placed on the capacities and specific needs of each patient, where an in-depth neuropsychological assessment is needed (to determine precisely which functions are preserved and which impaired) and where interaction is required with the patient's family. The family will help specify those difficulties that are most debilitating in their daily round and will support putting in place the chosen strategy of rehabilitation.

Acknowledgments

We thank the Fondation Médéric Alzheimer (30 rue de Prony, 75017 Paris, France) for financial support for the study by Moussard *et al.* (2008) described in this chapter and Barbara Tillman for kindly furnishing part of the material used with the patients in this study.

References

1. Andrewes D, Gielewski E (1999) The work rehabilitation of a herpes simplex encephalitis patient with anterograde amnesia. Neuropsychol Rehabil 9(1):77-99

2. Baddeley A (1992) Implicit memory and errorless learning: a link between cognitive theory and neuropsychological rehabilitation? In: Squire LR, Butters N (eds) Neuropsychology of memory. Guilford Press, New York

3. Balota DA, Duchek JM (1991) Semantic priming effects, lexical repetition effects, and contextual disambiguation effects in healthy aged individuals and individuals with senile dementia of the Alzheimer type. Brain Lang 40(2): 181-201

4. Berg L (1988) Clinical dementia rating (CDR). Psychopharmacol Bullet 24:637-639

5. Bier N, et al. (2008) Face-name association learning in early Alzheimer's disease: a comparison of learning methods and their underlying mechanisms. Neuropsychol Rehabil 18(3):343-371

6. Bier N, Vanier M, Meulemans T (2002) Errorless learning: a method to help amnesic patients learn new informations. J Cogn Rehabil 20(3):12-18

7. Bozoki A, Grossman M,Smith EE (2006) Can patients with Alzheimer's disease learn a category implicitly? Neuropsychologia 44(5):816-827

8. Clare L, et al. (2002) Relearning face-name associations in early Alzheimer's disease. Neuropsychology 16(4):538-547

9. Cleeremans A, Destrebecqz A, Boyer M (1998) Implicit learning: news from the front. Trends Cogn Sci 2(10):406-416

10. Colla M, et al. (2003) MR spectroscopy in Alzheimer's disease: gender differences in probabilistic learning capacity. Neurobiol Aging 24(4):545-552

11. Eldridge LL, Masterman D, Knowlton BJ (2002) Intact implicit habit learning in Alzheimer's disease. Behav Neurosci 116(4):722-726

12. Eustache F, Desgranges B, Messerli P (1996) Edouard Claparède et la mémoire humaine. Revue Neurologique 152:600-610

13. Ferraro FR, Balota DA, Connor LT (1993) Implicit memory and the formation of new associations in nondemented Parkinson's disease individuals and individuals with senile dementia of Alzheimer type: a serial reaction time (SRT) investigation. Brain Cogn 21(2):163-180

14. Fleischman DA, et al. (1999) Word-stem completion priming in healthy aging and Alzheimer's disease: the effects of age, cognitive status, and encoding. Neuropsychology 13(1):22-30

15. Gabrieli JD, et al. (1993) Intact acquisition and long-term retention of mirror-tracing skill in Alzheimer's disease and in global amnesia. Behav Neurosci 107(6):899-910

16. Glisky EL (1992) Acquisition and transfer of declarative and procedural knowledge by memory-impaired patients: a computer data-entry task. Neuropsychologia 30(10):899-910

17. Glisky EL, Schacter DL, Tulving E (1986) Computer learning by memory-impaired patients: acquisition and retention of complex knowledge. Neuropsychologia 24(3):313-328

18. Grafman J, et al. (1990) Implicit learning in patients with Alzheimer's disease. Pharmacopsychiatry 23(2):94-101

19. Halpern AR, O'Connor MG (2000) Implicit memory for music in Alzheimer's disease. Neuropsychology 14(3):391-397

20. Hopper TL (2003) "They're just going to get worse anyway": perspectives on rehabilitation for nursing home residents with dementia. J Commun Disord 36(5):345-359

21. Howard DV, Howard JH (1992) Adult age differences in the rate of learning serial patterns: evidence from direct and indirect tests. Psychol Ageing 7:232-241

22. Hughes CP, et al. (1982) A new clinical scale for the staging of dementia. Br J Psychiatry 140:556-572

23. Kéri S, et al. (2001) Are Alzheimer's disease patients able to learn visual prototypes? Neuropsychologia 39(11):1218-1223

24. Kessels RP, De Haan EH (2003) Implicit learning in memory rehabilitation: a meta-analysis on errorless learning and vanishing cues methods. J Clin Exp Neuropsychol 25(6):805-814

25. Knopman DS, Nissen MJ (1987) Implicit learning in patients with probable Alzheimer's disease. Neurology 37(5):784-788

26. Knowlton BJ, Ramus SJ, Squire LR (1992) Intact artificial grammar learning in amnesia: dissociation of category-level knowledge and explicit memory for specific instances. Psychol Sci 3:172-179

27. Knowlton BJ, Squire LR (1993) The learning of categories: parallel brain systems for item memory and category knowledge. Science 262:1747-1749

28. Knowlton BJ, Squire LR (1996) Artificial grammar learning depends on implicit acquisition of both abstract and exemplar-specific information. J Exp Psychol Learn Mem Cogn 22(1):169-181

29. Knowlton BJ, Squire LR, Gluck MA (1994) Probabilistic classification learning in amnesia. Learn Mem 1(2):106-120

30. Kuzis G, et al. (1999) Explicit and implicit learning in patients with Alzheimer disease and Parkinson disease with dementia. Neuropsychiatry Neuropsychol Behav Neurol 12(4):265-269

31. Lekeu F, et al. (2002) Training early Alzheimer patients to use a mobile phone. Acta Neurol Belgica 102(3):114-121

32. Meulemans T (1998) L'apprentissage implicite: Une approche cognitive, neuropsychologique et développementale. Solal, Marseille

33. Meulemans T (2001) Rééducation du fonctionnement mnésique: perspectives actuelles. Arobase 5(1-2):91-103

34. Meulemans T, Van der Linden M (2002) Artificial grammar learning in amnesia. In: Cleeremans A, French R (eds) Implicit learning and consciousness: an empirical, philosophical and computational consensus in the making. Psychology Press

35. Meulemans T, Van der Linden M (2003) Implicit learning of complex information in amnesia. Brain Cogn 52:250-257

36. Milner B (1968) Disorders of memory after brain lesions in man. Neuropsychologia 6:175-179

37. Milner B (2005) The medial temporal-lobe amnesic syndrome. Psychiatr Clin N Am 28:599-611

38. Moussard A, et al. (2008) Préservation des apprentissages implicites en musique dans le vieillissement normal et la maladie d'Alzheimer. 18(1-2):127-152

39. Nicolas S, Guillery-Girard B, Eustache F (2007) Les maladies de la mémoire. Editions In Press, Paris

40. Nissen MJ, Bullemer PT (1987) Attentional requirements for learning: evidence from performance measures. Cogn Psychol 19(1):1-32

41. Parkin AJ, Hunkin NM, Squires EJ (1998) Unlearning John Major: the use of errorless learning in the reacquisition of proper names following herpes simplex encephalitis. Cogn Neuropsychol 15:361-375

42. Perruchet P, Vinter A (1998) Feature creation as a by-product of attentional processing. Behav Brain Sci 21:33-34

43. Quoniam N, et al. (2003) Implicit and explicit emotional memory for melodies in Alzheimer's disease and depression. Ann N Y Acad Sci 999:381-384

44. Reber AS (1989) Implicit learning and tacit knowledge. J Exp Psychol Gen 118(3):219-235

45. Reber AS (1992) The cognitive unconscious: an evolutionary perspective. Conscious Cogn 1(2):93-133

46. Reber AS, Walkenfeld FF, Hernstadt R (1991) Implicit and explicit learning: individual differences and IQ. J Exp Psychol Learn Mem Cogn 17(5):888-896

47. Reber PJ, Martinez LA, Weintraub S (2003) Artificial grammar learning in Alzheimer's disease. Cogn Affect Behav Neurosci 3(2):145-153

48. Reber PJ, Squire LR (1994) Parallel brain systems for learning with and without awareness. Learn Mem 1(4):217-229

49. Reed JM, et al. (1999) Learning about categories that are defined by object-like stimuli despite impaired declarative memory. Behav Neurosci 113(3):411-419

50. Rosenbaum RS, et al. (2005) The case of K.C.: contributions of a memory-impaired person to memory theory. Neuropsychologia 43:989-1021

51. Saffran JR, Aslin RN, Newport EL (1996) Statistical learning by 8-month-old infants. Science 274:1926-1928

52. Saffran JR, et al. (1999) Statistical learning of tone sequences by human infants and adults. Cognition 70:27-52

53. Saffran JR, Newport EL, Aslin RN (1996) Word segmentation: the rôle of distributional cues. J Mem Lang 35:606-621

54. Sage JR, et al. (2003) Analysis of probabilistic classification learning in patients with Parkinson's disease before and after pallidotomy surgery. Learn Mem 10(3):226-236

55. Squire LR (1986) Mechanisms of memory. Science 232:1612-1619

56. Squire LR, Knowlton BJ (1995) Learning about categories in the absence of memory. Proc Natl Acad Sci U S A 92(26):12470-12474

57. Tillmann B, McAdams S (2004) Implicit learning of musical timbre sequences: statistical regularities confronted with acoustical (dis)similarities. J Exp Psychol Learn Mem Cogn 30(5):1131-1142

58. Van Halteren-Van Tilborg IA, Scherder EJ, Hulstijn W (2007) Motor-skill learning in Alzheimer's disease: a review with an eye to the clinical practice. Neuropsychol Rev 17(3):203-212

59. Vandenberghe M, et al. (2006) Can amnesic patients learn without awareness? New evidence comparing deterministic and probabilistic sequence learning. Neuropsychologia 44:1629-1641

60. Vanhalle C, et al. (1998) Putting names on faces: use of spaced retrieval strategy in a patient with dementia of Alzheimer type. ASHA, American Speech and Hearing Association, Special Interest Division 2. Neurophysiol Neurogenic Speech Lang Disord 8:17-21

61. Willems S, Adam S, Van der Linden M (2002) Normal mere exposure effect with impaired recognition in Alzheimer's disease. Cortex 38(1):77-86

62. Willems S, Salmon E, Van der Linden M (2008) Implicit/explicit memory dissociation in Alzheimer's disease: the consequence of inappropriate processing? Neuropsychology 22(6):710-717

63. Willingham BB, et al. (1997) Patients with Alzheimer's disease who cannot perform some motor skills show normal learning of other motor skills. Neuropsychology 11(2):261-271

64. Winograd E, et al. (1999) The mere exposure effect in patients with Alzheimer's disease. Neuropsychology 13(1):41-46

Learning processes and recovery of higher functions after brain damage

M. Barat, J.-M. Mazaux, P.-A. Joseph and P. Dehail

All brain damage, whatever its nature (usually vascular or traumatic), gives rise to serious deficiencies that are often interconnected. Some may be described as elementary to the extent that they result from changes to the sensorimotor cortex or primary sensorial cortex (rolandic areas, visual cortex, or primary auditive areas), or nervous pathways originating from them or projecting out of them. Others concern the so-called higher functions based on the multimodal association cortex, of which, it should be remembered, the surface is phylogenetically most developed in the human species; the association cortex conforms to the now largely relativized principle of functional asymmetry of the hemispheres.

Changes in the great symbolic functions such as language, memory, praxias, gnosias, and executive functions make neuropsychological or cognitive handicap unique. Developmental psychology has long since shown the reality of changes in brain activity under the influence of intensive and systematic training and the influence of external stimuli on the structuring and function of the brain. Even if, as J. P. Changeux has underlined (11), knowledge is acquired by a process akin to unlearning because "to learn is to eliminate", the basis of our knowledge, which is constantly renewed, follows a permanent, dynamic process of synaptic reorganization or cerebral plasticity. The discovery of this idea of cerebral plasticity is basic in neuropsychology because it underlies the principle of recovery after brain damage. Today it can even be confirmed *in vivo* by the techniques of functional imagery (fRMN, PET scan, …). Neuroplasticity is a permanent phenomenon that provides the basis for the effectiveness of learning processes, memorization, and adaptation to the environment. It is precisely this neuroplasticity that comes into play during the recovery of abilities lost as a result of brain damage. Learning processes work on the brain in two different ways, both of which operate through brain plasticity. In response to a new experience or new stimulation, neuroplasticity induces either changes in an already existing structure or the creation of new connections between neurones. The latter process leads to an increase in the density of synapses, while the former simply reinforces the most efficient or best adapted of the existing pathways. In both cases, it is a matter of "remodelling" the brain in order to acquire these new data and, if required, to preserve them.

But the cognitive deficiency, whether of a selective type (language, praxia, gnosia, memory) or multimodal, intervenes after the brain has matured, on a preexisting cognitive structure, unique because it is intrinsic to that individual.

Damage may therefore be responsible for particular emotional and motivational behaviors that in turn influence the neuropsychological syndrome. Apart from the deficiency, it is appropriate to take into account the effect of pre-morbid factors such as personality variables (age, psychosocial stage of development, intellectual, cultural, and social levels), which will significantly affect the capacity for recovery after damage and the effectiveness of the training techniques offered to the patient.

What are the principles of training in neuropsychology?

Cognitive reeducation assumes a capacity for learning in the brain-damaged person with the aim of improving deficit and so providing greater functional competence in everyday situations (6).

This implies that, quite apart from the theoretical principles underlying the training technique offered to the patient to reduce deficiency, it appears just as important to personalize the therapeutic approach after investigation of the repercussions in the patient's personal and relational life. Anxiety, depression, apathy, reduction in motivation, and difficulties in communication and social interaction must never be underestimated. For the clinical practitioner, training is to be construed holistically to the extent that it implicates in parallel the empathy of the therapist, who relies constantly on the family and on others of significance in the life of the patient.

What are the theoretical bases of training in neuropsychology?

The reeducation of higher brain functions was born out of the treatment of language problems (aphasia) in the second half of the twentieth century. Training techniques and their scientific validation developed in three stages; these techniques are all based on the principle of operant conditioning and follow the same procedural method (45, 46):
   – evaluation **before therapy**, aiming to establish the "baseline" of the deficiency and to work out the programme;
   – **programmed** therapy with periodic measurements, during the program, of the effects of the treatment (analytical tests of the deficiency) and of the application of the acquired abilities in daily life (evaluation by functional profiles);
   – finally, progressive suppression of the training.

Training by the strategy of restoration of the function in deficit

This method postulates that the affected cognitive system retains a great capacity for restoration after lesion, once the period of spontaneous recovery is over (recovery from diaschisis); the aim is to restore the defective function as closely as possible to its state before the illness. The relevant techniques are based on the principles of hierarchical organization of function, from the automatic to the autonomic-voluntary, then to the volitional, from the concrete to the abstract ..., and are put into action procedures of facilitation by repeated and intensive training. This approach, largely inspired by formal pedagogy, may therefore be described as "empirical" to the extent that it assumes high levels of ability to recover, and therefore of neuroplasticity, relying at the same time on the inspirational and relational qualities of the therapist. Such symptomatic training has been described as "semiological reeducation" in the domaine of aphasia (22). Studies of groups of patients in whom neuropsychological matching is always variable and subject to numerous compromises have shown that this method of training is most certainly effective (5).

Training by the strategy of reorganization

This theoretical is developed by cognitive neuropsychology. The proposition is that the problems observed result from selective dysfunction in specific processing components, operating relatively independently, in one or more cognitive architectures (44). It may be said that cognitive neuropsychology proposes the hypothesis that undamaged or potentially reactivable processing units persist in the cognitive function involved.

Starting from detailed analysis of the problem in the cognitive architecture concerned, understanding of the dysfunction allows development of the various stages of treatment:
- to restore the component in deficit;
- to reorganize the cognitive operation using intact functions;
- to alter the environment by reducing constraints on the function in deficit.

This approach, which is very costly in terms of analysis, allows the development of a personalized retraining programme (the "unique case" technique introduced by Marshall and Newcombe (29)).

Pragmatic or "ecological" training

Growth of awareness by neuropsychological therapists of the impact of cognitive problems on the everyday life of patients is relatively recent. It has led to the development of methods of functional evaluation (communication, autonomy, quality of life, ...) and above all to a genuine neuropsychological ergonomy (47) and treatment strategies based on theoretical models of behavior, emotion, activity, and participation. Within this framework may be included the techniques of group work, sociotherapy, replacement techniques, ...

What are the neuropsychophysiological bases of training in neuropsychology?

Two schools of thought about learning are apparent in the neuropsychological reeducation of brain-damaged subjects:
- **Explicit learning**, which depends on the declarative, episodic, and semantic memory, i.e., the capacity, presumed intact, to encode and recover varied infor-

mation in an explicit fashion, with the aim of improving competence after damage ("knowing what"). Such learning is closely linked to the executive attention system. In the explicit form, when learning is activated, the threshold for its reactivation is temporarily reduced. This economical cognitive mechanism may be illustrated by the phenomenon of prompting (e.g., the presentation of a word will prompt similar words: in form, in phonology, in meaning); less effort and attention is then required to repeat the learning exercise: the effectiveness of the treatment increases according to its repetition (reduction in global fRMN activity). The aim of such training by explicit repetition is to automate the cognitive treatment progressively and to reduce the use of attention networks in favor of the temporary reorganization of other networks.

– **Implicit learning**, which depends on the procedural memory, i.e., the ability to acquire "savoir-faire" ("knowing how") or skills through implicit learning. Procedural memory and implicit learning overlap extensively (31). Whereas the procedural memory is built on the acquisition of S-S associations (stimulus-stimulus), procedural memory is the automation of S-R associations (stimulus-response) in conditions of required actions. Finally, implicit learning may be defined as "nonepisodic learning, incidental with respect to complex information, without consciousness of what has been learned" (42). Such "incidental and unconscious" learning occurs without the person being aware of it. The skill that is progressively automated is with difficulty accessible to the consciousness and cannot be expressed verbally; it concerns the acquisition of complex knowledge, sensitive to factors of regularity in the environment.

While these two forms of learning compete in the elaboration and development of our cognition, the practical issue for any given patient concerns the ability to use the declarative memory and/or the procedural memory.

Most techniques of reeducation in neuropsychology depended until recently on conscious, explicit training. For a little over 10 years now, the attention of research and reeducation has shifted to implicit training with the aim of promoting a generalized functional ability for the acquisition of motor and perceptual skills, the acquisition of cognitive skills, and the acquisition of new knowledge. But the question remains concerning the possible interactions between these two approaches (**Table 1**).

Assuming that the idea of anatomical-functional separation of learning processes is accepted, three methods of intervention may be envisaged:

– A **"top-down"** method favoring cognitive representation, bringing into play attention processes, possibly mental imagery, or mental imagery manipulated by virtual reality (cf. Chapter "Virtual reality for learning and rehabilitation" E. Klinger, *et al.*). The association with repetitive transcranial magnetic stimulation (rTMS) is currently being assessed. According to the way it is used, it operates by activating or inhibiting connections on the stimulated side, offering possibilities for modeling cerebral plasticity.

Table 1 - Two types of learning processes.

Explicit		Implicit
		Sensorimotor skills
Declarative memory Episodic memory		Repetition
Exposure to stimuli		Automation Nonconscious
Conscious		
Temporal cortex		Basal ganglia Cerebellum
Cognitive representation	<Interaction?>	Sensorimotor representation

- A **"bottom-up"** method acting on sensorimotor representations at the infra-conscious level, the aim of which is activation of cognitive representation. With the same objective, the recent approaches of constraint therapy, automation, and sensorimotor manipulations may also be cited. Repetition acting on senso-rimotor representations produces the same effects of reduction in activation threshold. For example, repetition of a movement is facilitated if the parameters of time, strength, and direction are kept the same.
- Finally, a combination of the "top-down" and "bottom-up" methods in the same patient.

The description of mirror neurones provided by Rizzolatti and Craighero (40) may drastically alter neurophysiological concepts of learning. Demonstrated in the fron-toparietal complex of subhuman primates, mirror neurones are activated both by the processes of execution and by the observation of actions carried out by a third party. The possible significance of this network system is that it is essential for the acquisition of language (38), understanding the actions of others (theory of mind), learning of new abilities by imitation and mental imagery. The idea of a shared perception-action neu-ronal substratum, the bases of which are the networks of activation linking the goals and consequences of an action or the continuity between planning, perception, and action, supports sensorimotor representations common to mental representation (evocation), performance of an action, and learning (observation), and reconciles the two approaches: top-down and bottom-up. These concepts appear to confirm that parallel treatment models may be substituted for serial treatment models.

Learning processes and reeducation of language disorders: development of ideas

Reeducation of acquired language disorders (aphasias) is the preferred model in the development of ideas about training after brain damage. The last decade of the twentieth century saw the end of the controversy surrounding the effectiveness of reeducation. This has now been firmly established by well-run clinical tests, based on sound methodology, and by functional neuroimaging studies showing the direct impact of reeducation on brain metabolism and cortical neuroplasticity.

Reconciliation of training techniques in aphasia

The empiricist (training by restoration) and cognitivist (training by reorganization) schools of thought are now reconciled. The development of a therapy localizes the disturbed processing levels (semantic, lexical, or phonological) as well as the cognitive components involved (processing mechanisms, conversions, psycholinguistic stocks, access to representations), referring to cognitive neuropsychological models. The most recent, neoconnectionist, types of model insist on the simultaneity and interaction of activations: undertaking a language task activates simultaneously and in a reciprocal fashion lexico-semantic and phonological representations, not merely of the targeted item but also of its "neighbors". The information therefore spreads instantly through parallel, complex, and interconnected networks. The phenomena of inhibition, allocation of attention resources and modification of synaptic charge, are of overriding importance. Although the evidence provided by functional neuroimagery gives weight to connectionist theories, seemingly closer to the organizational reality of brain networks than cognitive models, speech therapist practice has yet to model clear strategies in this area. Current techniques still depend largely on the principle of treatment by sequential rather than parallel models. Taking the example of techniques intended to reduce anomia, at the heart of the various clinical types of aphasia, the tasks demanded call into play, in the most specific way possible, the phonemic, graphemic, or semantic systems, or in reading the pathway of "addressing" or "assembling". Besides, more and better account is taken of the dissociations established in scientific literature: nouns/verbs, animated/manufactured nouns, access/stock disorders, and so on. The influence of semantic complexity (typicity) and syntactic complexity is also taken into account. As for learning through facilitation (cueing, priming, repetition, multimodal stimulation, mental imagery, use of missing words, introduction of a delay, use of computers), its effectiveness is difficult to establish because the symptom of anomia probably depends on different mechanisms from one patient to another. Hence, it is important to clearly identify the nature of the deficiency (46).

Anomia therapies during aphasia (45)

Two main forms of therapy could be proposed in accordance with cognitive analysis:

1. Semantic therapy to restore semantic/lexical representations. Various tasks ask the patient to perform the semantic treatment with the proposed material.

– Semantic judgment when asking a response "yes/no" to a question concerning categorization (*is an apple a fruit?*), function (*is an apple could be eat?*), or specific attributes (*is an apple have a stone?*)

– Matching two items with semantic functional link (*glass/bottle, tree/door/ arm-chair*). The pairing is proposed with pictures, writing words, or both

– Matching verbal or writing definition and a pictured information ("*point out the object which is used to gum*"/*gum, pencil, ruler, ink*)

– Matching between two representations with the same concept (verbal or written word, picture)

2. Phonological therapy to restore the accessibility of the phonological representation in order to decrease activation levels, which are too much high: serial tasks are needed inciting the patient to produce verbal form of the word. Repetitive verbal production of the word contribute to decrease the level.

– Loud voice lecture of a written word with facilitation by a "phonemic key"

– Repetition many times

– Verbal denomination with a "phonemic key" at the beginning or at the end of the sentence

The pragmatic approach and the psychosocial approach

These approaches are undergoing considerable development. The PACE (promoting aphasic's communication effectiveness) (20) has expressed great interest in involving patients in total communication training that is not solely verbal. The availability from clinicians of valid tools of communication (19) and the introduction of the techniques of analysis of conversation (conversational analysis, CA) represent remarkable progress. CA sets out to analyze the impact of aphasia on the natural interactions between the aphasic subjects and their usual interlocutors, and more precisely to identify how these partners collaborate in the success (or failure) of the conversation. On the one hand CA helps to pinpoint the most disabling aphasic deficiencies in everyday communication, which then become the priority targets of reeducation; on the other hand, it identifies the strategies adopted by the participants to improve communicational efficiency. Starting with this analysis, the therapist can:

a. provide information about the nature of the patient's difficulties;

b. offer advice for improved participation in the success of the conversation;

c. provide a lead in putting these into practice.

This technique demonstrably improves the practical efficiency of communication, even though the linguistic capacities of the aphasic subject remain unchanged (8). Such treatment methods are typically found where the priority is adaptation of the environment to reduce social disadvantage and improve participation.

In the same spirit, training in the use of communication notebooks for severe global aphasias has confirmed its superiority over computerized functional replacement therapies, which have never properly taken off. Finally, the adaptation to aphasia of training by constraint and without error should be mentioned. This takes the form of short consecutive sessions in which patients are made to practise intensively those language tasks that they find most difficult (37, 49).

The effectiveness of communication groups in the chronic phase of aphasia has also been demonstrated (23). The objective of such groups, led by volunteers and anchored in the natural environment of the patients, is to reinforce the initiation of communication, delivery of messages, awareness of problems, attention to personal objectives, and increase in confidence.

The question remains concerning the intensity and duration of the therapeutic process. The literature agrees on the principle of sustained reeducation, several hours per week during the first two years. But intermittent "intensive" courses, aimed at reducing particularly persistent symptoms (problems with written language, problems of naming) may prove effective many years after brain damage (4).

Learning processes and reeducation of perceptual gnostic disorders

Implicit learning, the principles of which were recalled above, has been defined as the "ability of the human being to detect and integrate unconsciously the regularities, even complex ones, which constitute his or her environment (physical, linguistic, social, ...) with the objective of interacting more efficiently with the environment" (10). In a sense, we learn about the regularity of the world, how it is organized, and how it is structured, without even noticing (30, 31). From the earliest stage of cognitive development, a large proportion of knowledge is acquired by nonconscious mechanisms. No training can exist therefore without implicit treatment of perceptual processes.

Recent experimental data have shown that "unified" perception develops according to parallel though different methods of neurophysiological processing. There is a functional segregation between the neuronal networks contributing to recognition ("what") and to localization ("where") both for visual (32) and for auditive data (14). This probably also applies to the sense of touch (21). Recognition (the "what" pathway) brings into play a ventral network, temporal for explicit processing in the semantic memory, which is picked up by the episodic declarative memory, whereas localization (the "where" pathway) depends on a dorsal network, parietal for implicit processing in the procedural memory.

This dichotomy in perceptual processing and its representation provides a fertile model for developing therapeutic strategies after brain damage, relying on assessment of the intact connections between perception and the different types of memory. Several questions present themselves (10):

- What remains of the perceptual representation system in the semantic memory and what effect does priming have on access to conscious representation?
- What is the content of representations remaining after damage and what ability remains to construct new ones? (Example of learning unconscious visually guided movements after cortical blindness or "blindsight")
- What level of mental imagery is preserved in agnosias according to the degree of change in the perceptual representation system and what access is available to this representation in the declarative memory? Or conversely, what potential is there for a deficit in the level of representation to develop into a semantic damage?

A current practical application is provided by the strategies of retraining undergoing validation in the reeducation of visuospatial hemineglect syndrome, relying in turn on the implicit or explicit idea that the capacity for learning has been preserved. The formulation of hypotheses for successful therapy develops according to the theoretical level of the cognitive dysfunction: disorder of selective attention on the hemispace, disorder of the implicit representation of this space, implicit directional bias of the subjective vertical position in the egocentric space, ….

1. By a "top-down" approach, the cognitive investing of the neglected space is approached through training for awareness of the bodily space, associated with mental imagery (perhaps manipulated by virtual reality), reinforced by voluntary correction of the deviation in the way of looking in favor of exploration of the neglected space (visual scanning), with the objective of restoring the automaticity of this exploration of the hemispace. Simultaneous hemisphere activation by rTMS is currently under evaluation.

2. In a "bottom-up" approach, implicit sensorimotor representation is reinforced or manipulated by methods aimed at correcting directional bias in space: prismatic adaptation, eye patch, vestibular or electrical stimulation of the neck, constraint therapy of the neglected, or underused hemibody.

3. In a combined approach, "top-down "-"bottom-up" can be associated in voluntary tasks of postural reeducation, attentional engagement in the exploration of space, visual cueing of the subjective vertical, and techniques of sensorial manipulation.

Unilateral neglect syndrome rehabilitation by trunk rotation and scanning training (58)

Using a specific device (Bon Saint Come's device) that consists of two parts:

– The first one is a polysar thoracolumbar vest to which is attached a vertical metal bar that projects forward horizontally just above the apex of the subject head. The extremity of the bar, or pointer, is situated 1.5 m in front of the patient to make an axial rotation of the trunk under visual control to displace the pointer laterally and explore the spatial field. This activity ensures a stimulation of the attention of the trunk posture activity.

– The second part consists of a series of targets attached to a mobile wooden panel placed in front of the patient. The targets, of different geometric form, are connected to a light bulb and to a buzzer. When the pointer is brought into contact with the target, audible and luminous signals are elicited, producing a biofeedback effect. The therapist can also emit these signals using a keyboard.

The initial exercises, carried out from a sitting position, are usually short according to the patient's capacities. During the first sessions, the spatial research is initiated from the right to the left, which is neglected. After gaining adequate control of the trunk (usually in three to five sessions), the patient is asked to perform the same exercises in a standing position with the help of the physiotherapist. The training program is usually applied one hour a day for one month.

Assessment uses a battery of unilateral neglect syndrome (UNS) tests (line bisection, line cancellation, Bell test) and activities of daily living (ADL) test as functional independence measure (FIM).

Comparing with a control group who received conventional therapy (occupational therapy and physiotherapy), patients who received this training improve better in UNS and ADL tests, and the results are maintained after the end of treatment.

This training combines "top-down" and "bottom-up" methods with a synergistic effect between trunk rotation and visual and auditory scanning. The method appears to have a direct effect on UNS and to involve an actual relearning of spatial scanning. The synergistic effect between axial rotation of the trunk, generating specific motor, vestibular, and cerebellar activation, and classic exploratory reconditioning that preferentially activates the cognitive and visual systems. It is suggested that our spatial referent is constantly building by multimodal stimulations (visual, motor, sensitive, vestibular, auditory, and/or cognitive).

Learning processes and memory disorders

The memory systems remain an object of passionate debate. If memory is an entity, the neuropsychological approach to it is based on a hierarchical principle illustrated by the structural-functional model of Tulving (52): a collection of subsystems including the working memory (or short-term memory); the system of perceptual representations (perceptual representation system), which underpins the effects of perceptual priming; the procedural or implicit memory; and the explicit and declarative memory, which brings together the semantic memory (memory of concepts and general knowledge) and the episodic memory (memory of events in their temporal-spatial context).

In the area of severe, long-lasting memory disorders, restrictions in activity and participation are linked essentially to the difficulty, or even the impossibility, of accessing the episodic and declarative memory of events that have happened since the onset of the illness.

Strategies of recovery

Recovery strategies (18) assume that residual memory skills persist, notably via efficient associative cueing strategies in the declarative memory, for example, to find people's names or for active learning of read or heard texts. In an approach of the "top-down" type, the aim is to facilitate encoding and recovery of information.

Verbal mnemotechnical or mental imagery-based procedures have been put forward (55): facilitation effect on the learning of patronymics with presentation of photographs of faces, a technique of the "key word" for learning new vocabulary (27). Yet the facilitating effects of imagery techniques do not appear unless the mnemotechnical link connecting the information to be learned is systematically given to the patient. Comparison of three methods of learning name-face associations has analyzed, respectively, the effects of a mnemotechnical strategy based on imagery, a method of cue reduction making use of abilities preserved in the implicit memory and a multimodal presentation on video (51). Imagery has been shown to be the most effective of these, provided the mnemotechnical link is given. The results emphasize that the effectiveness of mental imagery is a function of the capacity to encode material in the form of mental images and, in the long term, in the form of representations. Studies of the use of imagery and of mnemotechnical methods of facilitating long-term memory invariably insist on a satisfactory level of attentional resources, of good understanding ability, and above all on a high level of motivation. On the other hand, this underlines the failure of such strategies in cases of confirmed dementia or in patients suffering from executive problems (see below).

To date, lasting effects on severely amnesic patients have not been demonstrated using techniques of the "top-down" type depending on attentional processes, and consciousness of the problem. Mental imagery is therefore always uncertain, as is rTMS of the left frontolateral cortex with the aim of activating episodic verbal memory capacities (39).

Strategies using preserved memory capacities (57)

Training methods often rely on supposedly preserved capacities in the implicit procedural memory (48). Despite great variation in patients, some of them will have retained the memory skills necessary for unconscious retention and use of the rules governing the implementation of compensatory strategies. Surprising results may thus be observed in perceptual priming tests for word recognition, allowing acquisition of new material by the semantic memory (acquisition of a computer language, words of a foreign language, new concepts, …), which are not accessible in the declarative memory.

The factors determining the degree to which the acquisition of semantic and procedural information is effective may be expressed as follows (57):
  – concept of familiarity in relation to already known information;
  – suppression of associative interference;
  – pragmatic integration of the signifying context of the items.

In practice, two methods of implicit training are or have been the object of clinical research:
  – The technique of cue reduction (26). The cues provided about the information to recover according to the principle of perceptual priming are progressively reduced. Despite contradictory results, this method has proved to be effective for learning computer vocabulary, confirming the possibility of non-declarative procedural and semantic transition memories.
  – The technique of errorless training (3). The principle is to give the right answer immediately after presentation of the items (e.g., after presentation of the first letters of a target word). This improves learning and reduces the level of memory lapses. The therapist provides the right answer rather than asking for a guess. Encouraging results have been obtained by this method in the learning of politicians' names and the names of friends (34), in learning the names of people and objects, and also in programming electronic memory aids.

Errorless training is designed in such a way that the information presented reduces as far as possible the risk of confusion and works to reinforce the competence of the implicit memory (59). Training in organized note-taking (notebook, diary) and involvement in concrete and familiar situations calling on the memory in an automatic and involuntary fashion all conform to the same errorless principle and can facilitate the operation of procedural memory, allowing patients to recover a certain amount of autonomy in their daily life in well-defined routine areas.

Is training for the acquisition of complex knowledge possible?

Asking this question comes down to asking if the implicit learning of facts, concepts, relations between events, and new procedures can be generalized to procedures that are closely related though different, to help for example the return to professional life. Studies of individual cases suggest a tentative affirmative reply, whether treatment is by implicit training in word processing that may be generalized to allow the manipulation of other computer programmes (56) or by updating procedural and conceptual knowledge by means of previous familiarity with the sphere of activity in the case of a librarian's work (1). Yet in both cases, the inability to remember explicitly the newly acquired knowledge persists.

Learning processes and executive function disorders

Executive dysfunction, attributed to changes in the frontal systems, brings together complex deficiencies in varying degrees: state of alertness (arousal), behavioral vigilance (awareness), selective, divided attention and attentional displacement (focal, divided, and shift), working memory, planning, concept formation, mental flexibility, decision making, reasoning, …. Such dysfunction has major consequences for behavior and social autonomy. Patients suffering from multiple sclerosis, rupture of aneurism of the anterior communicant artery, and severe brain injury make up, though not exclusively, the groups suffering most from these deficiencies.

Among the executive functions, two basic processes play a major role in the global dysfunction: problems of attention and problems of working memory.

1. **Attention**

This is the ruling cognitive function in all forms of training that use the "top-down" model. Attention disorders are commonly addressed through exercises aimed at a specific domain: speed of information processing, training in sustained, focused selective and divided attention, and attentional displacement. Treatments in this area use paradigms of the stimulus-response type requiring patients to identify and solve relevant stimuli among a selection of visual or auditory stimuli presented at varying speeds. The aim is to restore the "basic" attentional capacities by intensive training. Several studies have sought to improve the effectiveness of such treatments by introducing techniques such as feedback and reinforcement by sequential and hierarchically organized training strategies. (33, 35). Yet it remains difficult to separate specific effects resulting from improvement in attentional functions from those related to other executive problems, even within structured techniques of attention training. For example, in the post-acute phase of cranial trauma, current recommendations (12, 13) advise specific training by stimulation tests on basic aspects of attention, notably sustained attention, hierarchical organization of exercises imposing regulation of attention, work on alertness, vigilance, and reaction time.

2. Severe working memory disorders

A defect in short-term memory, verbal and/or visual, alters storage and above all the temporary processing of information. It considerably reduces the speed of information processing with all that that implies for the full range of executive functions. Cognitive psychology suggests a model of the working memory with three components: a central executive, the phonological loop (verbal working memory), and the visuospatial sketchpad (visual working memory) (44). An original approach to retraining of the verbal working memory has recently been proposed (53, 54). Aimed at restoring by means of specific retraining, the exercises target the central executive and the phonological loop by means of storage and processing operations. The prisnciple of increasing mental load is respected: levels of difficulty are arranged hierarchically in terms of the length of items, the level of processing, degree of imagery, frequency of use, speed of presentation, ... The demonstration of its effectiveness and transfer of progress into everyday life has been confirmed (47).

3. Severe brain injury

In this case, the associated cognitive problems make up a mosaic of closely inter-acting dysfunctions that render the analytical approach well-nigh impossible. This observation provides the basis of the holistic neuropsychological reeducation movement (holistic neuropsychologic rehabilitation or comprehensive holistic neuropsychologic rehabilitation) developed by Prigatano (36). This is a global approach targeting therapeutic operations in several areas at once or in sequence: cognitive, emotional, motivational, and interactive. Particular attention is paid to the level of alertness, vigilance, the bases of attentional processes, awareness, emotional control, interaction by self-regulating strategies (self-instructional procedure) and by self-monitoring, retro-control, and self-evaluation (self-instructional training). Hierarchical exercises designed to resolve the problem according to the principle of "goal management technique" and categorization (15) allow action on planning abilities; individual work is associated with group activities and behavioral regulation. Taking responsibility for patients in this way, under contract, has confirmed its clear superiority, compared with standardized, multidisciplinary reeducation, in terms of social autonomy and resumption of work (12, 13).

Holistic training in dysexecutive syndrome after severe traumatic brain injury (TBI) (36)

Personal case

Case of a 24-year-old brilliant student who experienced a severe TBI (Glagow Coma Scale = 3, length of unconsciousness = 3 weeks, cerebral MRI: left frontal and corpus callosum concussions with diffuse axonal bleeding)

After 28 months: impairment of selective and divided attention, of working memory, verbal learning, problem solving, decision making, self-awareness. He had also some anosognosia and depression.

During a four-week training, we proposed:

– a personal rehabilitation program to improve his consciousness of the cognitive deficiencies. We used a strategy from a "global" activity to details. For example, before the TBI, he liked art, history, and architecture; he was asked to prepare a relation on Bordeaux city for which he had a good knowledge and to present it in front of other TBI patients. At the beginning, he was very anxious, and we required him to use a block note where the first data he putted in were strongly confusing and noninformative. We tried to help him to make inquiries. One member of the team proposed to make attendance with him to collect data from the Tourism Office and the City Library, and to visit some districts of the city. We helped him to organize and to order the information. As a rule many problems occurred during this stage: decrease of interest, loss of chronology, loss of the note book, ...

– a group rehabilitation program with other TBI patients. The program included each day one session to explain medical considerations on consequences of the TBI, cerebral functioning of memory and executive function, mood, awareness, behavior, ... and to ask patients what they have understood on their problems. Another session per day is the "newspaper group": all the patients have to participate under the supervision of a psychologist and an occupational therapist at a diary report on daily memory difficulties, on what kind of strategies they used during the daily life. In the same "newspaper group," the patients have to choose a topic they have seen on the TV or read in a newspaper, to make a writing synthesis and to follow the topic during some days. A third session is the "communication group" conducted by a speech therapist: this session uses a videotape during various discursive exchanges. The data of the video are analyzed by the patients with the speech therapist in order to point the adequacy of the transmitted information, coherent or not. The fourth session is oriented to problem solving: the problems to solve are in accordance with daily life and patients' wants: cooking, purchasing, preparing a trip, being aware to the money, writing a CV, ...

Do possibilities exist for training in dementias of the Alzheimer type?

In the past decade, patient suffering, just as much as the socioeconomic cost of these incurable conditions, has led to consideration not merely of simple accompaniment but also of therapeutic procedures other than drug-based ones, which might slow down the process of cognitive decline. The results remain contradictory.

– Certain approaches have favored training methods based on the "top-down" method (learning therapy), essentially in the case of mild cognitive impairment (MCI) or of mild dementia: exercises requiring mental arithmetic or recall of texts (43, 50, 51). Certain methods combine naming exercises with high-frequency rTMS of the prefrontal dorsolateral cortex, with the aim of activating both the rapidity and quantity of words restored. This has enjoyed some success (16, 17). The technique of space retrieval (41) sets out to test recall of the target information at progressively longer intervals. This method has been used in explicit training tests in Alzheimer's disease on problems of naming, object position memory, and name-face associations (9). Comparison of different training methods in explicit and implicit memory has not revealed differences in a test of face-name associations. However, the best results are obtained by patients in whom the episodic memory is still present and when the recall time is ignored (7). The use of structured computer programs does not appear to yield better results (25).

Other, more numerous approaches are based on a global patient treatment (comprehensive rehabilitation program). Among these, training in the activities of daily life (procedural memory) appears to be superior to stimulation of residual cognitive functions (24). Group occupational activities, leisure activities, social interaction, emotional control, and physical activity are favored though not to the exclusion of more cognitive exercises based on recreational computer programs. This combination seems to yield the best results in the maintenance of autonomy and control of psychiatric, behavioral, and emotional disorders (2).

Conclusion

Practitioners confronted by patients suffering from cognitive deficiencies are faced with many methodological constraints: evaluation and especially the impact of deficiencies on the functioning of daily life and restriction of participation, and the choice of retraining method. The issue at stake here is nothing less than the credibility of reeducation in neuropsychology. Theoretical models have developed remarkably, thanks to our knowledge of cerebral function and to the concept of post-lesional plasticity. The fundamental problem is to reduce the effect of fragmentation of the functions assessed by analytical or cognitive neuropsychology and to clarify the transfer of abilities derived from reeducation to everyday life, beyond simply measuring learning of the items involved. The issue at stake in such training, whatever the theoretical modality, is to facilitate the functioning of preserved capacities and means of substitution put into action by patients themselves and their entourage.

References

1. Andrewes D, Gielewski E (1999) The work rehabilitation of a herpes simplex encephalitis patient with anterograde amnesia. Neuropsychological Rehabilitation 9:77-99
2. Atri A, Shanghnessy LW, Locascio JJ, Growdon JH (2008) Long-term course and effectiveness of combination therapy in Alzheimer disease. Alzheimer Dis Assoc Disord 22(3):209-221
3. Baddeley AD, Wilson BA (1994) When implicit learning fails: Amnesia and the problem of error elimination. Neuropsychologia 32: 53-68
4. Barat M, Mazaux JM, Joseph PA (2000) Intérêt de la rééducation prolongée des aphasies en décours des accidents vasculaires cérébraux. La lettre du Neurologue 3(4):151-154
5. Basso A, Capitani E, Vignolo LA (1979) Influence of rehabilitation on language skills in aphasic patients: a controlled study. Arch Neurol 36(4):190-196
6. Ben-Yishay Y, Prigatano GP (1990) Cognitive remediation. In: Rehabilitation of the adult and child with traumatic brain injury. F.A. David, Philadelphia, pp. 393-409
7. Bier N, Van der Linden M, Gagnon L, et al. (2008) Face-name association learning in early Alzheimer's disease: a comparison of learning methods and their underlying mechanisms. Neuropsychol Rehabil 18(3):343-371
8. Booth S, Perkins L (1999) Individualized advice and evaluating change in aphasia. Aphasiology 13(4/5):283-303
9. Camp CJ (1989) Facilitation of new learning in Alzheimer's disease. In: Gilmore GC, Withhouse PJ, Wykle ML (eds) Memory, aging and dementia. Springer, New York
10. Ceccaldi M, Clarke S, Meulemans T (2008) From perception to learning. Rev Neurol (Paris) 164:S154-S163
11. Changeux JP (1979) Théories du langage. Théories de l'apprentissage. Le débat entre Jean Piaget et Noam Chomsky. Centre Royaumont pour une science de l'homme. Seuil (ed), Paris, 525 pp
12. Cicerone KD, Mott T, Azulay J, Friel JC (2004) Community integration and satisfaction with functioning after intensive cognitive rehabilitation for traumatic brain injury. Arch Phys Med Rehab 85(6):943-950
13. Cicerone KD, Mott T, Azulay J, et al. (2008) A randomized controlled trial of holistic neuropsychologic rehabilitation after traumatic brain injury. Arch Phys Med Rehab 12:2239-2249
14. Clarke S, Bellmann A, Thiran A (2004) Auditory reflect: what and where in auditory space. Cortex 40:291-300
15. Constantinidou F, Thomas RD, Scharp VL, et al. (2005) Effects of categorization training in patients with TBI during post acute rehabilitation: preliminary findings. J Head Traum Rehabil 20(2):143-57

16. Cotelli M, Manenti R, Cappa SF, *et al.* (2006) Effect of transcranial magnetic stimulation on action naming in patients with Alzheimer disease. Arch Neurol 63(11):1602-1604

17. Cotelli M, Manenti R, Cappa SF, *et al.* (2008) Transcranial magnetic stimulation improves naming in Alzheimer disease patients at different stages of cognitive decline. Eur J Neurol 15(12):1286-1292

18. Coyette F, Van der Linden M (1999) La rééducation des troubles de la mémoire: les stratégies de facilitation. In: La rééducation en neuropsychologie: études de cas. Solal (ed), Marseille, pp. 209-225

19. Darrigrand B, Mazaux JM (2000) Echelle de communication verbale de Bordeaux. Ortho Edition, Isbergues, France

20. David GA, Wilcox MJ (1981) Incorporating parameters of natural conversation in aphasia treatment. In R. Chapey ed. Language intervention strategies in adult aphasia. Baltimore: Williams et Wilkins: 169-193

21. De Santis L, Spierer L, Clarke S, Murray MM (2007) Getting in touch: segregated somatosensory what and where pathways in humans revealed by electrical neuroimaging. Neuro Image 37(3):890-903

22. Ducarne B (1988) Rééducation sémiologique de l'aphasie. Masson (ed), Paris, 1 vol., 350 pp

23. Elman RJ, Bernstein-Ellis E (1999) The efficacy of group communication treatment in adults with chronic aphasia. J Speech Lang Hear Res 42:411-419

24. Farina E, Mantovani F, Fioravanti R, *et al.* (2006) Evaluating two group programmes of cognitive training in mild-to-moderate AD: is there any difference between a "global" stimulation and a "cognitive-specific" one? Aging Ment Health 10(3):211-218

25. Galante E, Venturini G, Fiaccadori C (2007) Computer-based cognitive intervention for dementia: preliminary results of a randomized clinical trial. G Ital Med Lav Ergon 29(3):26-32

26. Glisky EL, Schacter DL, Tulving E (1986) Learning and retention of computer-related vocabulary in memory-impaired patients: method of vanishing cues. J Clin Exp Neuropsychol 8:292-312

27. Gruneberg MM, Sykes RN, Gillett E (1994) The facilitating effects of mnemonic strategies in two learning tasks in learning disabled adults. Neuropsychol Rehabil 4:241-254

28. Laforce R (2002) Revue des mécanismes d'apprentissage par lesquels le striatum participe à l'apprentissage implicite d'habiletés. Rev Neuropsychol 12(3):379-399

29. Marshall JC, Newcombe F (1973) Patterns of paralexia: a psycholinguistic approach. J Psycholing Res 2:175-179

30. Meulemans T (1998) L'apprentissage implicite. Solal (ed), Marseille

31. Meulemans T (2000) Neuropsychologie de l'apprentissage implicite et de la mémoire procédurale. Rev Neuropsychol 10:129-157

32. Mishkin M, Ungerleider LG, Macko KA (1983) Object vision and spatial vision. Trends Neurosci 6:414-417

33. Novack TA, Caldwell SG, Duke LW, Berquist T (1996) Focused versus unstructured intervention for attention deficits after traumatic brain injury. J Head Trauma Rehabil 11(3):52-60

34. Parkin AJ, Hunkin NM, Squires EJ (1998) Unlearning John Major: the use of errorless learning in the reacquisition of proper names following herpes simplex encephalitis. Cogn Neuropsychol 15:361-375

35. Ponsford JL, Kinsella G (1988) Evaluation of a remedial programme for attentional deficits following closed head injury. J Clin Exp Neuropsychol 10:693-708

36. Prigatano GP (1999) Principles of neuropsychological rehabilitation. Oxford University Press, 1 vol., 374 pp

37. Pulvermuller F, Neininger B, Elbert T, et al. (2001) Constraint induced therapy of chronic aphasia after stroke. Stroke 32(7):1621-1626

38. Ramachandran VS, Oberman LM (2006) Broken mirrors: a theory of autism Sci Am; 295(5):62-9

39. Rami L, Gironch A, Kulisevsky J et al. (2003) Effects of repetitive transcranial magnetic stimulation on memory subtypes: a controlled study. Neuropsychologica 41(14):1877-1883

40. Rizzolatti G, Craighero L (2004) The mirror-neuron system. Annu Rev Neurosci 27:169-192

41. Schacter DL, Rich SA, Stampp MS (1985) Remediation of memory disorders: experimental evaluation of the spaced retrieval technique. J Clin Exp Neuropsychol 7:79-97

42. Seger CA (1994) Implicit learning. Psychol Bullet 115(2):163-196

43. Sekiguchi A, Kawashima R (2007) Cognitive rehabilitation – the learning therapy for the senile dementia. Brain Nerve 59(4):357-365

44. Séron X (1997) La Neuropsychologie cognitive. "Que sais-je" PUF, Paris, 3ème éd

45. Séron X (1997) Rééducation des déficiences cognitives: perspectives théoriques actuelles. In: Ravaud JF, Didier JP, Audilloux C, Aymé S (eds) De la déficience à la réinsertion, pp. 67-86. Editions INSERM, Paris

46. Séron X (1999) Efficacité de la rééducation en neuropsychologie. La rééducation en neuropsychologie: etude de cas. Solal (ed), Marseille, pp. 19-40

47. Séron X, Rossetti Y, Vallat-Azouvi C, et al. (2008) Cognitive rehabilitation. Rev Neurol (Paris) 164:S154-S163

48. Soliveri P, Brown RG, Jahanshabi M, Marsden CD (1992) Procedural memory and neurological disease. Eur J Cogn Psychol 4:161-193

50. Sunderland A, Tuke A (2005) Neuroplasticity, learning and recovery after stroke: a critical evaluation of constraint-induced therapy. Neuropsychol Rehabil 15(2):81-96

51. Talassi E, Guerreschi M, Feriani M, et al. (2007) Effectiveness of a cognitive rehabilitation program in mild dementia (MD) and mild cognitive impairment: a case control study. Arch Gerontol Geriatr 44(1):391-399

51. Thoene AT, Glisky EL (1995) Learning of name-face associations in memory impaired patients: a comparison of different training procedures. J Intern Neuropsychol Soc 1:29-38

52. Tulving E (1995) Organisation of memory: Quo vadis? In: Gazzaniga MS (ed) The cognitive neurosciences, pp. 839-847. MIT Press, Cambridge, MA

53. Vallat C, Azouvi P, Hardisson H, et al. (2005) Rehabilitation of verbal working memory after left hemisphere stroke. Brain Injury 19:1157-1164

54. Vallat-Azouvi C, Azouvi P, Pradat-Diehl P (2007) Rééducation cognitive de la mémoire de travail. In: Aubin G, Coyette F, Pradat-Diehl P, Vallet-Azouvi C (eds) Neuropsychologie de la mémoire de travail, pp. 195-209. Solal, Marseille

55. Van der Linden M, Van der Kaa MA (1989) Reorganization therapy for memory impairments. In: Séron X, Deloche G (eds) Cognitive approaches in neuropsychological rehabilitation, pp. 105-158. Laurence Erlbaum Associates, New York

56. Van der Linden M, Coyette F (1995) Acquisition of word processing knowledge in an amnesie patient: implications for theory and rehabilitation. In: Campbell R, Conway M, Gathercole S (eds) Broken memories: neuropsychological case studies, pp. 54-80. Blackwell, Oxford

57. Van der Linden M, Coyette F, Majerus S (1999) La rééducation des patients amnésiques: exploitation des capacités mnésiques préservées. Ici- La rééducation en neuropsychologie: études de cas. Solal (ed), Marseille, pp. 227-248

58. Wiart L, Bon Saint Corne A, Debelleix X, et al. (1997) Unilateral neglect syndrome rehabilitation by trunk rotation and scanning training. Arch Phys Med Rehabil 78:424-429

59. Wilson BA (2002) Towards a comprehensive model of cognitive rehabilitation. Neuropsychol Rehabil 12(2):97-110

PART III

LEARNING, MEDICAL TRAINING, AND REHABILITATION PRACTICE

Benefits of learning technologies in medical training, from full-scale simulators to virtual reality and multimedia presentations

J.-M. Boucheix, E. Bonnetain, C. Avena and M. Freysz

Introduction

The rapid growth of technology provides a wide range of new learning tools such as multimedia presentations of materials, interactive animated images for anatomy learning, 3-D models, full-scale (FS) patient simulators, and microworld training software, which are virtual reality tools that include high-level interactive haptic properties. These new learning approaches have been recently used in medical training and education.

The use of full-scale simulators for emergency medical training or in anesthesia is becoming a topic of great interest in Europe. Yet, Chopra (15), Gaba (21, 22), Nyseen (39-42), and Murray (43) have shown that anesthesiologists trained on mannequin-based simulators perform better than those not trained on the simulator when handling simulated crisis situations a second time. Simulators have been used since the 1960s to teach crisis management skills to personnel in the military, aviation, space flight, and nuclear power plant operations. Full-scale simulators have also been used to train professionals to perform tasks presenting a high level of risk to human life, which cannot be learned on the job, with a high level of accuracy. Recently, the human simulator has provided educators with a unique opportunity to extend this educational tool to physicians.

Until now, training with full-scale simulators was often limited to senior or expert anesthesiologists for high-risk crisis situations (e.g., anaphylactic shock or malignant hyperthermia (38)). With the recent improvement in technology, new applications for full-scale training arose, particularly in emergency medicine (38) and surgery. Full-scale simulators for emergency medical training could be of great interest for undergraduate medicine students who progressively start working in hospitals. In particular, in France, the manner in which medical studies are organized does not provide for any real specific learning phase between the theoretical classroom sessions that focus on the declarative aspect of knowledge (2) and the real on-the-job situations involving a high level of procedural knowledge (2).

Moreover, it has been well known for a long time in cognitive science that procedural learning requires an extensive amount of practice and that theoretical knowledge is not enough to be able to supervise complex emergency situations. These latter situations require a great level of "situation awareness" (27) during the evolution of a dynamic situation, including time pressure. Full-scale simulators in medical education provide a relevant way to train and enhance the link between the declarative-theoretical aspects of knowledge and the procedural aspects (2) of medical skills (**Fig. 1**).

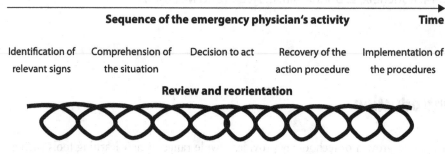

Fig. 1 - Basic process of the emergency physician's activity during medical care.

In the first part of this chapter, we will present our own experimental studies with a full-scale simulator in emergency medical student training. In the second part, we will move from a full-scale simulator to virtual reality. The conclusion will be focused on the future direction of learning technology in medical areas.

Learning complex emergency procedures with a full-scale patient simulator during student medical training

An experimental study with experts and novices

Many previous studies on full-scale simulators or on virtual reality were often limited to the description of the potential of new software, materials, or methods and emphasize the promise of such tools in medical education. However, in contrast, there are very few experimental studies showing the real benefits of full-scale simulation on performance in graduate medical education.

In the experimental study example presented in this part, advanced emergency medical students and experts were faced with a cardiac arrest scenario, with a full-scale patient simulator: SimMan (**Fig. 2**).

This "patient" simulator makes it possible to perform a large variety of actions including taking a pulse, taking blood pressure, injecting drugs (in the mannequin's arm), cardiopulmonary resuscitation, intubation procedures, listening to cardiac sounds, and so on. The mannequin responds in real time in exactly the same way as a "real patient" would. The mannequin is also able to deliver messages in response to learner questions.

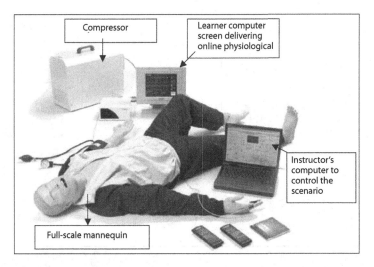

Fig. 2 - The full-scale simulator "SimMan" developed by Laerdal Medical Society.

We expected differences between the experts and the novices as far as how they managed the resuscitation task. These differences could be the fundamental basis for planning training sessions and scenarios particularly adapted to novices.

In an experiment involving 21 participants, we compared medical students (group novices, $N = 15$) and expert physicians (group experts, $N = 6$). The students were performing their fourth and fifth years (out of 10 in French medical studies). They were considered as "novices" in emergency medical skills. The "expert physicians" were seniors with more than 10 years of practice in emergency medicine. The physicians we labelled as experts in this experiment were experienced physicians with extensive emergency medicine practice who had graduated in emergency medicine and were recognized by colleagues as experts. Because the hospital took into consideration their input when defining the "good practices" procedures, these physicians appeared to be closer to a group of experts than just an experienced-only group.

Each participant (accompanied by a nurse and an ambulance driver) was placed in a situation that was identical to a real pre-hospital medical emergency situation in France. The main experimental framework was composed of two rooms: the full-scale simulator room 1, and the control and debriefing room 2 (**Fig. 3**).

In room 1, a high-tech camera was used in order to record all behaviors (verbal and nonverbal) during the task. The medical instructor and the experimenter were in the second room managing the cardiac arrest scenario from a computer linked to the full-scale simulator. The two rooms were separated by a wall (one-way mirror). The film recorded by the camera in the simulator room was projected in the second room by a video projector (in real time) and can be used for a debriefing phase.

All materials and machinery usually needed in such an emergency situation were available: emergency bag, reparatory system, oxygen, physiological measures on a screen, laparoscope ECG, and so on. Each participant was first given the same information just

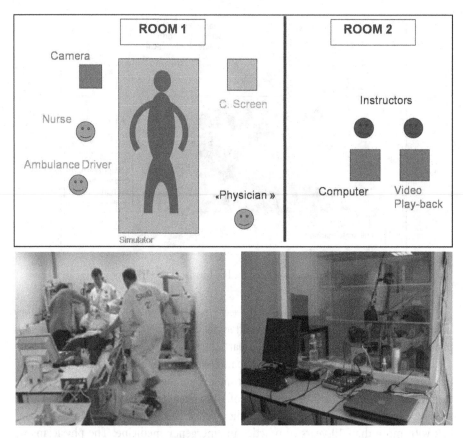

Fig. 3 - (a) Experimental design of the simulation situation.
(b) Example of participants in the simulation task.

before the beginning of the simulation scenario: "emergency services have been called (a specific phone number) by a 50-year-old man who is complaining of chest pain."

The scenario to be managed was a cardiac arrest (**Fig. 4**). However, they were not told that it was cardiac arrest. Each participant's task was to resolve the problem presented by the patient as quickly as possible. Two minutes passed between steps one and two during which the participant was expected to search for the right clinical and physiological information and build the right "mental model" of the problem (from the patient and the computer screen) in order to plan the following correct behaviors.

Each participant's prior theoretical knowledge about heart diseases (including cardiac arrest) was assessed a few weeks before the experiment with a multiple choice questionnaire. The results did not show any difference between experts and medical students, as both groups achieved high scores.

The experiment followed a four-step procedure. First, several weeks before the simulation session, each participant's theoretical knowledge about cardiac arrest procedure was assessed with a paper-based test. This was done in order to check that the two

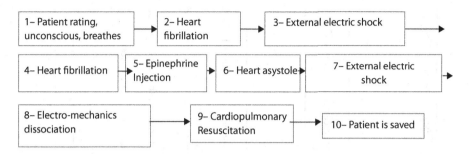

Fig. 4 - Steps in the scenario and expected actions.

groups (novice and expert) had the same theoretical background level. The second step was to spend time getting familiar with the simulator. This was done using a simple scenario constructed by the simulator designer in order to give every participant the same amount of prior experience with the simulator. The third phase consisted of the core of the experiment itself. Each participant entered the simulator room accompanied by two assistants: the nurse and the ambulance driver (which is the real situation in France). These two people (who were former instructors) were the same for each participant, and they were told to do nothing except what the medical student or the expert ordered them to do. During the task, all behaviors (including verbal messages) were recorded. At the end of the simulation (time constraint), the fourth phase of the task began: each student went to the debriefing room for the debriefing phase. The debriefing phase included a cognitive debriefing and a medical debriefing. For the cognitive debriefing, each participant was faced with his or her own actions during the task with the simulator (by replaying the recorded film) and had to justify each of the actions taken during the simulation phase. The subsequent medical debriefing consisted of a strictly medical analysis of the simulation phase conducted by the participant's medical instructor.

A quantitative analysis of the simulation phase and of the cognitive debriefing was carried out with specific dependant measures. For the simulation phase, the coding criterion covered the accuracy of the diagnosis (cardiac arrest and recognition of heart fibrillation), the number and the order of the correct procedural actions, the delay (time in seconds) between the actions, as well as the overall time to resolve the problem and the nature of the physiological information (heart rate, respiration, oxygen, blood pressure, and so on) taken or checked on the patient or on the screen. For the cognitive debriefing phase, each justification (argument) given for each procedural action was categorized. This categorization was done in order to obtain a quantitative analysis of each category for each group. The scoring system for the scenario leads to a 30-point grid. Each participant received a score out of 30 (**Table 1**). For each criterion, to be credited with one point, the participant had to carry out each action accurately, at the right time and in the right order.

Data were processed with ANOVAs including the group (experts vs. medical students) as the independent factor and the different criterions (actions, order, time for good diagnosis, delays, physiological information) as dependant factors.

Table 1 - Scoring criteria

SimMan State	Diagnosis Phase	Treatment Phase: "Procedure"	Treatment Effect Evaluation Phase
Cardiorespiratory arrest	*5 points* – Verification of breathing: BR* – Verification of consciousness: CS – Verification of airways: ARw – Pulse taken: P1	*5 points* – Oxygen: O – Machines and objects installations: INST= SCOPE+INST, Oxygen+INST, TENSION+INST, INJECTION+INST	
Fibrillation 1	*1 point* – Fibrillation noticed: F1	*1 point* – Defibrillation: D1	*2 points* – Verification of screen trace: TRACE C1 – Pulse taken: P2
Asystole	*1 point* – Asystole noticed: ASYSTOLE	*3 points* – Epinephrine demand: EPINE – Cardiopulmonary massage: CPR1 – Correct chain of action: CCA	
Fibrillation 2	*1 point* – Fibrillation noticed: F2	*1 point* – Defibrillation: D2	*2 points* – Verification of trace on the scope: TRACE C2 – Pulse taken: P3
Electromechanics dissociation:	*3 points* – Pulse taken: P4 – Oxygen saturation or blood pressure taken: O/T	*1 point* – Cardiopulmonary reanimation: CPR2	*4 points* – Pulse taken: P5 – Verification of trace on the scope: TRACE C3
EMD	– Electromechanics dissociation diagnosed: EMD		– Resumption of cardiac activity seen on the scope: RA – Confirmation of resumption of cardiac activity by taking pulse: CONFIR

* Abbreviation for each criterion used in Fig. 6.

The result showed significant differences between the two groups for actions, order, and time for good diagnosis, delays, and physiological information taking. The time spent by students was longer than the medical criteria for cardiac arrest, so it was often too late. Novice students took irrelevant actions, in the wrong order. They were quickly overloaded and could not plan or anticipate future actions and their effects on the patient. Novices did not consider the same information, as the experts, as being relevant for the diagnosis. Novices were less able than the experts to explain the rationale for the actions they took.

In summary, a full-scale simulator in medical education provides a relevant way to train and enhance the link between the declarative-theoretical aspects of knowledge and the procedural aspects (2) of medical skills.

Figure 5 shows that experts (global score, $m = 28.67/30$) performed better than novices $(16.14/30)$; $F(1,19) = 67.24$, $p < .001$.

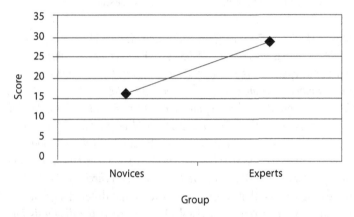

Fig. 5 - Global score for each group.

Many omissions can be observed in the novice group. Less correct actions were performed when compared to the experts. Novices performed less good actions than experts. However, novices spent on average much more time than the experts did ($M = 325$ s for experts and 380 s for the groups of students). The time spent by many novices was longer than the medical criteria for cardiac arrest, so it was often "too late."

Novice students undertook irrelevant actions and in the wrong order. It seems that experts are more capable than students of quickly constructing an exhaustive, accurate, and relevant mental model of the problem and of the right procedure at the beginning of the scenario. So they are able to plan a series of actions as well as quickly infer their expected consequences (**Fig. 6**).

Statistical analysis showed significant differences between the groups regarding the different criteria during the scenario phase (F(28,532) = 3.18, $p < .001$). Univariate comparisons between the groups made for each criterion on the grid (Kruskal-Wallis nonparametric H test) showed significant differences between experts and novices ($p < .05$, at least) for many criteria, particularly the following: CS *(consciousness not checked)* $H = 6.87$;

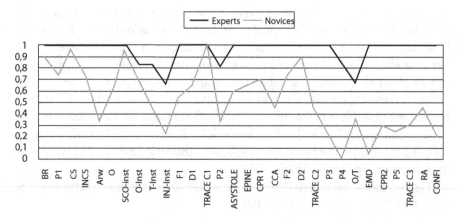

Fig. 6 - Mean rate of execution of the expected action relative to the scoring criteria.

ARw *(airway checked)* H = 7.16; F1 *(fibrillation noticed)* H = 11.07; P2 *(pulse checked)* H = 8.59; ASYSTOLE *(asystole noticed)* H = 15.05; EPINE *(order for epinephrine)* H = 7.02; CCA *(correct chunk: order epinephrine + cardiopulmonary resuscitation + injection)* H = 3.2; CPR1 *(correct cardiopulmonary actions after electric shock and systoles noticed)* H =7.57; TRACE C2 *(checking heart graph profile on the computer screen after shock)* H = 7.16; P3 *(pulse checked)* H = 8.92; P4 *(lack of pulse noticed)* H = 15.62; TS *(no blood pressure noticed)* H = 6.13; EMD *(electromechanics dissociation noticed)* H = 16.14; CPR2 *(cardiopulmonary resuscitation restarted)* H = 9.3; P5 *(pulse checked)* H = 11.83; TRACE C3 *(checking heart graph profile on the computer)* H = 9.3; CONFIR *(normal restart of the heart checked)* H = 15.15.

It is interesting to note that most of the criteria that differed significantly between the students and expert groups (see **Table 1**) concerned *the diagnosis phase* (which involved continuously taking precise physiological information from graphs and numbers on computer screen or about the state of the patient, e.g., notice fibrillation, systole, electromechanics dissociation) and also the *evaluation of the treatment effects* (e.g., the consequence of the actions) along the dynamic sequence of events but not actually doing the procedure itself and the good gestures.

This is an important result from a cognitive point of view. It means that the correct memorization, correct recall, and application of a procedure by students *is not enough* to give them the ability to manage correctly a complex dynamic and very risky situation such as a cardiac arrest. The good execution of the procedure itself has to be included inside a broader supervision activity. Supervision is driven by medical knowledge of the state of the patient along the sequence of events and actions (including an accurate dynamic mental model of how the biological system functions and reacts) (27, 1, 13). The physiological data concerning the patient needs to be continuously updated. Experts are more likely than novices or students to simultaneously performing "two activities": the execution of the procedure (good gestures, right actions in the right order) and the supervision of the state of the patient (supervision is guided by regular physiological information search and checking).

Acquiring a "clever" linkage between procedural knowledge and the supervision of the state of the patient looks like a dual task for a novice. Such dual task is cognitively very resource demanding. There can be a point where the processing demands of the task for attention and cognition (reasoning) become excessive and go beyond the limits of the working memory quantitative capacities (6). So, in such a situation, students were rapidly overloaded and could not plan or anticipate future actions and their effects on the patient. They could only focus their attention on a local action at the precise moment they were doing it and manage their actions by a trial-error "strategy." They were less able than experts to manage the physiological consequences of their actions and gestures at the same time. This means that students do not consider the same information, as the experts, as being relevant for the diagnosis. Also as we will see in the debriefing results, novices were less able than experts to explain the rationale for the actions they took.

These observations were reinforced by a specific study on the following criterions: information taking, time between actions, and the number of actions.

Table 2 shows that the experts took information much more frequently than the students $(F(1,18) = 4.73, p = .04)$.

Table 2 - Mean number of times information was taken for each group.

	Experts	Novices
Number of times pulse was taken	7	4.85
Number of times blood pressure was taken	3	2
Number of times oxygen saturation was taken	3.17	2.1

Also, **Table 3** indicates shorter times (delays) for experts than students when starting important actions.

Table 3 - Time before starting actions.

	Experts	Novices
Time (s) before first pulse was taken	13	166
Time (s) before first oxygen saturation	109	88
Time (s) before fibrillation noticed	43.5	224
Time (s) before delivering first electric shock	80	249.4
Time (s) before ordering epinephrine injection	178	254.4

Finally, **Table 4** shows a typical behavior in learning procedure, which reveals a tendency in novices to perform too much micro-segmented actions. This strategy is time and attention consuming and is an indicator of cognitive overload.

Table 4 – Number of actions taken during the procedure.

	Experts	Students
Number of different actions taken during the procedure	28	41.4
Number of disrupted actions	4	7.8
Number of un-achieved actions	2.5	5

Due to the limitations of this chapter, we will not detail the analysis of the debriefing. The main result of the cognitive part of the debriefing indicates that novices did not know precisely how to justify their actions despite the fact they were applying a compulsory procedure for resuscitation.

Conclusion, future direction, and recommendations in full-scale simulator

In summary, as the previous example showed, a full-scale simulator in medical education provides a relevant way to train and enhance the link between the declarative-theoretical aspects of knowledge and the procedural aspects of medical skills.

However, this study also showed that the use of a single scenario training session in novice students' professional training is not enough to provide trainees with skills that allow them to be able to manage complex procedures in a dynamic situation. Much more training is needed, with repeated exposure to scenarios, including a series of varied scenarios for the same kind of emergency problem. It could be expected that such professional didactics would help trainees build accurate abstract mental models of the problem to be resolved and acquire automated procedures. Another future direction is to gain more scientific knowledge about how mental models are built from intensive training. This goal implies focusing more on "online" measures of how trainees process information during a training session. Eye tracking method could bring about interesting information. For example, in our recent research, we used a mobile eye-tracking system during a medical student training session (**Fig. 7**).

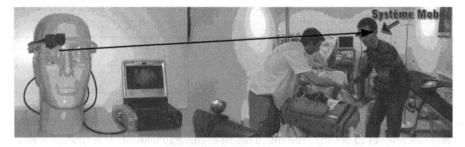

Fig. 7 - A mobile eye tracker used with the full-scale simulator SimMan.

From a full-scale mannequin-based simulator to computer screen-based microworld simulators in medical training

Limits of full-scale mannequin-based simulators

A limit on the use *of full-scale mannequin-based simulators* concerns their educational constraints. A first constraint is purchasing them and the maintenance costs. They also require the presence of a permanent professional instructional team. Another potential difficulty is that their systematic use is impossible with a large number of students (e.g., in the case of students undertaking their first years in medical studies). For example, in France a regular class of newly recruited medical students (via a competitive examination) includes anywhere from 100 to 500 students each year, depending on the size of the university.

In contrast, *computer screen-based microworld simulators* do not exhibit the same constraints as those of the *full-scale mannequin-based simulators* described above. They are less expensive, do not require the presence of a permanent professional instructional team, and can be used by students either in computer services (of the university) or at home with their own computers. As a result, their use could be highly recommended in the case of a large number of students. Such computer screen-based simulators are becoming more and more widely available in medical training areas.

Potential benefits of microworld simulators

Yet, in a well-controlled experimental study, Nyseen (39) compared the training value of two types of anesthesia simulators: a computer screen-based and a mannequin-based simulator. Experts and novices were tested. The results showed no significant differences between the two types of simulator.

However, the fidelity with real-life situations of computer-based simulators is low compared to full-scale mannequin simulators. They do not involve motor execution of specific actions on a mannequin but rather simply using a mouse to select and command available actions. Time pressure can be modulated and even excluded from a given simulation session. Such significant restrictions can really impair training sessions capable of preparing for real-life situations, but they are counterbalanced by other properties of computer screen-based simulators. These properties could be very useful to active learning and storing needed procedural knowledge beforehand in one's long-term memory, which is highly required in order to benefit from training with *full-scale mannequin-based simulators*. Indeed, new *computer screen-based simulators* are "serious multimedia games."

In the field of emergency medical training, new computer screen-based simulators have been recently developed. For example, a computer screen-based simulator called MicroSim was recently developed (by Laerdal Medical Society, 31) (**Fig. 8**).

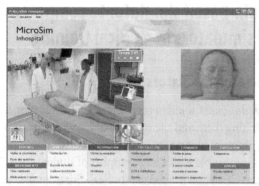

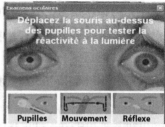

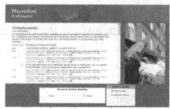

Pupil reaction self-test

Main screen, you are the physician (in white)

Text-based procedure

Fig. 8 - MicroSim. In hospital is a learning tool developed by Laerdal Medical Society.

It consists of a standard personal computer with a graphic and video interface that displays several teaching components, all related to resuscitation: breathing and respiration, cardiac arrest, arrhythmia, thoracic pain, and so on. Each component offers five different simulated scenarios. The learner is the physician and has to take charge of the patient's care. The learner can complete different actions (as with a real patient), conduct physical examinations, administer drugs and fluids, execute cardiopulmonary resuscitation, and so forth, by using mouse-controlled input and menu navigation and by clicking on a menu of actions displayed at the bottom of the screen. The learner can supervise the health of the patient (in real time) by using pop-up windows. The scenario speed can be user controlled (pause, play, stop, reverse, forward). At the end of the scenario, MicroSim delivers a written "debriefing," which is a report of the right and wrong actions, decisions, or knowledge used. The software automatically calculates the proportion of correct actions and the learning time. As far as we know, no empirical study has yet been published that aims to test the benefits of such computer-based simulators, which are real tutorials, on real-life skills in emergency medicine. In contrast to full-scale mannequin-based simulators, computer-based simulators do not allow motor execution of gestures. This limitation could be crucial to several fields or tasks in medical training that involve precise professional gestures such as surgery or complex intubation in emergency medicine.

Virtual reality, haptic, and depth perception properties

Compared with simple computer-based simulators, new training devices using virtual reality involve extensive interactivity, a real-world feeling, interactive and haptic properties, 3-D views (see **Fig. 9**).

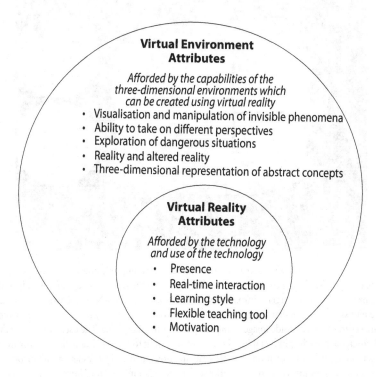

Fig. 9 - Attributes of virtual reality technology and virtual environments that are suitable for learning and training (17). Reprinted with permission from the University of Nottingham.

Instead of featuring a *physical fidelity* with the real-life situation, as do full-scale simulators, virtual reality environments aim to emphasize *psychological fidelity* with the real-life situation.

Examples in medical training

Haptic properties, high-level real-time interactivity, and depth feeling with 3-D environments dote virtual reality with great potential for learning with "ecological situations." So a very good transfer of training to the real-life situations is expected. In medicine, virtual environments have been developed in different fields and particularly in surgery, a domain in which direct interaction with objects or organs is needed. These environments and, particularly, simulators have been designed in order to train professionals on helping and assisting with actions (18) as well as guiding complex gestures (4, 5); see the examples of orthopedic surgery (**Figs. 10, 11**).

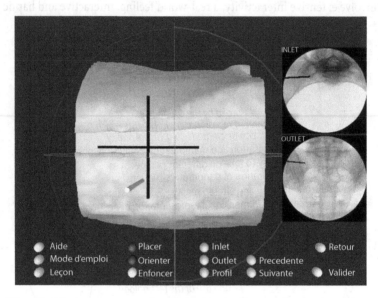

Fig. 10 - The goal of the (computer screen-based) simulator is to improve how one learns the correspondence between the 2-D image provided by the radiography and the real 3-D image of the body in the case of percutaneous orthopedic surgery (http://www-sante.ujf-grenoble.fr/SANTE/voeu/visfran/index.htm). Using the mouse, the user implants a pin in a 3-D pelvis volume hidden by a skin envelope marked with an X, which corresponds to a side image of the sacrum over the skin tissue. The user can control the position and progression of the pin by taking x-rays corresponding to the classical incidences for this movement (inlet, outlet, profile). For most surgical unit situations, two incidences are simultaneously visible (the current one and the preceding one). Reprinted with permission from the University of Grenoble, and from the authors Dubois, Vadcard & Luengo, 2008.

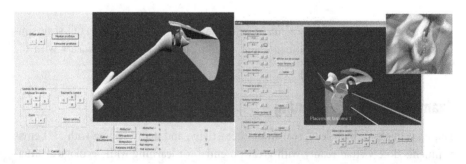

Fig. 11 - A simulator for shoulder prosthesis surgery (DUOCENTRIC®). Inserting holes for pin 1 and pin 2, following phantom 1. Reprinted with permission from the University of Dijon and ENSAM of Cluny, and from the authors Atmani, H., Merienne, F., Fofi, D., and Trouilloud, P., 2006.

An interesting recent evolutionary development consists in the development of more task-limited 3-D environments. Such simulators have been designed for endoscopic exploration or laparoscopy (8).

Some "difficult" limiting questions

Although the promises of virtual reality and virtual environments are great, there are some lively interesting and difficult questions about the effectiveness of such learning devices. It is quite possible to find a very large number of descriptions in the literature for different virtual environments in different professional domains. However, except for fundamental cognitive processes (16), there are very few empirical and experimental studies that aim to test their effectiveness for professional learning (3, 16). Another problem that is also relatively neglected is the transfer of learning in virtual environments to real-life situations.

Ergonomic analyses of virtual environments or virtual reality learning devices (3, 16) often underline a lack of psychological fidelity with real-life situations for haptic properties, presence, immersion feeling, and interactivity as well.

Spatial cognition and medical activities

A very interesting area for medical training and simulation is spatial cognition. Spatial learning has received more experimental attention than any other application where virtual reality is being used as a medium to investigate spatial cognition (20). There is accumulating evidence of the positive effect of the exploration of virtual environments on spatial navigation skills (16). Previous research showed the crucial role of 3-D presentation in navigation activities (44). Research is needed to examine whether skills learned in virtual environments transfer effectively to real-world environments, and also to examine whether spatial skills in the real world improve after practice and experience using a virtual environment (16).

Spatial abilities (including mental imagery, mental rotation, visuospatial reasoning, spatial memory, spatial visualization of objects, memorizing the relationships between objects) could be of crucial importance in medical training, e.g., in activities such as radiology and endoscopic organ exploration and for new surgery techniques such as minimally invasive surgical techniques (25, 26, 29, 31). Performance in surgery seems to be related to spatial abilities (25, 26). The anatomy could be very complex, with complex intrication of 3-D relationships in flexible structures.

Surgeons, but also radiologists, have to quickly build precise 3-D mental models from 2-D images, create mental representations of organs that cannot be seen, and use mental rotation, using allocentric perspectives. Hegarty and Waller (25) report a series of studies showing significant correlation (moderate to high) between standardized testing of spatial abilities and performance in surgical tasks. With noninvasive techniques, surgeons perform operations by watching a video image from an endoscope inserted through cannula. This situation can give rise to spatial problems (25, 26). Some research has been done on training surgical skills using virtual environments (46). For example, Tendick *et al.* (46), designed a virtual environment from an angled laparoscope. Learning rates of novices using the simulator were correlated from 0.39 to 0.58 with measures of spatial ability (19). Finally, recent research showed that spatial skills can be improved by using specific spatial training programs (14).

Multimedia learning, animated pictures, 2-D, and 3-D

Multimedia learning is defined as "learning from words (e.g., spoken as well as sprinted texts) and pictures (e.g., static illustrations, photos, maps, animations, graphs, and computer screen-based process simulation), or video" (36, 37). These materials create what we call "online instructional presentations." In medical education (as well as in other domains), a large number of educational or university websites show available multimedia presentations. Instructional online presentations, which can be used at home, are going to compete with traditional books, and even their use is going to rise above traditional books.

Previous research showed that in learning as well as understanding, multimedia presentations outperformed single modality presentations or texts versus Pictures, and so on (36, 37). Animations, interactive or noninteractive, videos, and 3-D objects have been increasingly introduced in instructional documents.

Animations versus static pictures to learn dynamic processes

Animations as well as videos can very realistically demonstrate or simulate biological dynamic processes. These processes can be invisible. In anatomy education for example, particularly in functional anatomy, animations could be superior to static pictures usually used in traditional paper-based images. In the case of an animated presentation, learners can observe the fine-grain microsteps of the depicted process in a realistic amount of time. Spatial as well as temporal aspects of a biological process can be depicted. Moreover, for complex and rapid processes, the speed can be slowed down. In contrast, for very slow biological processes occurring over long periods of tisme and for which it is difficult for a learner to gain access to available key steps, the processes could be sped up. Such transformation possibilities could have interesting learning potentialities, for example, in dermatology and skin disease (9-12). For example, in an animated presentation of the evolution of a skin disease, like skin cancer, the timescale of the progression of the features of the skin could be shortened in order to deliver a more expressive and apprehensible representation of the dynamic key transformations. Zoom techniques or cueing techniques could shed some light on some critical features that might appear on the skin at a precise stage of the disease.

Previous research about the effectiveness of animations showed that animated graphics, dynamic pictures, or video are clearly and intrinsically superior to their static counterparts only under specific presentation conditions (7, 9, 10, 11, 12, 28, 33, 47, 48). Previous research has led to animation design principles. We describe below three main principles for designing effective animated presentations of dynamic processes.

Interactivity and user control upon the speed of the process principle

A realistic presentation of a dynamic process, e.g., a biological or a technical process, can result in a very high-speed presentation of the microsteps of process. As a result, when a new event appears on the learner's screen, the previous event has not yet been completely perceived and processed by the learner. Many changes in the animation can occur simultaneously in different locations of the display involving split attention activities. So, realistic presentations could quickly overload learner's attentional and cognitive resources. This frequently impairs learning performances (6). Recent studies have shown that increasing the learner's level of interactivity with the animation could improve learning performances. The learner can be given the possibility of controlling the speed or acting upon the pace and the direction of the animation by using a control device. Controllability upon dynamic visualisations (videos or animations) gives the viewers and learners the opportunity to adapt a presentation's pace and sequence to their own cognitive needs and skills (7, 9, 10, 11, 12, 36, 37, 45).

The effects of giving learners more extensive control over the course of a dynamic depiction have also been investigated recently. Schwan and Riempp (45) conducted a study on how user control of video presentations affected participants' learning of knot-tying skills. Participants had to learn four knots of increasing complexity (double half-hitch, cleat wind, anchor bend, bowline) from a purely visual video clip. In the controllable condition, participants could stop, reverse, forward, or replay the video as well as change its presentation speed (slowing it down or speeding it up). In the non-controllable version, the speed and the duration of the videos were fixed and could only be restarted from the beginning when the learner had finished viewing it: an all or nothing type presentation. Compared with the noncontrollable videos, the controllable presentations required a much shorter learning period (viewing time as practicing time) to reach criterion performance: the procedure had to be demonstrated to the experimenter. Participants in the controllable condition often made use of the various control features to vary the way information was presented (particularly, stops, slow motions, time lapses, direction changes). These principles could be applied, for example, in learning to tie knots in surgery.

Also in the medical domain, Garg *et al.* (23, 24) studied the way medical students learn spatial anatomy with 2-D and 3-D rotating objects. Views of the carpal bones in the hand were presented as 3-D objects, the rotation of which could be either controlled or not by learners in the different experimental conditions. There was a significant positive effect when learners had control over rotation. The authors suggested that the use of self-controlled multiple-view representations, such as dissected samples, skeletons, and plastic and computer models, are an effective method for improving this type of learning. However, they found that spatial abilities affected performance within the 3-D condition. Controlling an animated rotating object has also been found to enhance the learning of those with low spatial abilities (23, 24).

More recently, Cohen and Hegarty (14) studied how students performed a novel spatial inference task that requires them to imagine and draw a cross section of a 3-D object, which looks like a "biological organ." While performing the task, participants could actively control two computer-animated views of the object, giving them different points of view on the objects. The results showed a high correlation *(.75)* between the use of interactive animation and drawing accuracy.

Cueing principle

Because of the transient aspect of animations, learners could find difficulties in selecting the relevant location of the picture accurately, e.g., where to look and when to look, at the right location at the right time. In order to help learners, cueing techniques have been developed that aim to properly guide the learner's attention. But it is not only a matter of attracting learner attention; a more crucial question is to guide learner's attention in a way that is spatially and temporally aligned with how the animation presents key information. Different types of cueing devices have been experimentally tested in previous research (10, 12, 34-37, 47, 48): verbal cues as well as visual cues.

Verbal cues consist in aural comments added to the visual presentation of the animation. Visual cues consist in a range of purely visual signals such as the traditional external arrows pointing to specific parts of the animation, or contrasting colors between different parts that highlight particular parts of the device, and highlighting spots so as to attract attention at the right time in a particular location of the process (30). New cueing approaches have recently been developed (12) and showed that an internal spreading color embedded in an interactive animation of a technical system was very efficient in improving the comprehension of the mechanical functioning of the causal chains of the technical system presented.

Segmentation principle

The detection or the recognition of the key steps of a continuous process presented with a realistically paced animation could be very difficult, particularly for novices and when the information delivered is fleeting. In order to avoid learning difficulties, an important ergonomic principle is to segment the animation into key microsteps, by using for example a series of key frames for the process. Another way to enhance important key instant processing of a complex and continuous dynamic process (e.g., the evolution of particular features of the skin in the case of a progressing skin disease) is to use temporal manipulation of the rhythm of the presentation. Critical features of the process can be slowed down. Thus, rhythm contrasts become very useful for focusing attention on key aspects of a dynamic phenomenon.

Conclusion

This chapter focused on the potential benefits of learning technologies in medical training. We mainly carried out studies in learning from full-scale as well as low-scale simulators, and then we described previous research on educational multimedia
presentations. These technologies could have great training and learning potential, in
particular for the development of expertise or to contribute to providing professionals
with competence and precise knowledge that helps them avoid human errors when
managing complex dynamic situations. The rapid growth of technology provided a
large number of new learning tools, some of them very innovative, as for example, virtual reality including highly interactive haptic properties. Many attractive descriptions
for these learning tools have been written in previous research. However, there are still
very few empirical and "scientific" evaluations of their real efficiency and transferability
in real-world situations. Current approaches to designing educational technology and
training simulators too often appear to be largely founded upon intuition rather than
research-based principles. In the future, more research is needed regarding their real
efficiency.

References

1. Amalberti R (2001) La conduite des systèmes à risques. PUF, Paris
2. Anderson JR (1993) The rules of the mind. Harvard University Press, Cambridge
3. Anastasova M, Burkhardt JM, Mégard C, Ehanno P, (2007) L'ergonomie de la réalité
    augmentée pour l'apprentissage: une revue. Trav Hum 70:97-125
4. Atmani H, Merienne F, Fofi D, Trouilloud P (2007) Computer aided surgery system for
    shoulder prosthesis placement. Comput Aided Surg 12:60
5. Atmani H, Merienne F, Fofi D, Trouilloud P (2007) From medical data to simple virtual
    mock-up of scapulo-humeral articulation. In: IEEE/SPIE 8th International Conference
    on Quality Control by Artificial Vision. May, Le Creusot, France
6. Ayres P, Paas F (2007) Can the cognitive load approach make instructional animations
    more effective? Appl Cogn Psychol 21:811-820
7. Bétrancourt M (2005) The animation and interactivity principles in multimedia
    learning. In: Mayer RE (ed) Cambridge handbook of multimedia learning, pp. 287-296.
    Cambridge University Press, New York
8. Blavier A (2006) Impact desimages en 2D ou 3D sur les processus cognitifs impliqués
    dans le traitement visuel et dans le contrôle de l'action: le cas de la chirurgie minimale
    invasive. Thèse de doctorat de l'Université de Liège
9. Boucheix JM (2003) Ergonomie et formation. Ergonomie cognitive des apprentissages
    en formation professionnelle. Psychol Fr 48(2):17-34
10. Boucheix JM, Guignard H (2005) Which animation condition can improve text
    comprehension in children? Eur J Psychol Educ 20(4):369-388
11. Boucheix JM (2004) Simulation and comprehension aid tool for complex technical
    documents. Advanced Learning Technology, ICALT, IEEE, pp. 898-900

12. Boucheix JM, Lowe RK (2010) Eye tracking comparison of external pointing cues and internal progressive cues in learning with complex animations. Learn Instr 20:123-135

13. Cellier JM, Eyrolle H, Mariné C (1997) Expertise in dynamics environments. Ergonomics 40(1):28-50

14. Cohen C, Hegarty M (In press) Spatial visualization training using interactive animations. Cogn Instr

15. Chopra V, Gesink BJ, De Jong J, et al. (1994) Does training on anesthesia simulator lead to improvements in performance? Br J Anaesthesiol 73:293-7

16. Cobb S, Stanton-Fraser D (2005) Multimedia learning in virtual reality. In: Mayer RE (ed) Handbook of multimedia learning: from multimedia to virtual reality, pp. 525-547. Cambridge University Press, New York

17. Crosier, J (2001) Virtual environments in secondary science education. Unpublished doctoral dissertation, University of Nottingham, England

18. Dubois M, Vadcard L, Luengo V (2008) Prise en compte de différents niveaux d'appropriation pédagogique dans la conception d'un simulateur d'apprentissage en chirurgie orthopédique. Congrès de l'AIPTLF (Association Internationale de Psychologie du Travail de langue française), 19-22 août 2008, Québec, Canada

19. Eyal R, Tendick F (2001) Spatial ability and learning the use of an angled laparoscope in a virtual environment. In: Westwood JD, et al. (eds) Medicine meets virtual reality, pp. 146-152. IOS Press, Amsterdam

20. Foreman N, Stanton D, Wilson P, Duffy H (2003) Successful transfer of spatial knowledge from a virtual to a real school environment in physically disabled children. J Exp Psychol Appl 9:67-74

21. Gaba DM (1999) The human work environment and anesthesia simulators. In: Miller RD (ed) Anesthesia, 5th ed, 2613-2668. Churchill Livingstone, New York

22. Gaba DM, Howard SK, Flanagan B, et al. (1998) Assessment of clinical performance during simulated crises using both technical and behavioral ratings. Anesthesiology 89:8-18

23. Garg AX, Norman GR, Sperotable L (2001) How medical students learn spatial anatomy. Lancet 357:363-364

24. Garg AX, Norman GR, Spero L, Maheshwari P (1999) Do virtual computer models hinder anatomy learning? Acad Med 74:87-89

25. Hegarty M, Waller DA (2005) Individual differences in spatial abilities. In: Shah P, Myake A (eds) The Cambridge handbook of visuospatial thinking, pp. 121-169. Cambridge University Press, New York

26. Hegarty M, Keehner M, Kooshabeh P, Montello DR (In press) How spatial abilities enhance, and are enhanced by, dental education. Learn Individ Differ

27. Hoc JM, Amalberti R (2007) Cognitive control dynamics for reaching a satisfying performance in complex dynamic situations. J Cogn Eng Decis Mak 1:22-55

28. Höffler TN, Leutner D (2007) Instructional animation versus static pictures: a meta-analysis. Learn Instr 17:722-738

29. Keehner M, Hegarty M, Cohen C, et al. (2008) Spatial reasoning with external visualizations: what matter is what you see, not whether you interact. Cogn Sci 32:1099-1132

30. Köning de BB, Tabbers HK, Rikers RMJP, Paas F (2007) Attention cueing as a mean to enhance learning from an animation. Appl Cogn Psychol 21:731-746

31. Lehmann A, Vidal M, Bülthoff HH (2008) A high-end virtual reality setup for the study of mental rotations. Presence 17:365-375

32. Sim-Man, Micro-Sim (2006).The full scale simulator "SimMan" and the computer screen simulator, developed by Laerdal Medical Society. Laerdal Medical France, Limonest, 69, France

33. Lowe RK, Schnotz W (2008) Learning with animation: research and design implications. Cambridge University Press, New York

34. Mautoné PD, Mayer RE (2001) Signalling as a cognitive guide in multimedia learning. J Educ Psychol 93:377-389

35. Mautone PD, Mayer RE (2007) Cognitive aids for guiding graph comprehension. J Educ Psychol 3:640-652

36. Mayer RE (2001) Multimedia learning. Cambridge University Press, New York

37. Mayer RE (2005) Handbook of multimedia learning: from multimedia to virtual reality. Cambridge University Press, New York

38. Messant I, Lile A, Avena C, et al. (2005) Evaluation sur simulateur multiple SimMan de la prise ne charge d'un choc anaphylactique préopératoire par des internes DES d'anesthésie réanimation. Ann Fr Anesth Réanim 24(6):698-699

39. Nyssen AS, Larbuisson R, Janssens M, et al. (2002). A comparison of the training value of two types of anesthesia simulators: computer screen-based and mannequin-based simulators. Anaesth Analg 94:1560-1565

40. Nyssen AS, De Keyser V (1998) Improving training in problem solving skills: analysis of anesthetist's performance in simulated problem situations. Trav Hum 61(4):387-401

41. Nyssen AS (2000) Analysis of human errors in anaesthesia: our methodological approach – from general observations to targeted studies in laboratory. In: Vincent C, De Mol BA (eds) Safety in medicine, pp. 49-63. Pergamon, London

42. Nyssen AS (2005) Simulateurs dans le domaine de l'anesthésie: outils de formation et de recherche. Réflexions sur la validité et la fidélité. In: Pierre Pastré (ed) Apprendre avec un simulateur. Octarès, Toulouse

43. Murray DJ, Boulet JR, Kras JF, et al. (2004) Acute care skills in anaesthesia practice: a simulation-based resident performance assessment. Anesthesiology 101:1084-1095

44. Stanton D, Foreman N, Wilson PN (1998) Uses of virtual reality in training: Developing the spatial skills of children with mobility impairments. In: Riva G, Wiederhold BK, Molinari E (eds) Virtual environments' in clinical psychology: scientific and technological challenges in advanced-patient therapist interaction, vol. 58, pp. 219-233. IOS Press, Amsterdam

45. Schwan S, Riempp R (2004) The cognitive benefits of interactive videos: learning to tie nautical knots. Learn Instr 14:293-305

46. Tendick F, Downes M, Gogtekin T, et al. (2000) A virtual test for training laparoscopic surgical skills. Presence 9:236-255

47. Tversky B, Bauer-Morrison J, Bétrancourt M (2002) Animation: can it facilitate? Int J Hum Comp Stud 57:247-262

48. Tversky B, Heiser J, Lozano S, (2008) Enriching animations. In: Lowe RK, Schnotz W (eds) Learning with animation: research implications for design, pp. 263-285. Cambridge University Press, New York

rhythm (16), the use of various materials is commonly encountered. Pitch concerns the variability of frequencies and constitutes, for example, the basis of the melody in music. In language, pitch corresponds to the fundamental frequency, and its variability plays an important role in tone languages (pitch is indeed linked to semantic as the same sound pattern means can correspond to four different words, function of the pitch and the direction of the variation of the pitch). However, the variation of pitch is also one component of the prosody, carrying information about the gender of the speaker, his or her emotional state, and so on. Variations of pitch in speech are linked to the grammatical role of groups of words, constituting an effective help for disambiguating the structures of certain utterances (4). However, even when all pitch information is suppressed from a speech in a non-tone language, the intelligibility stays high (16). Timbre is a property of sound that allows one to distinguish sounds when pitch, length, and loudness are equal. Using multidimensional analysis, Samson and Zatorre (21) have pointed out all perceptive dimensions underlying musical timbre processing. In their first experiment, the authors have digitalized nine isolated timbres, by selecting three levels of spectral content (number of harmonics) and three levels of temporal content (rise time). Their results showed that spectral features correspond to the first dimension (48% of the variance), while temporal information correspond to the second dimension (38% of the variance). A third dimension accounting for 12% of the variance isolated the four harmonic stimuli from the others (1 vs. 8). Thus, spectral features convey around half of the relevant information in a task commonly used in spoken language processing. From the linguistic approach of language, words are constituted of a set of minimal different units called phonemes. In French, the 36 phonemes can be shared in vowels (harmonic sounds) and consonants (noises). From the phonetic approach, the auditory difference between vowels is the result of the frequency of harmonics. They are selectively amplified in different parts of the vocal tract, constituting the four formants, but the two first formants are enough to discriminate vowels (5). As an example, the perception of an [a] differs from those of an [i] because the first formant is situated around 750 Hz and the second formant around 1500 Hz for [a], whereas it is around 300 Hz and 2250 Hz, respectively, for an [i]. From an acoustic approach, the succession of phonemes in an utterance can be considered as a succession of various timbres (16). On the other hand, consonants are commonly shared in two categories, relative to the addition of vibration of vocal folds, opposing voiceless or voiced consonants. In voiceless consonants, the timbre is composed of aperiodic frequencies. In voiced consonants, the vibration of vocal folds adds a further component in the frequencies: the fundamental frequency (F0) corresponding to the rate of vibration of the vocal folds. Then, always in terms of frequencies, constituents of vowels and consonants are fundamental for speech intelligibility. The term "rhythm" refers to the systematic patterning of sounds concerning timing, accent, and grouping. To speak a language with native fluency involves mastering the patterns of timing and accentuations that characterize the flow of syllables in words and sentences. The rhythm of a language is a product of its linguistic structure, which means that languages are rhythmically different because they differ in phonological properties that influence how they are organized as patterns of time. The structure of the syllables themselves (isolated vowel, consonant + vowel, or more complex structures) and particularly the frequency of these structures in the language play a great role. The duration of syllables is indeed linked to the number of phonemes. Second, speech rhythm depends also on vowel duration. In English, as an example, the word "bee," translated [bi:] in International Phonetic Alphabet (IPA), differs from the word "be," translated [bi] in the IPA, only because of the length of the vowel [i]. Some consonants are shorter than others. Considering the articulatory mode, we can divide stop consonants involving the closing of one part of the phonatory organs (lips, tongue, teeth, …) from fricative consonants in which the exhalation of breathing air is modulated by the position of the phonatory organs, producing then a particular noise (for instance, [f]). If fricative consonants can last as long as being out of breath, stop consonants last around 40 ms. So, in French, the discrimination of length differences helps to dispel perceptive ambiguities in consonants.

The second principle consists in the use of a supervised learning procedure and the most explicit representations of the characteristics of the sounds. Practically, the learning is shared between two phases where one characteristic of a sound is binary presented in two highly contrasted sounds. The therapist turns the child's attention to this contrast in the sensitization phase. As deaf children's auditory attention and knowledge are very poor, their first responses are due to chance. Then, the role of the therapist is to point out the errors, supporting the child until success. In the conditioning phase, the child learns to point out this difference of perception (in an identification task), giving in a bodily response (i.e., to represent a low-frequency sound in squatting down, or a high-frequency sound in stretching the body) (8). Later, the relevant difference of sounds is represented with a symbol. As an example, the difference of length is represented by a longer or shorter line. When the sound is delivered, the child is invited to point one of these two symbols. In the training of the differences of pitch (low-frequency and higher-frequency sounds) are commonly opposed and represented with a downward or a rising arrow. Thus, explicit learning and conditioning procedure ensure the automatization of the auditory feature processing. When the child recognizes these different dimensions, spoken sounds are used in receptive tasks and integrated in productive tasks, to support articulatory gestures.

However, this approach presents several weaknesses. First, in the Fu and Galvin review lead in deaf adults (9), the authors concluded that an approach centered on the acoustic properties of the signal was not enough for generalization: as an example, if auditory training significantly improved frequency discrimination with the trained stimuli, the improvement did not generalize to untrained stimuli (24). Second, it allows only the use of identification or discrimination tasks. McAdams (13) considers the process of auditory recognition as a succession of different steps, from the input to the complete recognition. The first one is under the dependence of the anatomy and the physiology of the ear, with a selective encoding of frequencies (tonotopy) and temporal features encoding. Then, in a pre-attentive step (11), the listener separates the components of the auditory signal, following the rules of the Gestalt theory. This process of grouping or separating the auditory flux is the basis of the constitution of separate auditory representations of the different sources present in the environment (2). The next step concerns processes analyzing relevant auditory features. The analysis occurs within a short period of time (microtemporal properties) or a longer period of time (macrotemporal properties). The analysis of microtemporal properties concerns simple auditory events, and depends on the nature of the structure that vibrates and how the vibration is produced. The characteristics of resonance bring information about the physical nature of the source. This category of properties constitutes the structural invariants of an auditory source, i.e., common auditory features of all the objects from the same category (like a prototype, allowing the identification of the category whatever the exemplar of the category producing the sound). The action produced at the level of the auditory object (hit, rubbing, …) brings other information called transformational invariants. These invariants convey information about the rhythm and the nature of the whole event and to assess if the variation of the sounds is attributable to the same source or to the intervention of another. Then, for McAdams (13), invariants are compared and adjusted to categories of auditory sources or events stored in memory. At this step, the stimulus is recognized as an exemplar of such or such category. The selection (or activation) of a representation stored in memory can ensure the activation of inputs in lexicon, concepts, or semantic associations linked to the previous knowledge. Auditory processes include also top-down processes (see 2). From this model, it appears that four cognitive operations occur in auditory perception: auditory scene analysis allowing, by the grouping or segregation of acoustic flux, the constitution of our environment in terms of auditory objects or events. Identification supposes that structural invariants are processed by the auditory system, allowing the phenomena of categorization. Discrimination concerns transformational invariants: in other words, the threshold in the differences in acoustic variations beyond which one considers that it concerns the same or another auditory object. At least, auditory memory works for the three other operations, allowing adjustment with representations stored in long-term memory. To train these four operations could enhance better auditory skills in deaf children.

Third, the learning procedure used is of explicit type. But this type of learning is considered as costly and requires attentional processes that are not always available in young children. However, the implicit learning paradigm could constitute another framework and offers different perspectives. In reference to its characteristics of generality and automaticity (see Chapter "Introducing implicit learning: from the laboratory to the real life", E. Bigand and C. Delbé), implicit learning processes are responsible for the continuous behavioral adaptation of humans during their entire life (17), implicit learning seems active very early in life from infancy. Laboratory experiment showed that some relevant aspects of first-language acquisition, i.e., segmentation (20), rest on implicit learning mechanisms. Because of its robustness characteristic, implicit learning still operates in elderly adults (10) and in pathologies of Alzheimer disease (14) and is weakly affected by age and personality differences. Following Vinter and colleagues in this volume, "*implicit learning covers all forms of unintentional learning in which, as a consequence of repeated experience, an individual's behavior becomes sensitive to the structural features of an experienced situation, without, at any time, being told to learn anything about this situation, and without the adaptation being due to an intentional exploitation of some pieces of explicit knowledge about these features.*" In the course of training time, the participants develop a behavioral sensitivity to the structure of the situation, so they become "familiar" to certain features. Implicit learning shapes the perceptions a participant develops of a situation through the direct and continuous tuning of the processes devoted to the treatment of incoming information. These processes provoke changes in the way information is encoded, and these changes directly affect the participant's phenomenal experience. The use of this learning procedure implies a lower cognitive cost from the learners.

Our experiment

To work out an auditory program implies to consider the learning procedure (including the duration and the quantity of training sessions), the type of tasks, and the kind of stimuli to use.

If explicit learning procedures are commonly used in traditional reeducation in deaf children (and also in most of the auditory training in adults (7-9), we assessed that an implicit learning procedure would also provide auditory benefits to children and allow a lower cognitive cost. But an implicit learning situation relies on four principles (see Chapter "Implicit learning, development, and education", A. Vinter *et al.*). The first one concerns the material to be learned, and it must be errorless. As participants learn regularities, the errors during the learning phase could interfere with correct responses (see Chapter "Implicit learning and implicit memory in moderate to severe memory disorders" A. Moussard and E. Bigard). Second, as attentional focus is limited in terms of time and space, regularities of the rule must be isolated and lie spatially and temporally. The third principle concerns training time: if the repetitions of the learning condition are considered as necessary, the duration and the number of the sessions must be considered in the function of each learning situation. The last principle refers to the design of the learning condition, including the fact that that the learner has to process the relevant information but without any explicit information.

As auditory perception rests on four cognitive operations – identification, discrimination, auditory scene analysis, and auditory memory – our training program comprises four types of exercises corresponding to the four perceptive operations. Thus, we built a game platform, and the child is invited to play. As an example, in the identification task, the child stays in front of a keyboard and has to place on the keyboard one of the six figurines corresponding to the listened sound. This action constitutes an auditory feedback, allowing the comparison between the source and the response (and to process structural invariants of the sounds). In the discrimination task, the child plays with another module: when introducing a magnet in a hole, the source is or is not modified in terms of frequency, timbre, or tempo. This exercise stimulates directly the process of the transformational invariants of an auditory event. In the auditory scene analysis task, the child plays with a checkerboard. Each square in filled with a red magnetic pawn. The action to remove one pawn can suppress one of the two (or three) auditory sources displayed. If the modification is perceived, the child has to replace the red pawn with a purple one. Even if the phenomenon of segregation or grouping of flux resulting of auditory analysis exists in very young children (23) and seems very primitive, their training is necessary (and difficult) in deaf children. Thus, this task implies the possibility for the child to exercise one major operation in auditory perception. At least, the memory task can be considered as a span task. The child uses the keyboard and has to match his or her responses to the source, making a choice between the six possibilities corresponding to the six active keys. The difficulty of the program is controlled in terms of cognitive operation, type of auditory stimuli, and length (memory task). In this procedure, the attention of the child is turned on the game (task) to realize but not on the auditory process, however essential to "win." In this perspective too, the type of auditory stimuli can be considered as an alibi to stimulate the perceptive operations. Their auditory characteristics are not presented in an "isolated way" as in the traditional approach. Instead, we consider that the variability of the auditory characteristics of the material, more ecological, ensures the training more perceptive operations. For this reason, we have used four types of auditory stimuli: environmental sounds, music, voices, and electroacoustic sounds, always in respect of a gradual level of difficulty (environmental sounds and music constituting the easier stimuli processed by deaf children and electroacoustic sounds the most difficult).

At least, the duration of the training and the interval between the sessions has not been experimentally studied, and the difference of stimuli and tasks does not allow any comparison. Busby and colleagues (3) observed minimal changes in speech performance in deaf adults after ten 1-hour training sessions in their experimental group while Dawson and colleagues (6)reported encouraging results for ten 50-minute vowel recognition training sessions in CI users. At least, Fu and Galvin's (9) training lasted two hours per day for five consecutive days. However, if these procedures are relevant in adults with prior auditory knowledge, no evidences of their relevance have been shown in prelingually deaf children. Moreover, in other fields (1), distributed learning seems more effective; for these reasons, our training lasts 20 half an hour sessions.

Four profoundly and two severely deaf children (mean nine years old) have been trained with this method. Five of them were hearing aid recipients, and one benefited of a cochlear implant. They were integrated in a specialized institution. Five of them were bilingual French Sign Language (LSF)/spoken French but demonstrate better abilities in LSF, and one is LSF user. During the training time, no auditory tuning has been led. To evaluate the effects of the training, we measured the children's auditory skills before training (pretest, T1), after training (T2), and six months later (T3) in trained tasks directly from our training program (18). In the identification task, performances were higher in T2 and T3, compared to T1 ($F(1,33) = 25.12$; $p < .0001$, and $F(1,33) = 29.64$; $p < .0001$), and processing times decreased significantly since T2 ($F(1,33) = 24.0$; $p < .0001$) and stayed stable in T3 ($F(1,33) = 31.3$; $p < .0001$). The performances in the discrimination task were also better in T2 than in T1 ($F(1,33) = 12.49$; $p < .001$) and in T3, compared to T1 ($F(1,33) = 5.27$; $p < .03$). The processing times decreased also since T2 ($F(1,33) = 5.8$; $p < .02$) and in T3 ($F(1,33) = 4.8$; $p < .03$), compared to T1. In the high-level tasks, like auditory scene analysis (ASA), the effects of the training were obvious in the decrease of the performances in T3 ($F(1,33) = 7.15$; $p < .01$) but not in the processing times. At least, the auditory training involved better performances in the memory task just after training ($F(1,33) = 30.18$; $p < .001$) but this effect was removed in T3. Processing times decreased significantly since T2 ($F(1,33) = 14.17$; $p < .001$) and were stable in T3 (**Table 1**).

We also evaluated the effects of the training on untrained task, as a phonetic discrimination test. This test was composed of 36 items and consisted in a similarity judgment of phonetic contrasts in oral/nasal vowels and voiceless/voiced consonants. As expected, the children showed better performances in T2 (just after training) than in T1. The results in the phonetic discrimination test were slightly lower in T3 but stayed significant compared to T1 (19).

Table 1 - Scores of our experimental group to the phonetic discrimination test.

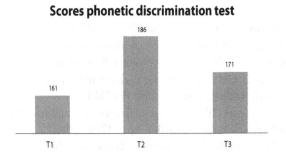

Scores phonetic discrimination test

Conclusion

Contrary to the traditional approach centered on the acoustic properties of the sounds, our program is based on the training of the cognitive operations in the perceptive processes. These processes are effective whatever the type of sounds and allow explaining the improvement observed in untrained tasks. Even if it seems that children are pre-equipped for the process of some of these operations, particularly auditory scene analysis (21), their accuracy is certainly linked to experience and likely to improve in prelingually deaf children. The implicit learning paradigm used here allows children to train these operations, paying attention to the tasks considered as games.

Moreover, from a clinical point of view, we have also observed an improvement of their motivation for sound processing in the training course. Using implicit learning paradigm in deaf children's therapy appears a relevant tool in auditory education, allowing the possibility to share out attentive effort in other tasks (i.e., articulatory exercises).

References

1. Baddeley A (1993). La mémoire humaine, théorie et pratique. PUG, Grenoble
2. Bregman AS (1990) Auditory scene analysis: the perceptual organization of sound. MIT Press, Cambridge, MA
3. Busby PA, Roberts SA, Tong YC, Clark GM (1991) Results of speech perception and speech production training for prelingually deaf patients using a multiple-electrode cochlear implant. Br J Audiol 25(5):291-302
4. Christophe A, Millotte S, et al. (2006) Perception du langagechez les nourrissons. Apprendre les mots. In: Guegen B (ed) Neurophysiologie du langage. Elsevier, Paris
5. d'Alessandro C (2006) Analyse des différents stimuli auditifs: muique, langage et bruit. Etude comparative. Le Cerveau musicien. D. Boeck, Bruxelles
6. Dawson PW, Clark GM (1997) Changes in synthetic and natural vowel perception after specific training for congenitally deafened patients using a multichannel cochlear implant. Ear Hear 18(7):488-501
7. Donaldson GS, Nelson DA (1999) Place-pitch sensibility and its relation to consonant recognition by cochlear implant listeners using the MPEAK and SPEAK speech processing strategies. J Acoust Soc Am 107(8W):1645-1658
8. Ferard D (2006) Rééducation de l'enfant sourd profond: oralisme. Précis d'Audiophonologie et de déglutition – Tome 1. Solal, Marseille, pp. 329-347
9. Fu Q-J, Galvin JJ (2008) Maximizing cochlear implant patients' performance with advanced speech training pocedures. Hear Res 242:198-208
10. Howard JHJ, Howard DV (1997) Age differences in implicit learning of higher order dependencies in serial patterns. Psychol Aging 12:634-656.
11. Jones MR, Yee W (1994) L'attention auxévènements auditifs: le rôle de l'organisation temporelle. In: Penser les sons, pp. 75-121. PUF, Paris
12. Kral A, Eggermont JJ (2007) What's to lose and what's to learn: Development under auditory deprivation, cochlear implants and limits of cortical plasticity. Brain Res Rev 56: 259-269
13. McAdams S (1994) La reconnaissance de sources et d'évènements sonores. In: Penser les sons, pp. 157-213. PUF, Paris
14. Moussard A, Bigand E, Clément S, Samson S (2008) Préservation des apprentissages implicites en musique dans le vieillissement normal et la maladie d'Alzheimer. Revue de Neuropsychologie 18:1-2
15. Nicholas JG, Geers AE (2004). Effects of age of cochlear implantation on receptive and expressive spoken language in 3-year-old deaf children. Int Congr Ser 1273:340-343
16. Patel AD (2008) Music, language and the brain. Oxford University Press, New York
17. Reber AS (1993) Implicit learning and tacit knowledge. Oxford University Press, Oxford

18. Rochette F, Pescheux P, Bigand E (2008) Entraînement auditif et éducation auditive des enfants sourds. Revue de Neuropsychologie 18:1-2
19. Rochette F, Bigand E (2009) Long-term effects of an auditory training. Ann N Y Acad Sci 1169(1):195-198
20. Saffran JR, Newport EL, Aslin RN (1996) Word segmentation: the role of distributional cues. J Mem Lang 35(4):606-621
21. Samson S, Zatorre RJ, *et al.* (1997) Multidimensional scaling of synthetic musical timbre: perception of spectral and temporal caracteristics. Can J Psychol 51:307-315
22. Tait M, Raeve LD, *et al.* (2007) Deaf children with cochlear implants before the age of 1 year: comparison of preverbal communication with normally hearing children. Int J Otorhinolaryngol 71:1605-1611
23. Trehub S, Trainor LJ (1994) Les stratégies d'écoute chez le bébé: origines du développementde la musique et de la parole. In: Penser les sons. Psychologie Cognitive de l'audition, pp. 299-347. PUF, Paris.
24. Wright BA, Fitzgerald MB (2005) Learning and generalization of five auditory discrimination tasks as assessed by threshold changes. In: Auditory signal processing: physiology, psychoacoustics and models. Springer, New York

Virtual reality for learning and rehabilitation

E. Klinger, P. L. (Tamar) Weiss and P.-A. Joseph

Introduction

Virtual reality (VR) offers a new paradigm for human-computer interaction, by providing to participants a space in which they become an actor in an environment that may be realistic and functional. Its goal is to allow cognitive and sensorimotor activities, performed in real time, in a simulated world, which can be imaginary, symbolic, or a replication of certain aspects of the real world (12, 27). Over the past 20 years, VR developed extensively, in parallel with overall technological advancements, leading to numerous applications, from industry to art, including architecture, vocational training, or psychotherapy. Rehabilitation is one of the domains that currently benefits from the potential of VR (43, 28,), and in particular, VR assets are exploited for learning and rehabilitation (53).

Learning after brain injury is difficult because it may involve different processes that are not used by the intact central nervous system. VR is able to provide opportunities to respond to and perform tasks in less complex ways that entail a simplified cognitive load, greater repetition, and progressive training in comparison to real-world tasks. This may lead to more salient data and better self-awareness. Cognitive training may be associated with physical training or may be performed with minimal motor involvement. Visual or other sensory modalities may be selectively involved, and cues or errorless learning may be used as necessary.

The objective of this chapter is to provide an overview of how VR has been applied to learning and rehabilitation for people with acquired brain injury. We begin by presenting the key issues concerning the use of VR tools, including both hardware and software. We then continue with some examples of VR applications in cognitive learning and physical activation for rehabilitation. VR assets and limits for these applications are discussed.

Fundamental VR basic issues

The concept of VR was introduced by Jaron Lanier in 1985. VR is a multidisciplinary domain that is based on both engineering science and social science, and whose possibilities and progress largely depend on technical developments (e.g., computing power, graphic cards, and screen resolution). In accordance with hardware characteristics, software, and task complexity, VR enhances the involvement of the user in a more or less immersive and interactive virtual human experiment.

Thanks to behavioral sensory and motor interfaces, the user is immersed within a computer-generated virtual environment that displays images and enables movement within the virtual world, interaction with the virtual 3-D entities, and performance of simulated tasks, all in real time. Immersion and interaction are thus two fundamental functionalities of VR (27) that can be exploited at different levels: sensorimotor, cognitive, and functional. Real-time interaction is ensured when users do not perceive any delay, or latency, between their motor actions within the virtual environment and the sensory response of the virtual world (**Fig. 1**). The level of immersion depends on the way the users' senses (usually visual and audio senses, less commonly haptic, vestibular, or olfactory senses) are augmented by information coming from the virtual world. Consequently, it depends on the quality of the performance of the technology.

VR refers to the use of interactive simulations to provide users with opportunities to engage in environments that may appear and feel similar to real-world objects and events and that may engender a subjective feeling of "presence" in the virtual world (52). This feeling of presence refers to the idea of being carried into another, "virtual" world (35). It is, to some extent, positively correlated to the number of stimulated sensory modalities, such as visual or audio feedback (52), and may be affected by various interdependent factors such as visual realism, display parameters, or corporal involvement of the participant (46, 62).

Another fundamental concept is cybersickness whose symptoms are close to motion sickness symptoms (e.g., headache, nausea, fatigue, dizziness). They may result, for example, from conflicts between the various centers of movement perception or from incongruity between the sensory signal and the corporal feelings (2, 54). These side effects mainly occur with head-mounted displays (HMDs) and large screen driving simulators, and are much less relevant for desktop or video capture systems that are mainly used in VR-based rehabilitation.

When designing virtual environments in order to achieve VR-based systems that offer learning experiences to people with acquired brain injury, it is necessary to consider all the previously evoked features, such as the risk of inconsistencies during multisensory solicitation. While reducing the risks and the costs, VR-based tools permit multiple and standardized repetitions, as well as a progressive improvement. They present many assets that have encouraged clinicians to investigate this domain for the past decade; these assets are explored further in this chapter.

Some VR tools

Participants experience VR-based systems by means of sensory interfaces (i.e., transfer of information from the system toward the participant, or perception) and motor interfaces (i.e., transfer of information from the participant toward the system, or action) (**Fig. 1**). Their choice is very important because it will impact the way people respond to the virtual system. It will influence the participant's level of interaction and immersion, his or her level of presence and the risk of cybersickness. An interface is considered to be an intuitive device if its function is natural to the users and if there is almost no necessity to learn its use.

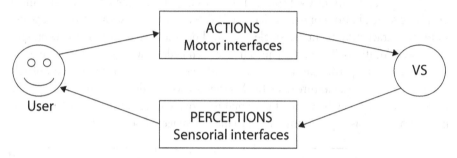

Fig. 1 - User's interfacing with the virtual system (VS).

We are now going to present the various elements that compose a VR-based system: the computer basis, the sensory and motor interfaces, and some software tools.

Computer basis of a virtual system

All VR-based systems include at least a computer that will, in real time, generate a virtual environment, modify this environment according to the participant's actions, manage the behavior of all the 3-D virtual entities, provide various sensory feedbacks, manage the interfaces and the sensors, and record data. Contemporary computers are able to run typical VR applications insofar as they have good graphics and audio cards. Clusters of computers may be required for more complex applications.

Visual sensory interfaces

Visual information is provided by means of visual sensory interfaces belonging to a wide range of devices, from low-immersive and low-cost ones (e.g., computer screen) to highly immersive and expensive ones (e.g., CAVE™: Cave Automatic Virtual Environment). The simplest and cheapest device is a computer screen that can be used alone. Sometimes a group of screens are placed around the participant to provide a panoramic view of the virtual environment (49). The low-immersion flat screen options are considerably less expensive and allow wide deployment of VR applications in health care settings and even in a patient's home.

The HMD facilitates visual sensory immersion, thanks to two small screens that are placed very close to the eyes (the field of view is almost fully occupied by the displayed virtual image). However, generally, thanks also to a tracker mounted on the HMD, the position of the image is displayed in accordance with movements of the head; the HMDs permit stereoscopic vision (each eye receives an appropriate picture leading to stereovision) when necessary. Often additional equipment that permits eye tracking or stereo audio is included with the HMD. One of the most commonly used HMD in therapy is the eMagin Z800 3Dvisor (www.3dvisor.com) (**Fig. 2**).

Other VR applications use projection systems that display the virtual environment on a large screen in front of the participant. Video capture VR uses a video camera and software to track movement in a single plane without the need to place markers on specific bodily locations. The participant's image is embedded within the simulated environment, and the participant may interact with the animated entities in a completely natural manner (e.g., GestureTek's IREX system; www.vividgroup.com) (**Fig. 3**). The projection screen may be placed horizontal to provide different planes of participant interaction, such as applications related to mental imagery (14) (**Fig. 4**).

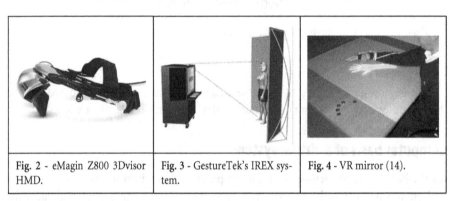

Fig. 2 - eMagin Z800 3Dvisor HMD.	Fig. 3 - GestureTek's IREX system.	Fig. 4 - VR mirror (14).

High-immersive, but also expensive, projection systems exist, such as the CAVETM, in which high-resolution projectors are directed to the walls of a room-sized cube (three to six). Standing inside of the CAVE and wearing special glasses for stereoscopic vision and head tracking, the participant interacts with a special joystick (a wand).

Other sensory interfaces

Audio information is commonly used in virtual environments either to enhance its overall ambience, or to inform participants about the events or about their performance. It can be provided by means of HMD earphones or loudspeakers using mono or stereo equipment (47, 57).

For the past decade, considerable efforts have been made to introduce haptic feedback in VR systems. Such interfaces allow the user to experience haptic (touch and force) sensation, leading to systems that are more similar to real-world behavior. For example, the haptic Rutger's Master II glove (www.caip.rutgers.edu/vrlab) (**Fig. 5**) provides force feedback during the manipulation of objects (21) or during finger motor training, and the PHANTOM® haptic device (www.sensable.com) provides force feedback to reach targets on a screen (5). The customized options are not commercially available. Some commercial options are expensive (e.g., the PHANTOM®, www.sensable.com) (**Fig. 6**), whereas others are more affordable (e.g., the PHANTOM® Omni™ or the Novint Falcon, home.novint.com). They are mainly used in motor rehabilitation. For cognitive and sensory rehabilitation (e.g., way finding for users with severe visual impairment (29,30)), haptic information may be transmitted by means of simplest interfaces such as force feedback joystick or steering wheel, joystick with vibration, or simply vibrators fixed at some specific body parts (10).

Very high immersion systems have also been developed to provide proprioceptive and vestibular information such as the CAREN platform (www.motekmedical.com). This moving platform, wide-screen display consists of a 2-m-diameter platform that can rotate around three orthogonal axes and translate in three directions along these axes; it is used in balance and gait research (8, 13, 31).

In specific applications, notably those involving the use of VR-based therapy to combat addiction, olfactory feedback is used (3). The principle is still very simple; the scents are provided from aromatic bottles, and their diffusion is managed by the computer according to the task or the participant's position in the virtual environment (www.biopac.com) (**Fig. 7**).

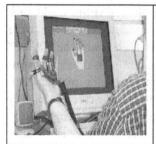
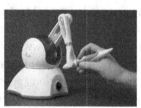
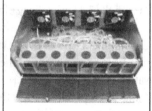

Fig. 5 - Rutgers Master II haptic glove.	Fig. 6 - PHANTOM® Omni™ haptic device.	Fig. 7 - Biopac scents delivery system.

Motor interfaces

Motor interfaces are used by the participant in order to navigate within the virtual environment, to handle virtual entities, or to carry out tasks. These devices may engage the user in direct or indirect interactions.

Direct approaches are based on participant's natural gestures and behavior that are tracked by the virtual system. They entail the use of visual tracking or motion sensors, such as the InterSense InterTrax2 inertial sensor (www.isense.com), which provides three degrees of freedom and can be fixed on an HMD to track head movements. In the GestureTek's GX system, visual tracking is carried out by means of a camera that tracks the movements of the participants while they stand or sit in front of a chroma key backdrop. The software detects the shape of the participant and introduces it within the virtual environment such that each movement of the body interacts with the animated graphics in a natural manner (59). It is also possible to restrict interaction to a single body part such as the hands by giving the user a red glove to wear. In order to increase participant immersion and to provide a feedback about the actions, vibrators may be added inside the gloves.

Indirect approaches include the use of the computer keyboard, mouse, joystick (26), or pads equipped with accelerometers such as the Nintendo Wii remote (www.nintendo.com). Interaction with a tactile surface has also been used (15).

Software tools

In addition to the hardware devices, a virtual application also comprises software tools. Some products were developed in the video games domain, e.g., the Sony Playstation2 (www.playstation.com), the Eyetoy (www.eyetoy.com), or the Nintendo Wii (wii.nintendo.com), and are used in rehabilitation (11, 40). However, their limits should be considered; since these tools were not explicitly designed for rehabilitation, the games cannot be modified to levels suitable for many patients, and they have not yet been validated for use in rehabilitation.

But, generally, the design of a virtual rehabilitation system requires the use of specific development software. They permit the design of the physical virtual world, such as with the 3-D modeling software Autodesk® 3ds Max® (www.autodesk.com), and the behavioral modeling or the integration of scenarios or tasks, such as with the 3DVIA™ Development solution of Dassault Systèmes (www.3dvia.com). This design process may be long, according to the complexity of the applications; it benefits from the innovative ideas of the engineers to reach rehabilitation applications. The current tendency is the development of tools that could be easily adapted and individualized by the therapists. Some examples can be reported like the NeuroVR system (www.neurovr.org) (42), whose current version allows only the construction of virtual situations, and the VR Worlds system of Psychology Software Tools (www.pstnet.com), which includes about 15 virtual places with virtual humans and allows the connection of various physiological sensors (1).

In summary, it is important to note that VR rehabilitation systems are designed according to an anthropocentric approach: the system is dedicated to the patient and is developed in order to involve the patient in determined tasks. This design process is punctuated by a lot of questions related to: the required patient activities, the triggered sensory modalities, the position of the patient during the experiment, the place and the role of the therapist during the sessions, the interfaces that should be chosen, or the data to record. Decisions should take into account several factors such as budget aspects, the size of the experiment place, the required level of sensorimotor immersion, or the capacities of the considered patient population. Depending on the characteristics of hardware, software, and task complexity, VR-based therapy aims to provide users with a meaningful experience within the context of the user's therapeutic objectives.

VR applications in cognitive learning for rehabilitation

There is considerable potential for using VR in cognitive learning rehabilitation, which is only just beginning to be realized. PC-based virtual environments are currently preferred for this purpose than more immersive virtual environments because they are relatively inexpensive and portable, and easy to use for patients. VR provides a new human-computer interaction paradigm in which users are no longer simply external observers of images on a computer screen but are active participants within a computer-generated virtual world. Patients may have some motor impairment relative to the controls but are still able to perform the virtual tasks (6). The studies that have so far been performed indicate that VR involvement would be usefully directed toward improving memory remediation using reorganization techniques. In memory assessment, the use of VR could provide more comprehensive, ecologically valid, and controlled evaluations of prospective, incidental, and spatial memory in a rehabilitation setting than is possible using standardized assessment tests. VR applications that are Internet deliverable could open up new possibilities for home-based therapy and rehabilitation. If executed thoughtfully, they could increase client involvement, enhance outcomes, and reduce costs (44).

Consequences in daily life of memory deficits are still difficult to identify, and VR testing is promising in that way. Few tests investigate prospective memory, which is a key process for autonomy, and real-world training did not show much efficiency (61). The additional knowledge gained from these assessments could more effectively direct rehabilitation toward specific impairments of individual patients. Brooks *et al.* reported a trial assessment involving 41 stroke patients, 1 week to 2 months post-stroke, who practiced in 4-room bungalow virtual environment (7). In a prospective memory task, participants were first informed that the owner of the virtual bungalow was moving to a larger house with a hall and seven rooms and that he had put "to go" labels on the furniture and objects to be moved. VR proved a useful medium to test stroke patients' prospective memory ability. The results indicated that stroke patients have particular problems with both the content and retrieval of prospective memory tasks, i.e., what to remember and when to remember it.

In memory remediation, VR training has been found to promote procedural learning in people with memory impairments, and this learning has been found to transfer to improved real-world performance. Rather than train underlying processes, another approach that shows promising results in a few small studies is training clients on specific functional skills, such as driving or vocational duties. Finally, modifications to the environment, implementation of strategies, provision of emotional support, and introduction of external supports/aids are important parts of a rehabilitation program, especially as the client returns to their home environment (36).

Only a few studies have assessed the impact of exercise and VR on the memory rehabilitation of persons with brain injury. Stanton *et al.* concluded that spatial information of the kind required for navigation transfers effectively from virtual to real situations (55). Spatial skills in children with disabilities showed progressive improvement with repeated exploration of virtual environments. Grealy *et al.* assessed cognitive function after a four-week intervention program in a traumatic brain injury (TBI) rehabilitation unit (16). A random allocation of crossover assessed changes in reaction and movement times after a single bout of non-immersive VR exercise and a no-exercise control condition. Subjects were supported in a sitting position on a recumbent VR exercise bicycle with the virtual environment presented on a color graphics screen mounted at eye level. During each exercise session, the subject had to steer a course around a virtual world or participate in a race against other virtual riders. The path's degree of incline in the virtual world was simulated visually and by a corresponding change in pedal resistance, and the bicycle was equipped with 15 gears operated by a hand switch. Airflow was simulated using a fan with vents placed below the visual display, and sounds relating to elements in the world were played through stereo speakers. After the four-week intervention, patients performed significantly better than controls on the digit symbol, verbal, and visual learning tasks. Significant improvements in reaction times were gained following a single bout of VR exercise. In another study (45), 30 students with learning disabilities were sequentially allocated to an active or a passive experimental group. Active participants explored a virtual bungalow searching for a toy car. Passive participants watched the exploration undertaken by the preceding active participants and searched for the toy car. All participants then performed spatial and object recognition tests of their knowledge of the virtual environment. In a further study, the errors of 45 participants on a real steadiness tester task were noted before they were randomly allocated to three groups – a real training group, a virtual training group, and a no-training group. After training, the participants performed a second test trial on the real steadiness tester. It was found that active participants, who controlled their movements in the virtual environment using a joystick, recalled the spatial layout of the virtual environment better than passive participants, who merely watched the active participants' progress. Conversely, there were no significant differences between the active and passive participants' recall or recognition of the virtual objects, nor in their recall of the correct locations of objects in the virtual environment. In the further study, virtual training was found to transfer to real task performance. VR demonstrated efficiency in developing the spatial skills of children with mobility impairments.

Brooks *et al.* reported prospective memory and route-finding memory training in a single case brain injury study (6). After stroke, a woman suffered from very severe spatial memory deficit and did not improve route-finding learning in the care facility even after diary practice with therapists. So a similar virtual environment was developed, and she was allowed 15 minutes of joystick training per day. A backward training method was adopted that involved the patient being instructed to withdraw backward from the target location for a short distance and then to advance forward again to the target location. After a three-week VR training, the patient showed improvement in both virtual and real conditions. Then the patient was trained in two different roads in virtual and real environments. She did not show any learning in real world, but she progressed successfully in the virtual condition. This result was maintained after training stopped. Differences in real and virtual training modalities may be explained first by shorter times to move in VR training than in real moving, second by the ability to go back and to show errors in a structured way, and last, but not least, by lack of interference in VR, which did not allow the patient to divert during the learning process. Nevertheless, this single case study needs confirmation by larger population-based comparative trials.

In a recent study, Lloyd *et al.* explored the benefits of errorless learning in an ecologically valid route learning task (32). A series of 20 patients with acquired brain injury learned two routes of equivalent difficulty in a virtual town. For one route, full guidance was provided throughout the learning trials in errorless learning paradigm; the other route was learned in a procedure allowing for trial and error. Route recall after errorless learning condition was significantly more accurate than recall after errorful learning.

Similar results in Alzheimer disease (AD) patients have been shown (18). Digital photographs of a shopping route were implemented in a close-to-reality simulation on a computer touch screen. The task was to find a predefined shopping route, to buy three items, and to answer correctly 10 multiple-choice questions addressing knowledge related to the virtual tasks. Within a 4-week training period including 12 sessions, however, substantial training gains were observed, including a significant reduction of mistakes. Training effects were sustained until follow-up three weeks later. Self-reported effects revealed that the training was well perceived. Thus, the task performance of AD patients improved substantially, and subjects appeared to have liked this computerized approach.

Current studies are carried out to explore the potential of VR in executive functions rehabilitation. For example, the Virtual Action Planning Supermarket (VAP-S) (**Fig. 8**) was designed by Klinger *et al.* to assess executive functions, and results among various populations (Parkinson disease, stroke, or mild cognitive impairment) confirmed its feasibility and its discriminative potential (23, 26). A study is currently carried out to test the rehabilitation assets in instrumental activities of daily living during a graduated shopping task within the VAP-S.

VR technology can also address the problems encountered in training elderly people to learn how to handle a mobility device. Some studies pointed out a promising transfer of training in a virtual environment to the real-life use of mobility devices (9).

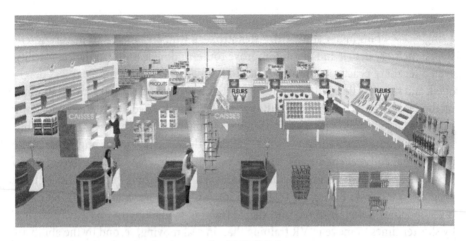

Fig. 8 - The Virtual Action Planning Supermarket (VAP-S) (26).

All these results are encouraging, especially regarding spatial learning, but have to be confirmed in larger controlled studies.

VR applications in functional evaluation and training

VR shows promise for training activities of daily living, such as street crossing or driving, with different populations.

Safe street crossing is a major concern for many patients with neurological deficits as well as for elderly people, and is thus an important goal in rehabilitation. The desktop VR system of street crossing used a simple graphic display to present vehicles of varying speed and direction to the user who viewed himself or herself represented as an avatar about to cross a street at a zebra crosswalk (24, 58). The aim of this VE was to test the effectiveness of virtual training for patients with stroke who had unilateral spatial neglect (USN) or other deficits of spatial perception, and to determine whether these skills transferred to performance in the real world. As with other VR-based interventions, this simulation has ecological validity and can be easily graded to elicit progressively improved patient performance.

Application of VR to driving assessment and training has had, to date, very promising results. A VR-based driving assessment system using an HMD was developed and tested at Kessler Medical Rehabilitation. The rehabilitation of driving skills following TBI is one example where individuals may begin at a simple level (i.e., straight, non-populated roads) and gradually progress to more challenging situations (i.e., crowded, highway roads, night driving) (51). The first study compared the VR-based driving system with the BTW (behind-the-wheel) evaluation, the current "gold standard," and found comparable results for the two approaches (50). Next, an analysis of the demands for safe driving was carried out, and the issue of divided attention was studied by adding a task of calling out digits appearing on the screen while maintaining driving at differing speed levels. The comparison of three patients with TBI to matched healthy controls showed that the speed of driving was consistent and similar for the two groups, but the patients failed to call the digits, while the healthy performed this task significantly better than the patients. Thus, the patients with TBI showed a serious problem in dual tasking. The results on the divided attention task were highly correlated with neuropsychological tests, validating the method of testing during VR driving. An extensive research project is underway to test the system for different neurological populations. As in the case of the street crossing program, described above, both cognitive variables that may explain the difficulty of performing the actual task (crossing streets or driving) and the functional evaluation and training for transfer and generalization to the daily tasks are combined. This provides for ecological validity of VR systems, which is missing in traditional standard measures.

VR applications in motor learning for rehabilitation

The same VR assets described above for cognitive learning are relevant to its use for motor learning. Specifically, the opportunities for active learning of tasks of varying levels of difficulty that motivate a patient are used to encourage multiple repetitions of high intensity exercise (43).

Recent studies of neural plasticity and motor function retraining suggest that multiple repetitions of movement are essential to regain function (37). However, it is difficult to achieve sufficient opportunities for practice in traditional clinical settings, and the opportunities decline still further once clients finish their active rehabilitation programs. Increasing the intensity and duration of rehabilitation in order to improve the quality of life of individuals with chronic diseases such as stroke can be achieved through physical activity since it reduces morbidity and prevents the development of secondary chronic diseases (41). Novel methods are needed to provide opportunities for functional activities that will increase the number of repetitions of purposeful movements during therapy and will support the implementation of home exercise programs. Maintaining the motivation of people to exercise independently at home is a related challenge since many exercise programs are monotonous and boring.

These principles of intervention for motor rehabilitation are highly suitable to the assets of VR reviewed in the first part of this chapter, and will be illustrated in this section with examples taken from a number of clinical studies on patients who have had a stroke. Piron et al. used a virtual environment to train reaching movements (38), Broeren et al. used a haptic device for the assessment and training of motor coordination (4), and Jack et al. have developed a force feedback glove to improve hand strength and a non-haptic glove to improve the range of motion and the speed of hand movement

(22, 34). Based on the results of the latter study, which included three patients who had a stroke, it appears that training within a virtual environment may lead to improvements in upper extremity function (greater range of motion, strength, endurance) in this population even when at a chronic stage.

Since many of the VR applications for rehabilitation have used desktop VR systems wherein the user interacts within the virtual environment via a keyboard, mouse, or joystick, the focus of intervention has often been cognitive, meta-cognitive, or functional or limited to wrist, digit, or ankle movements as illustrated above. More recently the use of other methods of interaction has enabled applications that can also be used for the improvement of motor deficits. For example, individuals with acquired brain injury have been trained to perform specific arm movements within a virtual environment and have then been able to generalize this ability and engage in daily functional use of the affected arm (19). Holden *et al.*'s more recent work has substantiated these findings on larger numbers of participants with stroke (20). These applications take advantage of VR assets to enhance motor learning by providing tasks that are ecologically valid and that provide immediate feedback including both knowledge of results and knowledge of performance (17).

The VividGroup's Gesture Xtreme system (formerly known as GX, now referred to as IREX) was used to develop an exercise program for balance retraining in which users see their own mirror image. This system has been shown to provide users with a high sense of presence without any encumbrance and to be suitable for different neurological impairments, including stroke, spinal cord injury (SCI), and cerebral palsy (59). Following 6 weeks of training at an intensity of 3 sessions per week, improvement was found for all 14 participants who had posttraumatic brain injury in both the VR and conventional physical therapy groups (56). However, the VR group reported more confidence in their ability to "not fall" and to "not shuffle while walking." The same VR system has been used to explore its potential to train balance for patients with spinal cord injury (25). Such training for these patients is essential in order to help them achieve maximal independence, namely, remediation of motor deficits via compensatory strategies to maintain balance. It was also evident that the task was highly motivating for them.

More recently, off-the-shelf VR systems have begun to gain popularity for motor rehabilitation, including both the Sony PlayStation EyeToy and Nintendo's Wii and Wii Fit. For example, the effectiveness of a VR-based exercise program to improve the physical fitness of adults with intellectual and developmental disabilities (IDD) who are in need of effective physical fitness training programs has been tested (33). The incentive supplied by VR appears to be necessary for this population since they tend to be inactive and unmotivated by conventional techniques. A 5- to 6-week fitness program consisting of two 30-minute sessions per week included gamelike exercises provided by the Sony PlayStation II EyeToy VR system. Significant improvements in physical fitness were demonstrated for most of the tests for the research group ($N=30$) in comparison to the control group ($N=30$), who engaged in only conventional group home activities.

Yavuzer *et al.* also reported results from a randomized controlled study (63) where the EyeToy was used as an intervention tool for training movements of the paretic upper extremity during subacute rehabilitation after stroke, in addition to the conventional therapy. Ten subjects participated in daily 30-minute therapy sessions for 4 weeks, while another 10 participants in a control group only watched the EyeToy games. They reported a significant improvement in the upper extremity movement and in self-care of the participants in the experimental group only.

Nevertheless, the restricted ability to grade the level of difficulty of the EyeToy applications emphasized a key limitation when it is used with individuals with stroke who are still engaged in subacute rehabilitation (40). The EyeToy encouraged non-isolated movements of the upper extremity and trunk, especially for individuals with a moderate motor impairment. These movements can be corrected by a therapist located in the virtual environment with or behind the client, providing support and handling. However, this may limit its use by more severely involved clients. Indeed, some of the individuals with moderate hemiparesis who were in subacute rehabilitation expressed frustration, especially when they could not manage to interact with the EyeToy environments with their weaker hand.

Neck pain and limitations in cervical range of motion are common and constitute a major cause of disability in the Western world. To date, most methods have relied on voluntary subjective responses to assessor's instructions. However, in day-to-day life, head movement is generally an involuntary response to multiple stimuli, and there is a need for a more functional assessment method, using sensory stimuli to elicit spontaneous neck motion response. A VR-based method was developed to assess cervical motion using an HMD and electromagnetic tracking (48). Thirty asymptomatic and 24 symptomatic participants were assessed by both conventional and VR methods. Inter- and intra-tester reliability was supported for both virtual and conventional methods, and virtual reality was found more precise than conventional assessment.

VR assets for learning and rehabilitation

In summary, there are several features that highlight VR assets in learning and rehabilitation. Although this list is not exhaustive, it does highlight the most salient features:

- – Delivery and control of ecological and appropriate multimodal stimuli within a significant and familiar context (e.g., classroom, office, supermarket, or street). VR systems appear to be perceived to be closer to real activities than conventional exercises. Patients have to cope with more dynamic stimuli, as is the case for real world challenges.
- – Observation of patient behavior, thanks to various recorded data for performance review and construction of adapted interventions. The tasks in which the patient is involved allow clinicians to collect detailed information about the

process of patient performance rather than focusing primarily on a final product (e.g., the juxtaposition of types of errors to task requirements vs. only an overall total error score). An analysis of these "learning tracks" leads to suggestions for further intervention adapted to the patient's capacities or to the therapeutic challenge.

– Construction of new intervention paradigms. VR allows clinicians to manipulate a variety of features, such as space, 3-D entities, time, physical laws, information (via texts, icons, or sounds), leading to the provision of standardized and repeatable experiments, or personalized and gradable ones. Furthermore, alternate learning approaches (e.g., errorless learning, contingent behavior, opportunities to immediately repeat a trial or parts of a trial after making an error) may be easily implemented.

– Increase of patient's motivation to learn and to train, thanks to gaming aspects and to the feeling of presence in virtual environments. VR systems have the benefit of novelty and challenge for patients. They increase the motivation to continue to train, while the equivalent traditional exercise may appear boring and repetitive.

– Decrease of costs and risks. VR applications permit some containment of costs, in terms of staff time, and risks to both patients and staff, which are incurred when training in real-world situations. Remote-located VR systems also increase the patients' access to care (60).

Limitations

The wide range of VR applications and their continuing growth highlight the potential of this technology to familiarize healthy subjects with various kinds of tasks and to facilitate learning (e.g., pilot training in airplane simulators). The issues for people with disabilities and health problems are more complex. Despite all the assets summarized above, evidence on the use of VR for the rehabilitation of patients following brain injury is still limited (17). Indeed, this technology may present limitations and, in some cases, even contraindications. We briefly review these limitations according to three aspects: fundamental, technico-economical, and ethico-cultural.

From a fundamental point of view, total virtual immersion is impossible, and likely not even desirable; the immersion space always includes both real and virtual elements. Indeed, mixed reality, wherein elements from the real world are transparently integrated into those from the virtual world, is becoming more popular (39). The immersion of a participant in a virtual world may be accompanied by sensorimotor and/or cognitive incoherencies that need to be recognized and minimized when possible. Usually only a few sensory modalities are provided (most commonly visual and auditory); recent efforts aim to integrate other modalities including haptics, smell, and proprioception. But vigilance is required; contradictory multisensorial stimuli may lead to conflicts that, in turn, often lead to cybersickness side effects. Similarly, use of inappropriate or inadequately controlled interfaces (e.g., Nintendo's Wii), may be misused by a patient unless strictly guided by a therapist. Attention to such limitations is necessary to assure optimal effectiveness of virtual entities for neurological populations. From a technico-economical point of view, risks are due to the technology, such as cybersickness, and they may disturb the participant during VR use. They are the consequence of our limits in the reproduction of reality. Technically, they may be due to latency, in other words, the temporal delay between the acquisition of a signal and the integrity of its sensory restitution. Qualitatively, they may be related to modeling of the virtual worlds, in terms of their fidelity with regard to the real world. In addition, the cost of the production of a VR application may become an obstacle to development. It requires collaboration between technical and clinical teams for software development and hardware purchase. Even as costs of equipment have significantly declined over the past decade, prices of some devices are still prohibitive for many clinical settings.

Finally, from an ethical point of view, the potential of VR to be an asset for clinical use is justified only if its use is effective and does not disturb the patient. VR immersion during and following patient care must be accompanied by an assessment of any of the risks. For example, is it reasonable and helpful to experiment with virtual driving before driving one's own real car? Will simulated training serve as an aid to the recovery process of CNS plasticity, or possibly act as a deterrent? The integration of these new technologies in clinical practice requires their validation via clinical trials. Reluctance and even apprehension on the part of some therapists is often counterbalanced by the favorable attitude of the patients. Nevertheless, the move toward evidence-based practice for VR is a positive step.

Conclusion

Over the past decade, the rapid development of VR-based technologies has been both an asset and a challenge for learning and rehabilitation. VR provides interactive functional simulations with multimodal feedback, task graduation, and review of performance, thanks to various recorded data. VR allows the clinicians to immerse the patient in a spatial and temporal context that is difficult to provide via conventional therapy in order to create novel clinical paradigms of learning and rehabilitation. The use of VR for cognitive and motor intervention is still at the stage of exploratory research with prototypes, although a number of single case studies, group comparisons, and even randomized clinical trials are now underway. Clinicians have begun to use the less costly and more accessible lower end VR systems. Application of VR for health care is expected to continue to grow due to the unanimous and urgent need for improved assessment and rehabilitation tools. This growth is being driven by a push-pull phenomenon. The push emanates from the continuing development of novel technologies, their more ready availability in clinical settings, and lowered costs. The pull stems from patients, clinicians, and third-party payers who recognize the need for treatment that goes beyond conventional therapy. Given the importance of aging in modern society and its impact on the need for health care, VR applications in learning and cognitive and motor rehabilitation will continue to strive to establish its scientific basis.

References

1. Baumann S, Neff C, Fetzick S, et al. (2003) A virtual reality system for neurobehavioral and functional MRI studies. Cyberpsychol Behav 6(3):259-266

2. Berthoz A (2003) Conflits sensoriels: la perception du mouvement. In: La décision, pp. 221-234. Odile Jacob, Paris

3. Bordnick PS, Graap KM, Copp HL, et al. (2005) Virtual reality cue reactivity assessment in cigarette smokers. Cyberpsychol Behav 8(5):487-492

4. Broeren J, Bjorkdahl A, Pascher R, Rydmark M (2002) Virtual reality and haptics as an assessment device in the postacute phase after stroke. Cyberpsychol Behav 5(3):207-211

5. Broeren J, Rydmark M, Sunnerhagen KS (2004) Virtual reality and haptics as a training device for movement rehabilitation after stroke: a single-case study. Arch Phys Med Rehabil 85(8):1247-1250

6. Brooks BM, McNeil JE, Rose FD, et al. (1999) Route learning in a case of amnesia: A preliminary investigation into the efficacy of training in a virtual environment. Neuropsychol Rehabil 9(1):63-76

7. Brooks BM, Rose FD, Potter J, et al. (2004) Assessing stroke patients' prospective memory using virtual reality. Brain Inj 18(4):391-401

8. Elion O, Bahat Y, Sela I, et al. (2008) Postural adjustments as an acquired motor skill: Delayed gains and robust retention after a single training session within a virtual environment. In: Proceedings of the 7th International Conference on Virtual Reality Rehabilitation, pp. 50-53. Vancouver, Canada

9. Erren-Wolters CV, van Dijk H, de Kort AC, et al. (2007) Virtual reality for mobility devices: training applications and clinical results: a review. Int J Rehabil Res 30(2):91-96

10. Feintuch U, Raz L, Hwang J, et al. (2006) Integrating haptic-tactile feedback into a video-capture-based virtual environment for rehabilitation. Cyberpsychol Behav 9(2):129-132

11. Flynn S, Palma P, Bender A (2007) Feasibility of using the Sony PlayStation 2 gaming platform for an individual poststroke: a case report. J Neurolog Phys Ther 31(4):180-189

12. Fuchs P, Burkhardt JM, Lourdeaux D (2006) Approche théorique et pragmatique de la réalité virtuelle, Chapitre 2 du volume "L'interfaçage, l'immersion et l'interaction en environnement virtuel". In: Fuchs P, Moreau G, et al. (eds) Le Traité de la réalité virtuelle vol. 2, pp. 19-59. Les Presses de Ecole des Mines de Paris, Paris

13. Fung J, Richards CL, Malouin F, et al. (2006) A treadmill and motion coupled virtual reality system for gait training post-stroke. Cyberpsychol Behav 9(2):157-162

14. Gaggioli A, Morganti F, Walker R, et al. (2004) Training with computer-supported motor imagery in post-stroke rehabilitation. Cyberpsychol Behav 7(3):327-332

15. Gal E, Bauminger N, Goren-Bar D, *et al.* (2009) Enhancing social communication of children with high functioning autism through a co-located interface. Artif Intel Soc. in press.

16. Grealy MA, Johnson DA, Rushton SK (1999) Improving cognitive function after brain injury: the use of exercise and virtual reality. Arch Phys Med Rehabil 80(6):661-667

17. Henderson A, Korner-Bitensky N, Levin M (2007) Virtual reality in stroke rehabilitation: a systematic review of its effectiveness for upper limb motor recovery. Top Stroke Rehabil 14(2):52-61

18. Hofmann M, Rosler A, Schwarz W, *et al.* (2003) Interactive computer-training as a therapeutic tool in Alzheimer's disease. Compr Psychiatry 44(3):213-219

19. Holden MK, Dettwiler A, Dyar T, *et al.* (2001) Retraining movement in patients with acquired brain injury using a virtual environment. Stud Health Technol Inform 81:192-198

20. Holden MK, Dyar TA, Dayan-Cimadoro L (2007) Telerehabilitation using a virtual environment improves upper extremity function in patients with stroke. IEEE Trans Neural Syst Rehabil Eng 15(1):36-42

21. Jack D, Boian R, Merians AS, *et al.* (2001) Virtual reality-enhanced stroke rehabilitation. IEEE Trans Neural Syst Rehabil Eng 9(3):308-318

22. Jack D, Boian RF, Merians AS, *et al.* (2001) Virtual reality-enhanced stroke rehabilitation. IEEE Trans Neural Syst Rehabil Eng 9(3):308-318

23. Josman N, Hof E, Klinger E, *et al.* (2006) Performance within a virtual supermarket and its relationship to executive functions in post-stroke patients. In: Proceedings of International Workshop on Virtual Rehabilitation, pp. 106-109

24. Katz N, Ring H, Naveh Y, *et al.* (2005) Interactive virtual environment training for safe street crossing of right hemisphere stroke patients with unilateral spatial neglect. Disabil Rehabil 27(20):1235-1243

25. Kizony R, Raz L, Katz N, *et al.* (2005) Video-capture virtual reality system for patients with paraplegic spinal cord injury. J Rehabil Res Dev 42(5):595-608

26. Klinger E, Chemin I, Lebreton S, Marié RM (2006) Virtual action planning in Parkinson's disease: a control study. Cyberpsychol Behav 9(3):342-347

27. Klinger E, Marié RM, Fuchs P (2006) Réalité virtuelle et sciences cognitives: Applications en psychiatrie et neuropsychologie. In Cognito – Cahiers Romans de Sciences Cognitives 3(2):1-31

28. Klinger E, Joseph PA (2008) Rééducation des troubles cognitifs par réalité virtuelle. In: Froger J, Pélissier J (eds) Rééducation instrumentalisée après cérébrolésion vasculaire, pp. 149-165. Masson, Paris

29. Lahav O, Mioduser D (2004) Exploration of unknown spaces by people who are blind, using a multisensory virtual environment (MVE) J Spec Educ Technol 19(3)

30. Lahav O, Mioduser D (2008) Haptic-feedback support for cognitive mapping of unknown spaces by people who are blind. Int J Hum Comp Stud 66(1):23-35

31. Lees A, Vanrenterghem J, Barton G, Lake M (2007) Kinematic response characteristics of the CAREN moving platform system for use in posture and balance research. Med Eng Phys 29(5):629-635

32. Lloyd J, Riley GA, Powell TE (2009) Errorless learning of novel routes through a virtual town in people with acquired brain injury. Neuropsychol Rehabil 19(1):98-109

33. Lotan M, Yalon-Chamovitz S, Weiss PL (2009) Improving physical fitness of individuals with intellectual and developmental disability through a irtual Reality Intervention Program. Res Dev Disabil 30(2):229-239

34. Merians AS, Jack D, Boian RF, *et al.* (2002) Virtual reality-augmented rehabilitation for patients following stroke. Phys Ther 82(9):898-915

35. Mestre D, Fuchs P (2006) Immersion et présence. In: Fuchs P, Moreau G (eds) Traité de la Réalité Virtuelle 3ème édition, vol. 1, pp. 309-338. Presses de l'Ecole des Mines, Paris

36. Michel JA, Mateer CA (2006) Attention rehabilitation following stroke and traumatic brain injury. A review. Eura Medicophys 42(1):59-67

37. Nudo RJ (2007) Postinfarct cortical plasticity and behavioral recovery. Stroke 38(2 Suppl):840-845

38. Piron L, Cenni F, Tonin P, Dam M (2001) Virtual Reality as an assessment tool for arm motor deficits after brain lesions. Stud Health Technol Inform 81:386-392

39. Pridmore T, Cobb S, Hilton D, *et al.* (2007) Mixed reality stroke rehabilitation: interfaces across the real/virtual divide. Int J Disabil Hum Dev 6(1):87-95

40. Rand D, Kizony R, Weiss PL (2008) The Sony PlayStation II EyeToy: low-cost virtual reality for use in rehabilitation. J Neurolog Phys Ther 32:155-163

41. Rimmer JH, Braddock D (2002) Health promotion for people with physical, cognitive and sensory disabilities: an emerging national priority. Am J Health Promot 16(4):220-224, ii

42. Riva G, Gaggioli A, Villani D, *et al.* (2007) NeuroVR: an open source virtual reality platform for clinical psychology and behavioral neurosciences. Stud Health Technol Inform 125:394-399

43. Rizzo A, Kim GJ (2005) A SWOT analysis of the field of virtual reality rehabilitation and therapy. Presence Teleoper Virtual Environ 14(2):119-146

44. Rizzo AA, Strickland D, Bouchard S (2004) The challenge of using virtual reality in telerehabilitation. Telemed J E Health 10(2):184-195

45. Rose FD, Brooks BM, Attree EA (2002) An exploratory investigation into the usability and usefulness of training people with learning disabilities in a virtual environment. Disabil Rehabil 24(11-12):627-633

46. Sanchez-Vives MV, Slater M (2005) From presence to consciousness through virtual reality. Nat Rev Neurosci 6(4):332-339

47. Sanchez J, Zuniga M (2006) Evaluating the interaction of blind learners with audio-based virtual environments. Annu Rev Cyberther Telemed 4:167-173

48. Sarig-Bahat H, Weiss PL, Laufer Y (2009) Cervical motion assessment using virtual reality. Spine, in press

49. Schultheis MT, Mourant RR (2001) Virtual reality and driving: the road to better assessment of cognitively impaired populations. Presence Teleop Virt 10(4):436-444

50. Schultheis MT, Rizzo AA (2001) The application of virtual reality technology in rehabilitation. Rehabil Psychol 46(3):296-311

51. Schultheis MT (2009) Final thoughts and future directions. In: Schultheis MT, DeLuca J, Chute DL (eds) Handbook for the assessment of driving capacity, pp. 201-215. Academic Press, San Diego

52. Sheridan TB (1992) Musings on telepresence and virtual presence. Presence Teleoper Virtual Environ 1(1):120-125

53. Standen PJ, Brown DJ (2005) Virtual reality in the rehabilitation of people with intellectual disabilities: review. Cyberpsychol Behav 8(3):272-282; discussion 283-278

54. Stanney KM, Kennedy RS, Kingdon KS (2002) Virtual environment usage protocols. In: Stanney KM (ed) Handbook of virtual environments: designs, implementations and applications, pp. 721-730. Lawrence Erlbaum Associates, Inc., Mahwah, NJ

55. Stanton D, Foreman N, Wilson PN (1998) Uses of virtual reality in clinical training: developing the spatial skills of children with mobility impairments. Stud Health Technol Inform 58:219-232

56. Sveistrup H, McComas J, Thornton M, et al. (2003) Experimental studies of virtual reality-delivered compared to conventional exercise programs for rehabilitation. Cyberpsychol Behav 6(3):245-249

57. Vastfjall D (2003) The subjective sense of presence, emotion recognition, and experienced emotions in auditory virtual environments. Cyberpsychol Behav 6(2):181-188

58. Weiss PL, Naveh Y, Katz N (2003) Design and testing of a virtual environment to train stroke patients with unilateral spatial neglect to cross a street safely. Occup Ther Int 10(1):39-55

59. Weiss PL, Rand D, Katz N, Kizony R (2004) Video capture virtual reality as a flexible and effective rehabilitation tool. J Neuroeng Rehabil 1(1):1-12

60. Weiss PL, Klinger E (2009) Moving beyond single user, local virtual environments for rehabilitation In: Gaggioli A, Weiss PL, Keshner EA, Riva G (eds) Advanced technologies in neurorehabilitation: emerging applications in evaluation and treatment. in press pp. 263-276

61. Wilson BA (1997) Cognitive rehabilitation: how it is and how it might be. J Int Neuropsychol Soc 3(5):487-496

62. Witmer B, Singer M (1998) Measuring presence in virtual environments: a presence questionnaire. Presence Teleop Virt 7(3):225-240

63. Yavuzer G, Senel A, Atay MB, Stam HJ (2008) "Playstation eyetoy games" improve upper extremity-related motor functioning in subacute stroke: a randomized controlled clinical trial. Eur J Phys Rehabil Med 44(3):237-244

Augmented feedback, virtual reality and robotics for designing new rehabilitation methods

J.V. G. Robertson and A. Roby-Brami

Introduction

Neuro-rehabilitation is currently undergoing a technological revolution! Groups of engineers and rehabilitation specialists are working on designing and testing a great variety of rehabilitation devices and systems. The reason for this is that, although it is generally accepted that rehabilitation improves outcome after stroke, patients are still left with impairments causing various levels of handicap and limiting their integration in community life. Comparison of traditional rehabilitation techniques has failed to show superiority of one over another (15), and concepts for rehabilitation have been changing over the last 20 years, with the biggest change being evaluation. There is a move to make rehabilitation techniques more evidence based. As such, numerous research teams have set about to create more effective rehabilitation techniques based on principles of motor control and learning and incorporating new technology to fulfil the principal goals of rehabilitation: increased functional ability and increased participation in the community. The aim of this chapter is to discuss applications for augmented feedback (AF) in rehabilitation of motor skills of patients with neurological disorders, in particular within virtual reality (VR) environments associated or not with mechatronic devices (robotics). First, we will examine some motor learning principles relevant to rehabilitation and how AF fits into these concepts. We will then go on to review applications of AF used for rehabilitation of specific movement parameters. We will also discuss the use of feedback distortion to manipulate action-perception coupling and systems based on movement observation.

Motor learning in patients with cerebral lesions

It has previously been established that patients with central neurological lesions are able to learn (71). Recovery is associated with the mechanism of **plasticity**. The plastic capacity of the nervous system has been demonstrated in numerous studies [see (45) for a review], and it is now accepted that plasticity is dependent on activity (use) and learning.

Clinical studies have shown that certain factors are essential for the optimization of neuro-rehabilitation techniques. Although evidence is reasonably limited, it does seem that **intensity** of therapy can affect outcome. Several studies have shown greater improvements in patients who spent more time in therapy (30). However, it is not just the *amount* of therapy that is important; the *type* of therapy is also important. Learning seems to be specific to what is practiced and is also influenced by the context. Indeed, plasticity of cortical areas following rehabilitation has been found to be **task specific** (63). There is evidence that for carryover from the therapy setting to activities of daily living to occur, exercises must be task oriented. This means that the task itself or at least parts of it must be practiced (11). In addition to this, the exercise must be realistic and contain a real goal. The presence of an object has been shown to enhance kinematic performance, compared to carrying out the same movement with no object in both healthy and stroke patients (73). This reinforces the notion that movements are indeed goal directed. In a review of intensity versus task specificity, Page (47) concluded that the most important factor was task specificity. **Strength** training seems to have little effect in comparison with task-oriented practice (43). Within task-oriented practice, exercises must be **varied**. Hanlon (20) showed that practicing reaching movements in different parts of the workspace was more effective when the position of the targets was randomized rather that blocked. In other words, repeating the same exercise in the same part of the workspace before changing is less effective than varying the target at each repetition. Over the length of rehabilitation time, therapy techniques must also be varied in order to overcome the "plateau" phenomenon (48). The number of **repetitions** carried out seems to be linked with outcome (46). However, patients must be given feedback and must practice "correctly" since repetition alone does not produce learning. The movements must be meaningful and involve tasks that require attention. Neurophysiological changes have been observed both at the spinal cord level (51) and in the brain (9) following visuomotor tasks, compared with controls who merely repeated movements. Each repetition must be an attempt to solve a goal-related problem by building on the previous attempts (5).

A problem in stroke recovery is the development of **compensatory strategies**. These strategies, such as the use of the "good" arm in place of the hemiparetic arm or trunk movements that limit the need for elbow extension during reaching tasks, have the benefit of rapidly increasing the capacity to achieve functional tasks. However, there is some evidence to show that the use of compensations may actually prevent patients from reaching their "true" capacity (41). Impairment-orientated training is important in order to promote "true" recovery and prevent learning of compensations. Platz and coworkers (51) demonstrated how an impairment-orientated training regime could have greater effects than traditional therapy.

The acquisition of new motor skills or reacquisition of "lost" skills requires **feedback**. Feedback occurs in many forms. Intrinsic feedback refers to a person's own sensory-perceptual information that is available as a result of the movement being performed. It is proprioceptive, resulting from the movement itself, or exteroceptive (auditory, visual, and haptic – sense of touch), due to the consequences of movement. Feedback also includes information related to the completion of the task, for example, reaching a target (knowledge of results, KR), and performance of the movement (knowledge of performance, KP) (60). For people with neurological disorders, interpretation of intrinsic feedback can be difficult or incorrect due to impaired somatosensory pathways, increasing the need for additional feedback information, which is usually provided by therapists. While KR is important for learning as well as motivation (13), patients with neurological disorders require KP if they are to make improvements at the impairment level.

In order to be able to implement an intense rehabilitation program, a key element is **motivation** (24). Without motivation, the patient may not adhere as well to the treatment and as such will not benefit as much as he could. The provision of feedback of certain movement parameters has been shown to increase motivation (13). Motivation requires not only a sense of fun but also a sense of purpose. The feeling of progression is important. The provision of AF in different manners is an excellent way to motivate patients.

Training of upper limb function through the use of computers to provide fun, rewarding, motivating therapy was pioneered by Paul Bach-y-Rita in the 1970s (3). His group modified joysticks to provide a variety of grip types along with a modified exercise track to enable patients to play electronic pong games via a TV screen; the system was named CAMR (computer-assisted motivating rehabilitation). Two patients could even play together with individual joysticks. They found that patients participated wholeheartedly in playing and benefited from improvements in their motor abilities as a result.

In summary, according to current knowledge, therapy should be intense, repetitive, impairment oriented, task specific, and motivating; strength training should not be a priority; and exercises should be designed to promote *learning*. Technological systems are new means to enrich the environment in order to fulfil these requirements.

Augmented feedback for rehabilitation

For the purpose of this chapter, we will define **augmented feedback** (AF) as the provision of supplementary sensory information (visual, auditory, or haptic) brought by technological means, which would not normally be present in the usual environment. Since many activities of daily living involve technology, we shall restrict the term "augmented feedback" to specific devices based on *information technologies*. These systems are generally related to **virtual reality** (VR) technologies, but we shall focus on relatively simple new means of interactive coupling rather than more complicated immersive 3-D virtual environments that will be further detailed in Chapter "Virtual reality for learning and rehabilitation", E. Klinger *et al.* **Robotic** technology is often associated with VR, to ensure a mechanical support for the exercises and/or to provide haptic force feedback.

The provision of AF requires some type of sensor or motion capture device in order to record the parameter that is to be fed back, along with an emitter to provide the feedback. Some types of feedback such as for KP must be given in real time. KR, however, is usually provided at the end of the movement, exercise, or session. A simple example of an augmented reality (AR) device is one that provides an auditory feedback of one movement parameter, such as weight bearing on a paretic lower limb during gait (4). Sounds can also be coupled with movements of objects or a part of the subjects' own body in such a way that they "hear their own movement" (33). By **interacting** with the feedback, the patient becomes aware of the effects of the way he or she moves (KP), thus encouraging active problem solving.

So what is the **role** of AF in rehabilitation? AF often forms a part of a **stimulating environment**. Enriched environments have been shown to influence recovery in rats with cerebral lesions (21). The environments provided to the rats are regularly modified with new elements being inserted every few days. Indeed this may be the reason why more traditional rehabilitation methods failed to show superiority over each other; the effectiveness lay simply in the fact that patients were stimulated to move, and the method used was secondary. Based on this idea, with modern technologies, it is possible to increase the level of stimulation as well as to control the sensory modalities that are stimulated.

Thanks to technology, feedback can be manipulated. This can allow patients with neurological disorders to interact more successfully than in the real environment (49). For example, reality can be distorted so that a small movement of the arm can be seen as a large movement on the screen. Success following movement attempts is very important in order to prevent phenomena such as learned disuse from occurring (64).

The recordings of movement parameters by technological devices can also be used as an **objective evaluation tool** to follow patients' progress as well as to provide motivation by informing patients of their success (KR). Depending on the types of sensors used, systems can measure a variety of parameters such as accuracy, smoothness, velocity, stability, coordination, motivation, and strength.

Van Vliet and Wulf (68) carried out a review of the effectiveness of AF after stroke. They point out that if feedback is provided too frequently, it may actually have a negative effect, as the learner may become dependent on it. It would seem that reducing the proportion of trials for which feedback is provided enhances the learning effect. However, they also highlight the fact that many questions regarding exactly how feedback should be provided remain unanswered.

Rehabilitation

Task-oriented rehabilitation

A large variety of VR systems of different levels of sophistication and with different levels of immersion have been developed to provide functional rehabilitation for the upper limb, posture, balance, and gait. These systems are described in detail in Chapter "Virtual reality for learning and rehabilitation", E. Klinger *et al.*

Task-oriented rehabilitation at the impairment level

Rationale

The relationship between impairment and disability is not fully understood. Many treatment protocols result in improvements at the impairment level with little transfer to activities of daily living. Task-specific training seems to improve generalization of learned skills; however, it is not always easy to design task-oriented exercises that promote motor recovery at the impairment level and discourage compensatory strategies. Particular movement parameters that are altered following stroke have been demonstrated. These include decreased velocity, alterations in the shape of the velocity curve, loss of smoothness, and perturbations in inter-joint coordination (54, 57, 32). These deficits are difficult to rehabilitate in a normal setting because they are not necessarily visible to therapists and even less so to patients. Technology allows the development of new coupling systems that use measures made at the impairment level and convert them in a task-related application, combining the benefits of both "ismpairment-oriented" and "task-related" training (i.e., the performance, KP, can be used as a goal, KR).

Before using augmented or virtual environments for rehabilitation of particular movement parameters, it is essential to verify that the environment itself does not alter them. Such a study was carried out by Viau *et al.* (69). They compared reaching, grasping, and releasing a real and a virtual ball in stroke and healthy subjects. Although small movement differences were found between the environments and the study was limited to one type of environment, the authors suggest that movements may be similar within a virtual and real environment.

Studies using visual feedback

In order to improve endpoint control, a visual display may show an "ideal trajectory" that patients can try to copy with their own movement. This idea is being worked on by an Italian team (52) and a team from the MIT (23). Using a desktop display, patients view simultaneous views of their own arm trajectory and a "teacher" trajectory on a computer screen. Objects can also be instrumented so that patients can practice displacing or using them, such as pouring from a cup. Different features of the movement can be highlighted, such as distance and orientation error; the teacher speed can vary; sound cues can be added to enhance timing; and a static trace of the teacher trajectory can be used to enhance spatial learning. Improvements in Fugl-Mayer scores have been demonstrated in several pilot studies.

Zheng *et al.* use inertial sensors to track motion of the arm and replay it on a computer screen (76). Instead of displaying trajectories, a visual display of the patient's reconstructed arm is given along with a "template" arm whose movement the patient attempts to replicate. Templates can be varied; for example, it could be the first movement made by the patient or the best movement that he or she has previously made. In this way, the goal is always achievable, and the patient is encouraged to beat his or her own performance. Patients can choose between two types of template presentation

(**Fig. 1**): one displays the exercise movement and the target template movement in two separate windows and the other displays them in the same window with the template movement as a ghost layer. This system is still in the early stages of development.

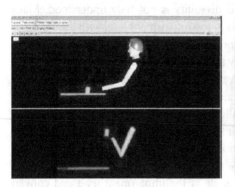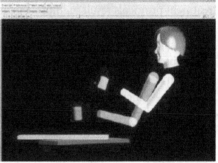

Fig. 1 - Display of exercise movement and target movement in same or separate windows. Reproduced from Zheng *et al.* 2006 (76) with permission.

Studies using auditory feedback

A disadvantage of visual feedback for KP is the dependence on the computer screen. This limits the activities that can be practiced. Auditory feedback appears, however, particularly adapted for the provision of KP or as a "kinematic guide" for uncon-strained movements since, for many types of reaching movements, the nervous system depends on visual and proprioceptive information and audition is a "redundant" sense. Because of this, it can be used as an augmented type of feedback without interfering with normal physiological processes.

Auditory feedback has been used to improve hand path straightness. Maulucci *et al.* (40) tested an auditory feedback that informed subjects of the deviation of their hand from the ideal trajectory by the use of a tone that was emitted if the hand strayed out with the "normal reach zone." In this controlled study, they showed that hand trajec-tory was significantly closer to the normal trajectory and that changes in movement direction were significantly decreased in the group who trained with the feedback.

A novel musical feedback has been used within a virtual environment to improve smoothness of reaching movements (25). The auditory feedback consisted of a musical phrase that was recognizable only if hand motion was smooth (**Fig. 2**). Interference of other instruments also occurred if patients used trunk movements. In a small pilot study, the authors found that hand trajectories became smoother with the feedback. The auditory feedback was not, however, tested alone. It is possible that a simpler AF environment based on the musical auditory feedback would have been as effective as the complex virtual environment that they used. This would be easier and less costly to implement in clinical settings than a virtual environment.

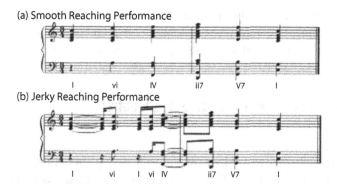

Fig. 2 - Hand motion can be linked to a musical phrase. The smoothness of the phrase depends on the smoothness of hand motion. Reproduced from Huang *et al.* (25) with permission (© 2005 IEEE).

Gait symmetry can also be trained with a musical feedback. Schauer and Mauritz (59) developed a device consisting of sensor insoles that detect the ground contact of the heels, and a portable music player. The music is played at an adjustable speed, which is estimated from the time interval between two consecutive heel strikes. The required time period to play a quarter meter is stretched or compressed instantly to coincide with the patient's present step duration. In a study of stroke patients, gait parameters such as velocity and stride length improved significantly in the experimental group (who used the feedback) but not in the control group (who received therapy without feedback). There was also greater stance time symmetry between limbs for the experimental group as well as foot rollover path length.

Augmented feedback and artistic practice

A very different system based on the concept of **creativity** is being developed based on the SoundScapes system, which was invented by Lewis-Brooks (33). The system consists of non-wearable sensors that register motion and transform the movements into sound, video, and light. In this way, the participants have the opportunity to see/hear their pattern of movement and to see/hear which parts of the body they are moving/not moving. They can create music and/or pictures and light with body movement. The author's philosophy is to use productive creativity to supplement the feeling of progression, or perhaps *be* the progression. The system is designed to be adaptable so that the users can choose the kinds of feedback they want. For example, one patient (who was a painter) never listened to music and was only motivated by visual feedback. He gave a catalogue of his work to the author who replicated it on the computer and created an exercise in which the movement of the patient's hands could recreate his own paintings! So far, the system has been tested on a limited number of subjects.

The above studies demonstrate how AF can improve movement quality. It would seem that AF enhances control of movement and can accelerate learning of a motor task by guiding subjects toward the most effective patterns of actions. Studies that evaluate the effect of a single type of AF are very useful, as it is important to understand the individual effects of stimuli and feedbacks prior to combining them in a more complex environment such as VR.

Activity workbenches and augmented feedback

Real objects

Several **systems that use real objects** coupled with motion sensors are being developed. They are designed to be used in the clinic or at home without the need for direct supervision; therefore, feedback is an essential component.

The AutoCITE was developed to provide automated constraint induced therapy (CIT) (38). It consists of a computer, eight task devices arrayed in a cabinet on four work surfaces, and an attached chair (**Fig. 3**). The computer provides simple one-step instructions on a monitor that guides the participant through the entire treatment session. Completion of each instruction is verified by sensors built into the device before the next instruction is given. Results of a study seem to show that training with the device is as effective as standard CIT (65).

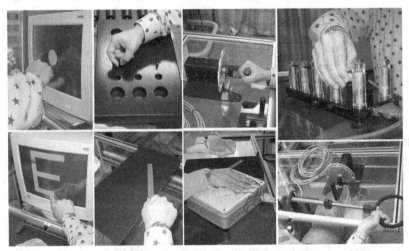

Fig. 3 - The AutoCITE consists of eight instrumented task devices. Reproduced from Taub *et al.* (2005) (65) with permission.

A similar system called the H-CAD (home care activity desk) consists of seven instrumented tools: a key, light bulb, book, jar, writing, checkers, and keyboard. In this way, reaching, grasping, lateral pinch, pinch grip, holding, manipulation, and finger dexterity can be practiced by the patient. A randomized multicenter clinical trial in patients with central neurological pathologies was carried out to compare the effect of home therapy with the H-CAD with usual therapy (26). Average test scores (ARAT and nine-hole peg test) were not significantly different in either group at the end of the intervention, but there appeared to be a link between the amount of improvement and the amount of time spent using the H-CAD. The authors suggest that some improvements should be made to the H-CAD regarding aesthetic aspects and difficulty of the tasks with more options of different levels. Both patients and therapists were, however, generally highly satisfied with the system.

Computer games and instrumented joysticks

Bach-y-Rita's work (3) was mostly ignored for practically two decades. Recently, however, other teams have taken up the idea. A system based on the same principle but more complex is now being developed in Wisconsin. It has been named the robot/CAMR suite (28). It consists of an adapted joystick (TheraJoy), which is almost 1 m in length allowing a large range of movement, as well as an adapted steering wheel (TheraDrive), which can be sensorized to measure grip force and tangential forces. The system is still in the early stages of testing.

Reinkensmeyer's team is developing a joystick system that can provide assistance or resistance to movement (55). It has been developed with specific tasks mostly for assessment purposes, but it also uses games. Because it has been designed particularly for home use, it consists of a cleverly designed feedback package. Three types of progress charts provide quantitative feedback of rehabilitation progress. The first chart keeps track of system usage. A "to-do list" is displayed upon logging in and compares the desired frequency of use with the actual frequency of use. When the actual frequency for an activity exceeds the desired frequency, the system places encouraging feedback on the "to-do list" by writing "Good job!" next to the activity. The second type of chart provides performance feedback immediately upon completion of an activity along with three references for comparison: a customizable target score, the average past performance on the activity, and the previous score achieved on the activity. A third type of chart, the "progress overview," displays a graphical history of the user's scores on a particular activity. The scores can be displayed either as a function of time or as a function of the number of times the activity has been performed. These charts are all designed to motivate patients to train more in order to beat their previous scores.

Combining AF with robotics

Robotics and mechanical support of the upper limbs

The results of many studies have led CIT to be accepted as being an effective rehabilitation method (70). This technique is, however, not available to all patients. A minimum functional level is necessary before patients can receive this type of therapy, making it inappropriate for severe to moderately impaired patients.

The recent explosion in the development of robotic devices for rehabilitation may offer a solution for patients who have not yet reached the functional level necessary to participate in CIT. Robots are tireless systems ideal for carrying out intensive, repetitive training. Their built-in mechanisms of fine detection can be used to constantly monitor the patient's performance and progress. The large variety of sensors that can be used with robotic devices allows feedback on a multitude of different kinematic and dynamic movement parameters to be provided to patients and therapists. The combination of robotic systems with AF or VR environments seems to be an excellent manner of fulfilling the currently accepted criteria for optimal rehabilitation.

The simplest mechanical interactions are provided by instrumented joysticks described above, which can produce force but do not provide support to assist the movement if needed. The first supportive devices developed for arm rehabilitation were **robotic manipulanda**. Initial focus was on technical developments of the robots themselves, such as the development of appropriate modes of control.

Hogan and colleagues at the MIT have great experience in robots for rehabilitation and have developed a method of adaptive impedance control (22). It consists of a "virtual" spring that guides hand motion in such a way as to allow errors but minimize their magnitude. Current robots function in three principal modes: passive (the robot does all the work), active-assisted (the robot provides assistance if the patient is unable to complete the movement), and active-constrained (movements are constrained so that the patient directs forces in a particular direction or uses particular patterns of coordination, for example). Research suggests that an "assist-as-needed" approach promotes the greatest learning.

The visual displays provided with these 'hi-tech' robotic systems are often very simple. For example, the visual display linked to the MIT-Manus robotic manipulandum consists of targets displayed in a circle that the subject has to touch with a curser via the movement of the robotic arm (62).

Other systems require the patients to reproduce shapes such as a circle (6, 36). These movements are often impaired in patients, and training of shape tracing may help to improve coordination; however, these exercises may lack a functional element. Some evidence suggests that improvements may occur following these training programs (70), but the effect on functional capacity has been little evaluated. The visual feedback provided by these systems allows the patients to see their errors through comparison of the nominal path with their own path. Feedback regarding direction of errors, timing, amount of assistance, and so on, can also be given, thus providing KP relating to kinematic parameters, although the exercises are less functional.

One study has evaluated the **benefits of adding virtual reality to robotic training**. Mirelman *et al.* (42) compared rehabilitation with the Rutgers Ankle Rehabilitation System, which is a 6-degrees-of-freedom platform force-feedback system that allows individuals to exercise the lower extremity by navigating through a virtual environment that is displayed on a desktop computer. Eighteen patients with chronic hemiparesis trained with the robot three times per week for four weeks in one-hourly sessions. Half of the group used the robot in combination with a VR environment displayed on a computer screen. Both groups carried out a similar number of movement repetitions. Interestingly, the patients who trained with the robot alone reported fatigue earlier and required more rests than the robot + VR group. The results showed a significantly greater transfer of learning into functional walking skills in the robot + VR group. The authors suggest that the problem-solving nature of the VR games promoted greater motor learning. They suggest that the presentation of AF provided KR of action outcome and KP, helped direct subjects' attention to the relevant features of the action to improve the next attempt, and is crucial for motor learning and skill acquisition.

Manipulanda only allow constrained movements of proximal joints, usually only in two dimensions. Quite recently, **robotic orthoses** have begun to emerge. These are exoskeletons that attach to the arm and allow control of the whole arm instead of just the endpoint. The hand may be fixed if holding a handle is required, or it may be free, allowing retraining of arm and hand function together. The GENTLE/S system uses a more complicated interface with a selection of virtual rooms within which the patient can work, including a home environment and a supermarket environment (2). In a similar manner, the T-Wrex system (which is not actually a robot, as it has no motors but contains sensors and uses elastic bands to compensate the weight of the arm) uses a variety of games that aim to be functionally relevant (58). Each game is designed to use a task in order to train a particular aspect of movement.

Rehabilitation of hand function

Rehabilitation of hand function can be particularly challenging, and recovery of hand function can be a real problem for stroke patients. The power grip synergy is often preserved, but patients may have difficulty in opening the hand and also in differentiating finger movements. Differentiation of finger movements is essential for many daily activities. It is very difficult to design "task-oriented" exercises when patients have little movement of their hands, so a variety of systems have been developed to assist hand opening and closing. Because of the fragile nature or the position of actuators on the palmer surface of the hand, it can be difficult to practice taking real objects when wearing these systems. VR is therefore well suited in combination with these assistive devices. Many different systems are currently being developed; we will describe a few different types.

The Rutgers Master II-ND glove is an exoskeleton consisting of pneumatic actuators that are capable of exerting up to 16 N of force. It has been coupled with a VR display via a desktop computer. Thanks to sensors, the patient sees a virtual hand that gives an exact representation of his own movement in space. The glove provides resistance while the patient attempts to push down a piston with each finger. The virtual pistons on the screen fill with a color proportional to the displacement of the real pistons. This type of system is more fun than the traditional strength training devices used in therapy consisting of springs or putty.

The "cyber glove" developed by the company Immersion (http://www.immersion.com/3d/products/cyber_glove.php) is a different type of system. It is a sensitized structure worn on the hand that contains strain gauge sensors to measure hand movement. On its own it is used to measure the joint range of movement for games involving training of the range of motion and finger fractionation, and a desktop display of a virtual hand can be provided. It can be coupled with a type of exoskeleton named the "cybergrasp," which provides force feedback.

Some pilot studies have been carried out on the effectiveness of these devices for stroke hand rehabilitation. Adamovich *et al.* (1) report the results of a pilot study that combined the Rutgers Master II-ND and the "cyber glove" used for 8 hemiparetic patients who were able to extend the wrist at least 20° and the fingers at least 10°. They were trained for 2 to 2.5 hours per day, 5 days per week, for almost 3 weeks. Such intensive training is facilitated by the use of a virtual environment in which exercises can be greatly varied and motivation sustained. Most subjects showed improvements in the range of finger and thumb movement and speed as well as finger fractionation capability. Performance also improved according to the Jebsen hand function test. The combination of the two gloves appears highly useful for training certain parameters of hand function that may otherwise be difficult to train. It is also useful for the measurement of hand kinematics, which can otherwise be limited using clinical tests or quite complicated using motion analysis systems.

A very different type of rehabilitation "glove" was developed by a team from Northwestern University (38). It contains an air bladder on the palmar surface to push the fingers into extension. It is coupled with electromyography (EMG) sensors on hand flexor and extensor muscles. Assistance to movement is controlled by a combination of the EMG signal and the difference between present hand opening angle and desired hand opening angle. EMG-triggered muscle stimulation has been shown to have some effectiveness on recovery (72). This device does not stimulate the muscles but only assists the movement if the patient actively contracts appropriate muscles. Research in the development of robotics for rehabilitation seems to show that an "assist-only-as-needed" paradigm is most appropriate for motor learning in stroke patients.

The same team also developed a "body-powered orthosis." It is based on prosthetic technology and consists of a glove with cables on the dorsum of the hand activated by the non-paretic limb, which pull the fingers into extension. In this way, the user controls the amount of assistance provided for finger extension. An in-line force sensor is used to estimate the amount of assistance provided. This is converted into sound pitch in order to provide AF to subjects relating to the amount of help the system is giving them. This information is also stored so that progress can be monitored.

The latter two devices are combined with see-through head-mounted display (HMD) goggles, which allow the patient to see his or her own hand as well as virtual objects (augmented reality) (**Fig. 4**). They can also be used with real objects. A pilot study was carried out on three stroke patients, and some improvements were in functional test scores, particularly with the use of the assistive devices. Simply attempting to grasp the virtual objects without assistance from either of the hand opening devices did not seem to change test scores (38).

Takahashi *et al.* (63) describe a robotic system capable of adapting the level of assistance given to the patient's needs. The Hand Wrist Assistive Rehabilitation Device is a 3-degrees-of-freedom pneumatically activated device assisting the hand in grasp and

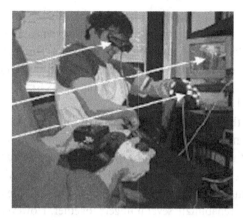

Fig. 4 - A subject using the body-powered orthosis. Reproduced from Luo *et al.* (38) with permission (© 2005 IEEE).

release tasks. Joint angle sensors within the robot's joints allow the control of a virtual hand displayed on a computer screen in front of the patient. Thirteen chronic stroke patients received fifteen 1.5-hour sessions over three weeks. Significant improvements were seen in impairment scales as well as functional scales.

VR and haptic technology

For rehabilitation of the hand, the provision of **haptic feedback** seems particularly important. Although all daily activities depend on the correct functioning of action-perception loops, this is even more the case for activities involving the hand where the sense of touch is particularly important. There is a very fine coupling between the response of mechanoreceptors in the skin and grip force (27).

Haptic technology is a branch of robotic producing devices able to apply mechanical stimulations (forces, vibrations, and/or motions) to the users in order to give them haptic illusions as they interact with virtual objects or environments. Haptic feedback is used to enhance the VR interaction and immersion and render the task more real, and has potentially large applications in rehabilitation. However, still few AF or VR systems currently incorporate haptic technology, which is costly. There are also complex problems such as calibration to synchronise haptic and visual feedback. If not well synchronized, then the user can feel disconnected from the virtual environment (10).

One commercially available haptic device is the PHANTOM developed by SensAble Technologies. It is used for a large variety of purposes and has been used for some studies in rehabilitation (8, 35). It consists of an articulated arm with 3 to 6 degrees of freedom. The user holds the end part, which is like a stylus.

Broeren *et al.* (8) tested the PHANTOM on five chronic stroke patients. The stylus was linked to a computer and coupled with stereoscopic shuttered glasses. The task was to move the stylus as a virtual "bat" to hit balls using a cylinder or pen grip. The subjects experienced force through the stylus when they hit a ball. Few improvements were found on clinical tests, although some kinematic improvements were found on the test developed by the authors, which involved using the stylus. This highlights the problems of such training that might be effective on the skill specifically trained but without any functional carryover. Perhaps this type of training needs to be more associated with "real-life" functional exercises.

A problem with the PHANTOM is that patients must be able to hold the weight of their arms as well as move them. This means it is only suitable for reasonably high-level patients. However, the work space may be too limited for this patient group.

A haptic interface for finger exercise (HIFE) has been designed in Slovenia (39). At present, only one finger can be exercised at a time, although the eventual aim of the team is to be able to rehabilitate several fingers together. However, the benefit of this system seems limited since fingers are never used in isolation in activities of daily living.

Cassadio et al. (12) incorporated a haptic representation of targets along with the visual representation on a screen. Subjects could practice with eyes open or closed, and in the latter case, they could feel the target via the haptic channel. The theory behind this is that enhanced use of proprioception may further decrease pathological patterns of movement. Few results are as yet available regarding the effects of this type of feedback.

So how important is it to include haptic feedback? Incorporation of haptics into AF systems appears interesting in order to complete the perception-action loop, particularly in patients with neurological disorders; however, this question has been little studied. Liu et al. (34) did not find an advantage to combining visual and haptic (proprioceptive) information compared with visual information alone for healthy subjects asked to follow a trajectory. This task is, however, of a different nature to those including haptic feedback in response to a virtual object.

The benefits and disadvantages must be carefully weighed up in the design of a system that could include cheaper methods to induce contact illusions, for example, vibrations. Indeed, very simple coupling systems involving vibration can give the illusion of virtual objects when actively moved (61). Feintuch et al. (16) are currently investigating the possibilities of using vibratory haptic discs that deliver tactile stimuli. The system appears to be feasible, and the next stage is to test how realistic these stimuli will be for healthy subjects and patients.

The combination of robotics and AF or VR appears to be currently the optimal non-invasive rehabilitation solution. For this reason, Patton et al. (49) have developed a system to "combine our knowledge of the nervous system with the tireless, precise, and swift capabilities of a robot." This system, called VROOM (virtual reality robotic and optical operations machine), is an AF system combined with a haptic-interface robot (Fig. 5). It has been developed for scientific exploration of motor control but with the eventual aim to be used for stroke rehabilitation.

The authors' experience suggests that in order to achieve significant practical application in rehabilitation, human-interface robots must safely operate in three dimensions with a large workspace and an appropriately designed visual interface. Moving

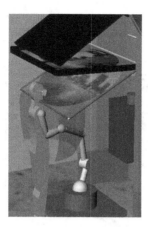

Fig. 5 - The VROOM system designed by Patton *et al.* (2004). Reproduced from Patton *et al.* (49) with permission (© 2005 IEEE).

targets and feedback of force and movement errors are essential. Equally, the instrumentation must superimpose images on the physical world, preserving the reality of everyday tasks.

VR and assisted gait training

Assisted gait training devices began to be developed in the 1980s. The initial approach was to suspend a patient in a harness over a treadmill, and two therapists assisted leg motion. Since then, technological devices have been designed to assist leg motion and coupled with AF systems. The Lokomat is probably, currently, the most technologically advanced type of gait training apparatus. It is a driven gait orthosis with 2 degrees of freedom per leg combined with a body weight support system and a treadmill. Thanks to the incorporation of force transducers into the system, the patient's activity relative to the activity of the motors can be estimated. This is a very important feature of such a device, as patients can easily become dependent on the assistance provided by a system, and as such, they do less work. The provision of biofeedback via a computer screen during Lokomat training has been shown to motivate patients as well as provide valuable information for therapists (37). The therapist can select the data shown in order to focus the patient's attention on different aspects of his gait.

Recently, attempts have been made to link the Lokomat to a VR system including a haptic display (**Fig. 6**) (29). This is complex because the Lokomat was not initially designed to be able to give haptic feedback, and this can only be given at the hip and knee joints. However, a recent study on healthy subjects showed promise, although the system is still being developed.

Four scenarios are being developed for different rehabilitation purposes. One is walking through water for strength training, and another is soccer in which if the subject does not exert a great enough effort then a virtual opponent takes control of the

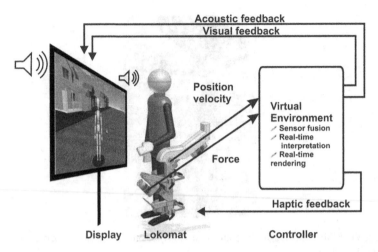

Fig. 6 - Linking the Lokomat to a virtual environment. Reprinted from Koenig *et al.* (28), Copyright (2008), with permission from IOS Press.

ball! There are also scenarios for obstacle crossing and crossing the road. These latter scenarios are not unlike some of those that have been developed by teams in Québec (18) and Taiwan (75), which also aim to train patients to cross the road or to pass obstacles. However, the main difference is that without a robotic orthosis, these systems cannot control "how" the movement is carried out. The advantages of combining virtual scenarios with an assistive device such as the Lokomat are the possibility of providing adapted levels of assistance to patients who require it while enabling them to participate in interactive and engagement therapy "games." It could, however, be argued that when patients are at the stage of learning to cross the road (i.e., increasing gait speed and judging the speed and distance of cars), the presence of an assistive device is inappropriate.

Use of augmented feedback to modify action-perception coupling

Visual-proprioception conflict and error management

AF can be used to **distort feedback** in order to motivate patients or to modify motor behavior. Studies indicate that subjects rely more on visual feedback than kinesthetic (17). Because of this phenomenon, visual feedback can be altered to produce illusions regarding movement, even though the visual feedback may be incongruous with proprioceptive feedback. For example, distortion of visual kinematic feedback given on a screen may be such that a small movement of the arm can be seen as a large movement on the screen. This can be used to increase task success and to motivate patients. This has been demonstrated by Brewer *et al.* (7) in a pinching task. Two PHANTOM robots were coupled to a visual display on which the number of bars highlighted increased with finger span. The distance mapped to the visual feedback bar was gradually altered so as to encourage the patients to produce a larger span. A pilot study on two patients showed improvements on the grasp and pinch subset of the ARAT after eighteen 90-minute rehabilitation sessions.

There is some evidence suggesting that **enhancing errors** may actually produce greater improvements than by reducing them. Patton *et al.* (50) demonstrated, in a preliminary single trial study using a robotic manipulandum with 18 stroke patients, that increasing initial direction error (via a "curl force") produces greater improvements in initial movement direction of the hand by the end of the trial. Although these results need to be confirmed over a longer-term trial, they are very interesting.

Optic flow

Optic flow is a typical pattern of visual motion generated at the eye as the person moves through the environment. It can be manipulated in order to create a sensation of walking faster or slower. Lamontagne *et al.* (31) evaluated the ability to modulate walking speed according to changes in optic flow speed. They used an HMD to create a virtual corridor through which healthy subjects and patients could walk by means of a self-paced treadmill. The advantage of a self-paced treadmill is that the user can modulate the speed simply by changing his or her own gait speed. Their results showed that both healthy subjects and stroke patients walk faster in response to slower optic flow; that is, the slow optic flow creates an illusion of slow walking, stimulating subjects to increase velocity. Increasing gait velocity is a frequent goal of rehabilitation.

Training regimens

Environments that provide AF (virtual or otherwise) offer an excellent research tool with which to **investigate training regimens**. For example, which types of feedback are most effective, and how much practice and what frequency are optimal? Use of technological-based rehabilitation techniques offers a useful mechanism to manipulate these factors to train, test, and record both healthy subjects' and patients' motor responses. This is essential if we wish to optimize rehabilitation techniques. For example, Todorov *et al.* (67) used a simulation of a table tennis game presented on a screen positioned to the side of a real table tennis table to test different types of feedback given by a "teacher paddle" on the screen. Subjects could see the trajectories of their swing and the effect on a simulated ball on the screen and, in this way, practice their technique. Performance was measured before and after the simulated training by the use of a real ball on the real table. They found that teaching temporal coupling between the flight of the ball and the execution of the swing was essential to the success of the training method.

Motor imagery and movement observation

Motor imagery is a cognitive process in which a subject imagines that he or she performs a movement without actually performing the movement or even tensing muscles (44). Studies have shown that the act of imagining a movement triggers activation in parts of the brain relevant for the movement [see Mulder (44) for a review]. This phenomenon has also been found for movement observation. The mirror neuron system is believed to play an important role in this process (56). Some studies indicate that both motor imagery and movement observation may improve the performance of actual motor acts, although large-scale randomised controlled trials on the subject are lacking, especially in patients. As a result of these findings, rehabilitation techniques based on movement observation have begun to emerge.

Mirror therapy involves the patient moving both limbs simultaneously while seeing the ipsilesional limb and its mirror image in place of the hemiparetic limb. In this way, the patient receives a type of "distorted" visual feedback since the vision he or she receives via the mirror is actually an illusion. Although it lacks a "fun" dimension, some functional improvements have been demonstrated (74). It has also been shown to enhance cortical reorganization (19).

This concept has been transferred to a VR environment. Eng *et al.* (14) developed a system based on the hypothesis that observation with intent to imitate is the optimal way of stimulating the action recognition system. The patient sees two virtual arms on a screen in front of him or her. Initially, movement of the virtual arm that corresponds to the paretic arm is actually controlled by the non-paretic arm so that the patient sees "correct" movements. Gradually, this control can be transferred to the paretic arm as the patient recovers. A controlled study is underway to evaluate the effectiveness of this technique in acute patients.

In video capture VR, which consists of camera-based platforms, the user stands or sits in a demarcated area and sees his or her mirror image projected on a large screen within a simulated environment. This type of system can be used for rehabilitation of the upper limb, gait or balance, as described by Klinger *et al.* in Chapter "Virtual reality for learning and rehabilitation", E. Klinger *et al.* One of the theories proposed to justify its use is that of action observation. However, there is an important difference between "mirror therapies" described above in which the patient observes movements which are actually performed by his "good limb" and as such are deemed to be normal and video capture rehabilitation in which the patient is able to observe his or her errors.

Conclusion

The incorporation of technology in rehabilitation means that AF can now be provided on a multitude of kinematic and dynamic parameters. Although few comparative studies have been carried out, evidence suggests that the provision of AF enhances the effect of rehabilitation techniques, by increasing motivation as well as facilitating motor learning. There may be a particular role for this type of feedback in distorting reality or increasing errors in order to further increase motor learning; however, more research on these questions is necessary. Systems which include feedback can be designed for independent practice, providing opportunity for repetitive but motivating training, developing problem solving abilities essential for motor leaning.

However, many questions remain unanswered. For example, is the complex stimulation offered by virtual environments more effective than simple AF of one movement parameter? Another question is the presentation of feedback. Is there a difference in effect between seeing a virtual hand or the patient's own hand? Many more questions remain. At present, technology is being explored to find its limits. As developments stabilize, research will be able to focus on particular motor learning questions and benefit from the use of technological devices.

References

1. Adamovich SV, *et al.* (2005) A virtual reality-based exercise system for hand rehabilitation post-stroke. Presence 14(2):161-174
2. Amirabdollahian F, *et al.* (2007) Multivariate analysis of the Fugl-Meyer outcome measures assessing the effectiveness of GENTLE/S robot-mediated stroke therapy. J Neuroeng Rehabil 4:4
3. Bach-y-Rita P, *et al.* (2002) Computer-assisted motivating rehabilitation (CAMR) for institutional, home, and educational late stroke programs. Top Stroke Rehabil 8(4):1-10
4. Batavia M, *et al.* (2001) A do-it-yourself membrane-activated auditory feedback device for weight bearing and gait training: a case report. Arch Phys Med Rehabil 82(4):541-545
5. Bernstein N (1967) The coordination and regulation of movements. Pergamon Press, Oxford, England
6. Bi S, Ji L, Wang Z (2005) Robot-aided sensorimotor arm training methods based on neurological rehabilitation principles in stroke and brain injury patients. In: 27th Annual International Conference of the IEEE Engineering in Medecine and Biology Society. Shanghai, China, pp. 5025-5027
7. Brewer BR, Klatzky R, Matsuoka Y (2008) Visual feedback distortion in a robotic environment for hand rehabilitation. Brain Res Bull 75(6):804-813
8. Broeren J, *et al.* (2007) Assessment and training in a 3-dimensional virtual environment with haptics: a report on 5 cases of motor rehabilitation in the chronic stage after stroke. Neurorehabil Neural Repair 21(2):180-189
9. Carey JR, *et al.* (2007) Comparison of finger tracking versus simple movement training via telerehabilitation to alter hand function and cortical reorganization after stroke. Neurorehabil Neural Repair 21(3):216-232
10. Carignan CR, Krebs HI (2006) Telerehabilitation robotics: bright lights, big future? J Rehabil Res Dev 43(5):695-710
11. Carr R, Shepherd J (1998) Neurological rehabilitation. Optimizing motor performance. Butterworth-Heinemann, Oxford
12. Cassadio M, Morasso P, Sanguineti V, Giannoni P (2006) Impedance-controlled, minimally-assistive robotic training of severely impaired hemiparetic patients. In: BioRob 2006. Piza, Italy
13. Colombo R, *et al.* (2007) Design strategies to improve patient motivation during robot-aided rehabilitation. J Neuroeng Rehabil 4:3

14. Eng K, *et al.* (2007) Interactive visuo-motor therapy system for stroke rehabilitation. Med Biol Eng Comput 45(9):901-907

15. Ernst E (1990) A review of stroke rehabilitation and physiotherapy. Stroke 21(7):1081-1085

16. Feintuch U, *et al.* (2006) Integrating haptic-tactile feedback into a video-capture-based virtual environment for rehabilitation. Cyberpsychol Behav 9(2):129-132

17. Flanagan JR, Rao AK (1995) Trajectory adaptation to a nonlinear visuomotor transformation: evidence of motion planning in visually perceived space. J Neurophysiol 74(5):2174-2178

18. Fung J, *et al.* (2006) A treadmill and motion coupled virtual reality system for gait training post-stroke. Cyberpsychol Behav 9(2):157-162

19. Giraux P, Sirigu A (2003) Illusory movements of the paralyzed limb restore motor cortex activity. Neuroimage 20(Suppl 1):S107-S111

20. Hanlon, R.E., Motor learning following unilateral stroke. Arch Phys Med Rehabil, 1996. 77(8): p. 811-5

21. Hoffman AN, *et al.* (2008) Environmental enrichment-mediated functional improvement after experimental traumatic brain injury is contingent on task-specific neurobehavioral experience. Neurosci Lett 431(3):226-230

22. Hogan N, Krebs HI (2004) Interactive robots for neuro-rehabilitation. Restor Neurol Neurosci 22(3-5):349-358

23. Holden MK, *et al.* (2001) Retraining movemsent in patients with acquired brain injury using a virtual environment. Stud Health Technol Inform 81:192-198

24. Holden MK (2005) Virtual environments for motor rehabilitation: review. Cyberpsychol Behav 8(3):187-211; discussion 212-219

25. Huang H (2005) Interactive multimodal biofeedback for task-orientated neural rehabilitation. In: 27th Annual International Conference of the IEEE Engineering in Medicine and Biology Society. Shanghai, China, pp. 2547-2550

26. Huijgen BC, *et al.* (2008) Feasibility of a home-based telerehabilitation system compared to usual care: arm/hand function in patients with stroke, traumatic brain injury and multiple sclerosis. J Telemed Telecare 14(5):249-256

27. Johansson RS (1991) How is grasping modified by somatosensory input? In: Humphrey DR, Freund H-J (eds) Motor control: concepts and issues, pp. 331-355. Wiley, New York

28. Johnson MJ, *et al.* (2007) Potential of a suite of robot/computer-assisted motivating systems for personalized, home-based, stroke rehabilitation. J Neuroeng Rehabil 4:6

29. Koenig A, *et al.* (2008) Virtual gait training for children with cerebral palsy using the Lokomat gait orthosis. Stud Health Technol Inform 132:204-209

30. Kwakkel G (2006) Impact of intensity of practice after stroke: issues for consideration. Disabil Rehabil 28(13-14):823-830

31. Lamontagne A, *et al.* (2007) Modulation of walking speed by changing optic flow in persons with stroke. J Neuroeng Rehabil 4:22

32. Levin MF (1996) Interjoint coordination during pointing movements is disrupted in spastic hemiparesis. Brain 119:281-293

33. Lewis-Brooks A (2004) HUMANICS 1 – a feasibility study to create a home internet based telehealth product to supplement acquired brain injury therapy. In: Proceedings

of the 5th International Conference on Disability, Virtual Reality and Associated Technologies, Oxford, UK

34. Liu J, Cramer SC, Reinkensmeyer DJ (2006) Learning to perform a new movement with robotic assistance: comparison of haptic guidance and visual demonstration. J Neuroeng Rehabil 3:20

35. Lövquist E, Dreifaldt U (2006) The design of a haptic exercise for post-stroke arm rehabilitation. In: Proceedings of the 6th International Conference on Disability, Virtual Reality and Associated Technologies. Esbjerg, Denmark, pp. 309-315

36. Lum PS, et al. (2002) Robot-assisted movement training compared with conventional therapy techniques for the rehabilitation of upper-limb motor function after stroke. Arch Phys Med Rehabil 83(7):952-959

37. Lunenburger L, et al. (2004) Biofeedback in gait training with the robotic orthosis Lokomat. In: Conference Proceedings – IEEE Engineering in Medicine and Biology Society, San Francisco, USA. pp. 4888-4891

38. Luo X, et al. (2005.) Integration of augmented reality and assistive devices for post-stroke hand opening rehabilitation. In: 27th Annual International Conference of the IEEE Engineering in Medecine and Biology society. Shanghai, China, pp. 6855-6858

39. Mali U, Goljar N, Munih M (2006) Application of haptic interface for finger exercise. IEEE Trans Neural Syst Rehabil Eng 14(3):352-360

40. Maulucci RA, Eckhouse RH (2001) Retraining reaching in chronic stroke with real-time auditory feedback. NeuroRehabilitation 16(3):171-82

41. Michaelsen SM, Dannenbaum R, Levin MF (2006) Task-specific training with trunk restraint on arm recovery in stroke: randomized control trial. Stroke 37(1):186-192

42. Mirelman A, Bonato P, Deutsch JE (2008) Effects of training with a robot-virtual reality system compared with a robot alone on the gait of individuals after stroke. Stroke 40(1):167-174

43. Moreland JD, et al. (2003) Progressive resistance strengthening exercises after stroke: a single-blind randomized controlled trial. Arch Phys Med Rehabil 84(10):1433-1440

44. Mulder T (2007) Motor imagery and action observation: cognitive tools for rehabilitation. J Neural Transm 114(10):1265-1278

45. Nudo RJ (2006) Mechanisms for recovery of motor function following cortical damage. Curr Opin Neurobiol 16(6):638-644

46. Nugent JA, Schurr KA, Adams RD (1994) A dose-response relationship between amount of weight-bearing exercise and walking outcome following cerebrovascular accident. Arch Phys Med Rehabil 75(4):399-402

47. Page SJ (2003) Intensity versus task-specificity after stroke: how important is intensity? Am J Phys Med Rehabil 82(9):730-732

48. Page SJ, Gater DR, Bach YRP (2004) Reconsidering the motor recovery plateau in stroke rehabilitation. Arch Phys Med Rehabil 85(8):1377-1381

49. Patton J, et al., (2004) Robotics and virtual reality: the development of a life-sized 3-D system for the reabilitation of motor function. In: Conference Proceetings – IEEE Engineering in Medecine and Biology Society, San Francisco, USA pp. 4840-4843

50. Patton JL, et al. (2006) Evaluation of robotic training forces that either enhance or reduce error in chronic hemiparetic stroke survivors. Exp Brain Res 168(3):368-383

51. Perez MA, Lungholt BK, Nielsen JB (2005) Presynaptic control of group Ia afferents in relation to acquisition of a visuo-motor skill in healthy humans. J Physiol 568(Pt 1):343-354

52. Piron L, *et al.* (2008) Satisfaction with care in post-stroke patients undergoing a telerehabilitation programme at home. J Telemed Telecare, 14(5):257-260

53. Platz T, *et al.* (2005) Impairment-oriented training or Bobath therapy for severe arm paresis after stroke: a single-blind, multicentre randomized controlled trial. Clin Rehabil 19(7):714-724

54. Regnaux JP, *et al.* (2008) Effects of loading the unaffected limb for one session of locomotor training on laboratory measures of gait in stroke. Clin Biomech (Bristol, Avon) 23(6):762-768

55. Reinkensmeyer DJ, *et al.* (2002) Web-based telerehabilitation for the upper extremity after stroke. IEEE Trans Neural Syst Rehabil Eng 10(2):102-108

56. Rizzolatti G, *et al.* (1996) Premotor cortex and the recognition of motor actions. Brain Res Cogn Brain Res 3(2):131-141

57. Roby-Brami A, *et al.* (2003) Motor compensation and recovery for reaching in stroke patients. Acta Neurol Scand 107(5):369-381

58. Sanchez RJ, *et al.* (2006) Automating arm movement training following severe stroke: functional exercises with quantitative feedback in a gravity-reduced environment. IEEE Trans Neural Syst Rehabil Eng 14(3):378-89

59. Schauer M, Mauritz KH (2003) Musical motor feedback (MMF) in walking hemiparetic stroke patients: randomized trials of gait improvement. Clin Rehabil 17(7):713-722

60. Schmidt R, Wrisberg C (2004) Motor learning and performance. Human Kinetics, Leeds, England

61. Sribunruangrit N, *et al.* (2004) Speed-accuracy tradeoff during performance of a tracking task without visual feedback IEEE Trans Neural Syst Rehabil Eng 12(1):131-139

62. Stein J, *et al.* (2004) Comparison of two techniques of robot-aided upper limb exercise training after stroke. Am J Phys Med Rehabil 83(9):720-728

63. Takahashi CD, *et al.* (2008) Robot-based hand motor therapy after stroke. Brain 131(Pt 2):425-437

64. Taub E, Uswatte G, Elbert T (2002) New treatments in neurorehabilitation founded on basic research. Nat Rev Neurosci 3(3):228-236

65. Taub E, *et al.* (2005) AutoCITE: automated delivery of CI therapy with reduced effort by therapists. Stroke 36(6):1301-1304

66. Taub E, Uswatt G (2006) Constraint-induced movement therapy: answers and questions after two decades of research. NeuroRehabilitation 21(2):93-95

67. Todorov E, Shadmehr R, Bizzi E (1997) Augmented feedback presented in a virtual environment accelerates learning of a difficult motor task. J Mot Behav 29(2):147-158

68. van Vliet PM, Wulf G (2006) Extrinsic feedback for motor learning after stroke: what is the evidence? Disabil Rehabil 28(13-14):831-840

69. Viau A, *et al.* (2004) Reaching in reality and virtual reality: a comparison of movement kinematics in healthy subjects and in adults with hemiparesis. J Neuroeng Rehabil 1(1):11

70. Volpe BT, *et al.* (2008) Intensive sensorimotor arm training mediated by therapist or robot improves hemiparesis in patients with chronic stroke. Neurorehabil Neural Repair 22(3):305-310

71. Winstein CJ, Merians AS, Sullivan KJ (1999) Motor learning after unilateral brain damage. Neuropsychologia 37(8):975-987

72. Woldag H, Hummelsheim H (2002) Evidence-based physiotherapeutic concepts for improving arm and hand function in stroke patients: a review. J Neurol 249(5):518-528

73. Wu C, *et al.* (2000) A kinematic study of contextual effects on reaching performance in persons with and without stroke: influences of object availability. Arch Phys Med Rehabil 81(1):95-101

74. Yavuzer G, *et al.* (2008) Mirror therapy improves hand function in subacute stroke: a randomized controlled trial. Arch Phys Med Rehabil 89(3):393-398

75. Yang, Y.R., et al., Virtual reality-based training improves community ambulation in individuals with stroke: a randomized controlled trial. Gait Posture, 2008. 28(2):201-206

76. Zheng H, *et al.* (2006) SMART project: application of emerging information and communication technology to home-based rehabilitation for stroke patients. In: Proceedings of the 6th International Conference on Disability, Virtual Reality and Associated Technologies. University of Reading, UK: Esbjerg, Denmark, pp. 215-220

Achevé d'imprimer sur les presses de la SEPEC
Dépôt légal : Mai 2010